DESIGNER CANCER KILLERS
& Orange Wunder

*God-Designed, God-Inspired
To Kill Your Cancer, Not You!*

Deanna K. Loftis, RN, BBA

All Scripture quotations, without exception, are taken from the AV 1611 King James Bible

Copyright © 2010 Deanna K. Loftis, R.N., B.B.A.

All rights reserved. No part of this publication may be reproduced, stored in a retrieval system, or transmitted in any form or by any means, electronic, mechanical, photocopying, recording, or otherwise, without the prior written permission of the publisher.

ISBN: 978-1-60383-348-6

Published by:
Holy Fire Publishing
717 Old Trolley Road
Attn: Suite 6, Publishing Unit #116
Summerville, SC 29485

www.ChristianPublish.com

Cover Design: Jay Cookingham

Printed in the United States of America and the United Kingdom

DEDICATION

Dedicated to "the high and lofty One that inhabiteth eternity, whose name is Holy;" and to His Son, The Lord Jesus Christ, "In whom are hid all the treasures of wisdom and knowledge."
(ISA 57:15 & COL 2:3 AV 1611 KJV)

DISCLAIMER

This book is neither a medical guide, nor a manual for self treatment. It is for informational purposes only and is not intended to be a substitute for medical diagnosis, treatment or health care, nor should it be construed as practicing medicine. None of the websites mentioned in this book consider themselves self-treatment medical guides, but are for informational purposes only. Nutrients given herein are dosage suggestions and are for your information only. You should always check with your physician for your own individual needs regarding any supplements, especially if you have a chronic disease or illness or if you have health questions regarding the use of any information in this book. The author and publisher do not prescribe and assume no liability for any adverse effects or consequences resulting from the use of any of the suggestions, preparations, recipes, therapies, or procedures discussed in this book, nor for the reliance thereon, nor for interpretation errors or transcription errors. Many of the statements and treatments regarding various therapies and substances herein have not been thoroughly evaluated by the FDA, and most websites referenced have the FDA disclaimer on them. It is always possible to have allergic responses to herbs, vitamins, minerals, and their preparations, so caution is advised. Be aware that some herbs and supplements can interfere with the action of prescription medications, or may be incompatible with certain drugs. What you choose to do with this information is up to you. The publisher and author of this book assume no liability for those decisions. Should you use products or therapies from those websites, or those described in this book, you do so at your own discretion and risk.

My Appreciation To:

I would like to express my deepest gratitude to the many people who have encouraged me, influenced me, inspired me, or shared some of the experiences that would one day prompt me to become a writer. First, to the one who saved me and redeemed me with His own blood, the Lord Jesus Christ, who gave me the imparted wisdom, direction, and perseverance that made this book possible; to my devoted and loving sisters, Chris and Shelby, who have always been there for me with their help, promotion, prayers, and encouraging steadfast confidence in me, without whom my writing probably would never have been anything beyond a mere dream; my dear sister, Patsy, for her opinions, prayers, and confidence in me; my loved ones who passed on after their valiant battles against this disease, who were all told that chemo and radiation were their only hope; my dear friends, Dee, Mary, Ann, Carol, Antoinette, Gwen, and Tina from the "old days," when we shared many triumphs and tribulations together; to determined warriors like MaryJo Siegel, Jason Merkle, Vernon Johnston, and so many others, who have fought and conquered this awful disease and given me permission to tell their stories; to brave, pioneering physicians like Dr. Stanislaw Burzynski, who has saved many lives, yet finds the time to write and thank me for my books; to other great pioneers in the medical profession like Dr. Thomas Levy, Dr. T. Simoncini, Rene Caisse, Dr. Mark Levine, Dr. Irwin Stone, Johanna Brandt, Dr. Mark Sircus, Dr. Frederick Klenner, Ewan Cameron, Dr. Robert Cathcart, Dr. Johanna Budwig, Dr. Matthias Rath, Dr. Abram Hoffer, Linus Pauling, Dr. Joseph Mercola, Dr. Julian Whitaker, and many others, who fought (and continue to fight) uphill battles against the entrenched conventional medical establishment, in order to boldly promote natural, non-toxic remedies for overcoming cancer, and to the Christian publishing specialists and others at Holy Fire, for their promptness, honesty, guidance, and integrity in dealing with their authors, and their consistent and patient care in turning out exceptional products.

TABLE OF CONTENTS

Introduction 9

Chapter 1
When Cancer Hits Home 15

Chapter 2
The Orange Wunder Formula & Others – God-Inspired Healing 27

Chapter 3
An Oil of Blessing – God's Natural Cancer Killing Machine 43

Chapter 4
Vitamin C – Premier Cancer Killer & Health Sustainer 61

Chapter 5
God's Healing Sunshine Gift – Vitamin D 101

Chapter 6
Magnesium & Zinc – Mineral Mania 113

Chapter 7
Selenium - Don't Fight Cancer Without It 141

Chapter 8
Iodine, Lost Treasure, Medical Marvel 159

Chapter 9
Glutathione (GSH) Cellular Warrior 177

Chapter 10
CoQ10 – Longevity Yardstick, Cancer Killer 185

Chapter 11
The Miracle of pH Balance 197

Chapter 12
God's Marvelous "Green Thumb" 221

Chapter 13
Other Life-Saving, Non-Toxic Cancer Killers 247

Chapter 14
Immune System Killers: The Worst Offenders 287

Chapter 15
Detox Steps – Getting the Toxins Out Safely 327

Chapter 16
The Greatest Help of All – Divine Intervention 339

APPENDIX I 349

APPENDIX II 351

REFERENCES 355

INDEX..385

If any of the *italicized* words in this book are direct quotes, they are always followed by a reference.

INTRODUCTION

With my newest book, *Gentle Cures for Tough Cancers,* barely off the press, I am basically taking part of that book, expanding on it and adding some new material that I have recently discovered as a result of the experiences a close family member of mine went through in beating cancer within the last few months, thus, my third book. For those of you who read my first book in 2005, which was 728 pages, and my second book (above), which is nearly 750 pages, this new book will seem short in comparison! Nonetheless, the information compiled in this smaller book is critical for those fighting cancer, or with loved ones battling this disease. Though I have chosen a few major cancer fighters to highlight in this book, in no way do I wish to detract from the importance of such amazing antioxidants as Poly-MVA, beta carotene, the cruciferous vegetables, Maitake D-Fraction, Ukrain, B17, the green drinks, or any of the other nutritional powerhouses discussed in my first two books. This new book would make a great companion book to my last book. Be sure to read the chapters in that book (above) that relate to the specific kind of cancer you have and the extra nutritional chapters that will help you, along with the amazing new discoveries I have written about in this book.

The more I research, the more I study, the more I am convinced that the primary secret to healing cancer (and other diseases) involves keeping the body well-supplied with powerful antioxidants as discussed in this book (many of which are incorporated into my new *Orange Wunder Formula* recipe), as well as keeping the human body in a state of alkalinity. Toxins cause stress and acidify the body. Chemo and radiation acidify the body. High protein diets acidify the body. White sugar, flour, fast food, meats, food additives, man-made chemicals, dyes, pollutants in the environment, every day stress – these can all create acidic levels that leave us vulnerable to cancer and other diseases. Overwhelming research has proven that raw green foods, raw fresh vegetables and fruits, minerals, oxygen, fresh air, fresh water, benevolence towards others, the right attitude, proper rest, exercise, prayer, worship, and trusting in God, can nourish and alkalize all cells in the body. Many books touch on the subject of alkalinity and acidity. I did so in my most recent book, *Gentle Cures for Tough Cancers that* was released in August of 2009 and was just announced a *FINALIST* in the National 2010 INDIE Excellence Book Awards in the Health & Well Being category. Some books have very long and labored instructions for converting the body from excess acidity to a refreshing alkaline state. This book will tell you about a handful of miracle ingredients that will help you get well, and also, how to become more alkaline in such a way that it won't take you weeks and months. It can be done within a matter of a few days, it won't cost you a small fortune, and it could very well save your life or the life of someone you love.

Those of you who read my first two books know that I lost three family members to cancer. Their struggles were partly what began me on the road to investigating alternative cancer therapies. All of them received standard conventional chemo and/or radiation for their cancer. All of them were dead within just a few months of their treatments. Think about how many people you know whose lives have been lost or forever altered by cancer. I have a half-brother who was diagnosed with colon cancer and refused chemo after having bowel surgery. His doctor insisted that he would be dead within six months without chemo. That was more than 25 years ago. He is still alive and well, he never had the chemo, and his cancer never returned.

Since my first book came out, I have also lost a cousin to cancer. She developed breast cancer after many years of being on prescription hormone replacement therapy (HRT) given to her by her family physician. (I wrote an entire chapter about the horrors of synthetic HRT in *Gentle Cures for Tough Cancers*). She took Tamoxifen (Nolvadex®) for the breast cancer, and then developed uterine cancer from the Tamoxifen (one of its many side effects). She then underwent a total hysterectomy and chemo afterwards; however, the cancer returned in her peritoneal area and liver. She underwent more chemo treatments and within a few months, she died right before Christmas. She had called me to ask me for my recommendations. This was after she had already taken several rounds of chemo. I sent her a copy of my book and discussed several items she could use. She never used any of my recommendations, not a single one. Instead, she allowed herself to be slowly poisoned with the same drugs that she was told would extend her life and help heal her cancer. She listened to the same advice that killed my mom, my father-in-law, and my brother-in-law. They never asked any questions. They believed that the drugs would cure them. They didn't. They gambled and lost their lives. That is four out of four people in my family who took chemo and lost their lives. Not very good statistics, are they?

Well, you can imagine my dismay when yet a fifth close family member of mine was recently diagnosed with Stage IV inoperable bladder cancer that had gone into his sacral bones. I'm sure that his record of smoking cigarettes for more than 40 years was a major contributing factor. This happened in the late fall of 2009, just a few months after my second book came out. When his urologist referred him to an oncologist, I knew that between the two of them, they would recommend chemo. In spite of the fact that I am not an advocate of chemo—I know that some cancers do respond well to certain chemo drugs—however, because of years of research, I also know that chemo can be like playing a game of Russian roulette. It might buy you time, but it will also depress the immune system and may actually cause the occurrence later in life of a secondary cancer more difficult to fight than the one you started with. This is actually one of the many side effects of chemo you may never be told about. These are known as *drug-resistant cancers*, some of which have been known to respond well to pawpaw, which I discussed in detail in Chapter 21 of my last book, *Gentle Cures for Tough Cancers*, which is available for order at most online websites and bookstores throughout the U.S. *(Amazon .com),* Canada *(Amazon.ca),* Europe *(Amazon.co.uk),* Japan, Australia, New Zealand, Asia, and the nations of the United Kingdom. Some of the bookstores in my local area, such as Barnes & Noble, stock my books.

I am an advocate of non-toxic antineoplastons (developed by Dr. Stanislaw Burzynski in Houston, Texas), Ukrain, and many other natural therapies that don't harm healthy cells, and I discuss many of these in my previous books and this book as well. Thousands of people have responded well to Burzynski's antineoplastons, Ukrain, and some of the newer cancer-fighting drugs coming on the market that are not even called chemo drugs because they are so non-toxic.

You can write about alternative medicine and be a strong supporter of it, but that is no guarantee that your closest family members are going to take up the banner as well. As a matter-of-fact, you may find a lot of resistance within your own blood relatives. I have close relatives who are not into alternative health, haven't read a single book I've ever written, and would never consider anything that isn't "conventional," however, that does not discourage me from continuing my research and writing. On the contrary, it makes me more determined than ever, probably because of the many people who DO write to encourage me, read my books, and tell me of their great results using items I've researched and recommended to them, and people like Dr. Stanislaw Burzynski in Texas and Dr. Steven Ayres, who send me letters thanking me for writing these books.

Most everyone in my family knows how I feel about chemo and radiation, but having said that, I also realize that you must allow adults to choose for themselves the treatments that they will be a part of. Doctors are very influential and even though I had an oncologist admit to me about five months ago that: "We doctors are not as smart as most people THINK we are," they are still very adamant about their belief that you can heal diseases by flooding the body with free-radicals and toxic substances that often kill the immune system (and sometimes the patient, before they kill the cancer)! Can you believe that this very same oncologist said to me, "Years from now people will probably be laughing with disbelief at the current way that we are treating cancer, but for now, this is all we have." Well, I am already in disbelief, but I don't think it's a "laughing" matter. The truth is that chemo and radiation are not *all that we have*. It's just that most conventional doctors are not trained in nutritional or alternative medicine and many have no idea what ELSE is out there that works without killing the immune system, or they do know of such treatments, but never speak of them.

My immediate concern wasn't so much for what might happen down the road from the suppression of my relative's natural immunity, but what kind of serious side effects he might have during the treatments. He isn't a book-reader, could care less about alternative therapies, and is from the "old school," that still believes the modern medical establishment couldn't possibly be steering thousands of people wrong when it comes to their pharmaceutical drug treatments— *could they? Possibly?*

I said all of that to say this: if you become interested in alternative therapies and start reading books like mine and others who write about non-toxic cures for disease, don't assume everyone in your immediate family is going to be overjoyed with your decision! Don't assume that because someone is interested in alternative health, every one of their relatives is on board with the program. In Mark 6:4 Jesus said *"A prophet is not without honour, but in his own country, and among his own kin, and in his own house."* Well, you can tweak that when it comes to many alternative health advocates. My enthusiasm for alternative therapies isn't shared in the least by my closest family members, apart from four of my sisters, a brother, and some fellow Christian friends, who have always supported my views and applauded my efforts and research. You can't force your opinions on others. You can only express your opinions and let others choose for themselves what risks they are willing to take. Most cancer patients are desperate and they soak up every word their physician tells them without ever asking any questions.

I can still remember my mom's oncologist telling her that chemo would extend her life. She was dead less than eight months later. Well maybe it did, because perhaps she would have lived six months, instead of eight without it, but how much better would her quality of life have been during that six months compared to what she went through because of the side effects of the chemo? She had all the typical immune-suppression side effects when she went through chemo. The thing is my mom had total faith in her physician. This was many years before I began researching alternative health remedies and natural therapies for cancer and other diseases. All I can do is present my own findings and let people decide for themselves what course they are going to choose. Most important of all, be informed and remember this, if you find all the choices in my books a bit overwhelming, you don't have to take everything. You only need a few powerful antioxidants to turn your illness around and heal your body! Everything does not work the same for everyone. You may have better results with some ingredients than others do. Others may have better results than you do with certain antioxidants. Just keep flooding your body with antioxidants and your immune system will heal itself and fight the disease for you!

By the time my first book was ready for print in 2005, I had spent years researching the material on alternative cures for cancer. I simply wanted people who have cancer to be able to have a quick, ready reference that they could check for current natural cancer therapies at their fingertips, so they would not have to spend years digging for the material like I did, besides, I knew many of them didn't have the luxury of *years* of research. Time was not on their side.

From the start, I decided that I would do everything I could possibly do to help my relative keep his immune system boosted regardless of his decision to allow his physician to use some of the same drugs which had already caused the deaths of other family members of mine. You can read exactly what I did in Chapters 1 and 2 of this book. You will be amazed at the results. I believe that through much prayer, God inspired me in developing the formulas I used. I also believe that you can use these same formulas for your own loved ones to bring them back to health and extend their lives, whether they are fighting cancer or some other life-threatening disease.

CHAPTER 1

When Cancer Hits Home

****

When yet another close family member of mine was diagnosed with Stage IV invasive, inoperable bladder cancer in early November of 2009, years before, I had already lost several other family members to various cancers, all of them to conventional medicine's chemo, radiation, and surgery regimen, as I discussed in my first two books. After my close family member had undergone a cystoscopy and bladder tumor biopsy, I recall the urologist giving him this little *speech* after the procedure. It went something like this:

> The cancer you have is very aggressive and has formed a large tumor in your bladder which has spread into your sacral bone. I tried to remove the bladder tumor, but it was too large. I could only get a small part of the tumor. I am not going to talk cure to you, but I believe we can help you maintain a good quality of life, so that you can take each day at a time and get the best out of the time you have left. Stay active, do the things you enjoy doing. Let each day count.

I always call these little "speeches," *terminal talks*. You know – *we can't really cure you, but you can live each day you have left to the very fullest you are capable of before the inevitable hits*. They didn't really give him a length of time prognosis, but I knew from the tone of voice and somber attitude, and with my nursing background, that the outlook was pretty dismal. He was also very negative about the entire outlook and flatly told him that "this cancer will eventually kill you." I wasn't surprised to hear such a statement coming from his mouth. Apparently, this physician knew nothing of the words from *Proverbs 18:21*: **"Death and life are in the power of the tongue."** I believe doctors have the ability to speak blessings (or curses) over people exactly by saying things like this to their patients! How many times do physicians tell their patients, *"there is nothing else we can do for you, you have six weeks left, get your affairs in order."* What happens? The patients lose all HOPE, believing these words. They go home, get everything in order, give up, accept these words and die. I know you have to be realistic, but nothing is impossible with God. When you take away all HOPE that people have, you leave them with nothing but despair and resignation. Well, when I was praying over him later, I kept telling my relative that he was going to beat this cancer and according to the Word of God, he could already claim his healing and I prayed healing verses over his life.

Of course the urologist referred him to an oncologist and the oncologist told him that (since the cancer had already gone into the bones), surgery was not even an option. He recommended two chemo drugs that he said, hopefully, would put him into remission and extend his life. The very first PET scan showed the actual cancer in his bladder and sacral bones. His urologist had already tried to remove the large tumor in the bladder through a cystoscopy, but could not do so. He said it was too large and only managed to biopsy it and remove a small section. Three of my relative's other family member's in the room had already decided that he was going to take chemo before he did. When I asked his physician about some of the newer, less toxic therapies, such as Burzynski's antineoplasons and Ukrain, and some of the newer immune-friendly drugs being developed for treating cancer, first I got a blank stare, then he dismissed what I said with a comment about getting a second opinion, then there was a moment of uncomfortable silence in the room. My relative's other three family members were livid with me and horrified that I had even questioned the oncologist's protocol, and told me later that they felt I was undermining the doctor's own self-confidence in his prescribed regimen. They even thought I wanted to send him to Europe for treatment! They had no idea that Ukrain is a cancer drug. They thought I wanted to send him overseas to the country of Ukraine for cancer therapy! I kid you not, this really happened! They didn't know what Ukrain or antineoplastons are (neither did his physician), and none of them had ever been around nurses long enough to know that that is exactly what nurses do. We don't blindly accept everything we are told, especially when it comes to treatment plans for a close family member. It is just the nature of nurses, especially those of us who have been in the profession for many years!

Decisions...Decisions

The oncologist decided on using *Cisplatin* and *Gemzar* for my relative's bladder cancer, two very powerful chemo drugs with potentially serious side effects. One very positive note is that when his labs showed that he was low on Vitamin D, his physician started him on high-doses of vitamin D, 50,000 units a week. I was also glad to see that he was hanging intravenous magnesium before his first chemo round. I discuss magnesium at length in Chapter 6 of this book. I know how important magnesium is.

I had often tried to get my relative (and other family members) to use higher supplements apart from a single multi-vitamin pill daily; however, he has never shared my enthusiasm for alternative health therapies, hates taking pills, would much rather have a hamburger or hot dog for dinner than salmon and salad, and isn't much of a book-reader. He will read newspapers for hours, but not books.

Multi-vitamin-mineral pills are good for getting trace amounts, but they hardly provide the dosage needed to maintain health in our ever-increasing polluted world. Some of them contain 400 U of vitamin D and you don't always know if it's synthetic D2 or natural D3, and even most Naturopaths today will tell you that you need 1000-10,000 U of vitamin D3 a day (if supplementing and not able to get pure sunshine). Also, you might get 60 mg of vitamin C in a daily multi-vitamin pill, when what you really need (to bring you out of subclinical scurvy and prevent colds, heart disease, chronic illness, cancers, and flu) is closer to 8,000—10,000 mg a day! Most people just do not get enough vitamin C, magnesium, iodine, CoQ10, selenium, alpha lipoic acid, chlorophyll, beta carotene, B vitamins, and most other nutrients with a single compressed multi-vitamin pill a day.

Seeking God in Prayer

Because I was determined that my recently diagnosed family member not become chemo victim #5 in my family, I sought God in prayer and fasting about exactly what he would have me do to help keep him well, in spite of his decision to take chemo. I wanted him to be able to keep his immune system at top level throughout the process, despite the fact that he continued to smoke cigarettes, though he had cut down drastically to 2 or 3 cigarettes a day. I did not want him to wither away, dry up and die like my other relatives had done! I literally prayed and asked God precisely what he would have me do to help get my loved one well and cancer-free. I knew I had a great "arsenal" of immune-boosting items in both books I had written, but there were many to choose from. My relative and I talked about the 7 steps of *Harmony Healing* that I discussed in my last book, *Gentle Cures for Tough Cancers,* and I encouraged him to keep a positive attitude, to memorize healing scripture verses, and to picture himself well, to claim healing for himself (as we both did), and we praised God for his healing, even when it was not yet evident. Even with the alternative therapies, there were a lot of choices. God answered those prayers in a most amazing way!

Though he was diagnosed the first week of November 2009, circumstances worked out so that my relative did not actually start receiving chemo until several weeks later. This gave me prayer time and time to develop a strategy to help him fight the disease and the side-effects of the treatment.

He chose the conventional protocol recommended by the oncologist (which is what I knew would happen because that is all oncologists know). Patients are so overwhelmed by their diagnosis and so filled with fear that they are completely at the mercy of oncologists, who are only trained in chemo and radiation. Most of them know absolutely nothing about alternative therapies and those that do, wouldn't dare mention them for fear of being ostracized by their peers, or they read about them in the privacy of their own homes, surfing the internet, or from books like this one.

Strategically Planning & A God-Inspired Formula

My relative ended up going through the chemo, which was his choice, but he also used all the alternative nutritional formulas that I developed and recommended to him during the process. He ended up using a combination of conventional and alternative "medicine". Many people use this treatment approach and have excellent results with it. Such was his case. What actually happened was that God inspired me to incorporate many natural treatments into some very powerful nutritional formulas, one of which he drank every single morning before his chemo program. The others he drank later in the day. While I did not develop these formulas overnight, they did come to me within a matter of days during the time I was praying and fasting, and I can only give God the credit that is due him for his guidance and direction during this time! I am not even sure what day I could point to and say "that was the day God inspired me to create this formula," but what happened was not instantaneous. Did I hear an audible voice directing me? Certainly not. I simply prayed, fasted, and the information was mentally imparted to me. I believe this is what is known as *God-inspired.* I simply acted by faith and these formulas were the result of that action.

I call the first formula, **Orange Wunder,** because the German word for **miracle** is **wunder**, and this drink truly is a healing miracle! Not only that, but two of the ingredients I used are partly from the Budwig diet, developed by a famous German biochemist who cured her own cancer patients with two of the ingredients that I incorporated into my *Orange Wunder Formula*, which you can read about in Chapter 2. If you or someone YOU love is fighting cancer, or any chronic illness, what can this formula do to help YOU or them get well? I believe that prayer and this formula (and the other two that I developed) is what boosted my family member's immunity, kept the chemo drugs from causing severe side effects, and helped bring about his total cancer remission. He also went on the prayer list at my local church, and many relatives and friends who knew him were praying for him.

Before he even started the chemo and during the time he was taking it, we prayed together and occasionally took communion, using grape juice and crackers. This is completely scriptural. Many families do not take advantage of celebrating communion as explained in the Bible, yet communion among believers has great healing power and should be done more often. You do not have to be in a church filled with 300 people to take communion. Jesus tells us in *Matthew 18:20: "For where two or three are gathered together in my name, there am I in the midst of them."* If there are only TWO of you, the presence of God is there. You can participate in taking communion on a daily basis. All believers are "kings and priests" before God, so this ordinance should be practiced more often by families, especially if you are praying over someone who is sick. You can also anoint your sick family member with anointing oil while you are praying over them. Use any fresh olive oil, or another vegetable oil you have on hand.

I started giving my family member nutritional supplements that he would never take before. He has never been much of a natural health enthusiast, even though he's related to someone who writes books on the stuff! In the past, he would always take a simple multi-vitamin/mineral and that is about the gist of his *nutritional regimen*.

I began giving him extra vitamin C every day (2,000 mg to start) and I developed three nutritional drinks for him, the first one (***Orange Wunder***), discussed earlier, was what I believed to be the most important of the three, mostly because it had such potent ingredients for boosting the immunity. He took it every single morning without exception. After describing this amazing health drink, I will discuss in the following chapters some of the individual items that are found in this drink and why they are so important for maintaining and restoring health. This drink, the others I formulated, and the items I discuss in the following chapters (some of which are in these drinks) are what I consider God's most important natural, ***Designer Cancer Killers!***

GOOD NEWS!

The results were amazing. My relative began chemo in December 2009, and I can tell you that December and January were very long, cold, and dismal months! We had some of the coldest, most miserable weather we have had in many winters. He started chemo 4 weeks after he received his diagnosis. The first chemo infusion was on December 2nd, 2009. After only two rounds of chemo (the last dose on January 26, 2010), he was told on February 11, 2010 (less than 14 weeks after his diagnosis), by his happy (and rather surprised oncologist) that he was in TOTAL REMISSON! His second PET scan was normal; the tumor was gone from his bladder and bones. During the chemo, he never developed a single episode of nausea or vomiting, no hair loss, no serious neutropenia or thrombocytopenia, no weight loss, no exhaustion and fatigue, no mouth sores, no throat or stomach ulcers, no skin rashes, no fevers, and he actually gained 26 pounds during the two rounds of chemo! This was during the coldest part of the winter of 2009-2010, and he even ate spicy chili TWICE a week while taking chemo (sometimes 3 times a week) without having any abdominal discomfort whatsoever! He loves chili in the winter. The weight he gained was "good" weight. It was not edema. It was subcutaneous fat and muscle mass that he needed. One early complication that he did develop was blood clots in his legs, which his physician said was caused by the cancer. He was placed on blood-thinners, and did not have any serious problems, or hospitalizations from the clots. He had some slight edema in his feet from the clots, but nothing that slowed him down or prevented him from being totally independent as was usual for him, nor anything that caused him pain, discomfort, or loss of sleep, and the swelling in his feet eventually went away. Sometimes, after being up and about for several hours, he will get some slight swelling in his ankles. The fact that he had to go on blood-thinners narrowed down the availability of many excellent alternative nutrients. He was not able to use any CoQ10, mushroom formulas, green drinks, or herbals that I would have suggested otherwise.

The Disbelief

Needless to say, my family member's oncologist and urologist were both incredulous that he was in complete remission after only 2 rounds of chemo, and it is even possible that he was in remission BEFORE that (possibly even after only one round) had they taken the PET scan sooner, they would have known. His oncologist even kidded about the fact that many times doctors, such as him, often make the mistake of putting patients on chemo drugs, then just keeps dosing them and forgets to check for results as soon as they should. (I didn't say anything at the time, because I remember thinking that, as long as I was around, he wouldn't be forgetting, because I would be reminding him!) As a matter-of-fact, they repeated the PET scan, I think because they simply could not believe the results! His oncologist told him he had never seen anyone respond so rapidly and positively to the treatment the way he had, with a total remission after only 2 rounds of chemo. He kept telling him how amazed he was that he had no side effects, had gained 26 pounds, never lost his hair, looked great, and never missed a beat. His urologist said the same thing. I merely told his doctor that I had been giving him some nutritional vitamin drinks (which was absolutely true), but no details. I kept all of his records just to compare the before and after labs and PET scans, so I have the proof. What happened truly was a miracle! Not only that, but he had many people praying for him. I believe it was a combination of all these factors that got him well.

I would like to point out that before he began chemo and before he began the nutritional drinks; my relative used a soda bicarb, blackstrap molasses solution that I mixed for him to help alkalize his body, because most cancer patients are very acidic. He took the formula for 10 days. That recipe is very similar to the one used by Vernon Johnston ("Vito"), that is given later in this book, except that Vito used a stronger dosage. Before he began chemo, my family member needed stents in his ureters because the bladder tumor was so large that it was pushing against one of the ureters and blocking his urine from getting to the bladder, plus the fact that his prostate was enlarged. He would not have tolerated the high salt (soda bicarb) level that Vito used in his formula.

Whether you choose to go the conventional medicine route, the alternative medicine route, or a combination of both, will have to be your decision. I cannot make that decision for you. Just as I stated in my first two books, I have spent many years collecting the data, but the final choice is yours. While my relative was fighting cancer using chemo, I was determined to help him keep his immunity at an optimum level and minimize the harmful side effects that chemo drugs can cause. My protocol succeeded in doing exactly that. (I would also like to point out the fact that he is the only person out of FIVE of my family members within the last 25 years who survived chemo!) He is the only one who had access to the formulas in this book. I discuss several medical marvels in this book, which truly can be considered **Designer Cancer killers** from God. My *Orange Wunder Formula* in Chapter 2 uses many of these natural life saving, non-toxic ingredients.

Though his urologist was convinced that the tumor would return and wanted him to be scheduled for a very radical bladder removal surgery, my family member's oncologist disagreed and said that he could find no evidence to convince him that he should have this radical surgery, and that he was in total remission. The urologist scheduled him for another cystoscopy to replace the stents that had been placed in the ureters, and even included in the surgery consent form, permission for him to biopsy and try to remove (resect) any new tumor growths. I told him this would not be necessary, that his cancer was gone and there would be nothing to biopsy. With his surgical cap and gown on and a glance over his shoulder in my direction as he walked toward the surgery suite, his only comment to me was, "I hope you're right." After the cystoscopy, when he came to discuss how it went, he sat down at a small table that was reserved for family meetings, and said that he had good news! He admitted that no biopsy was done because there was no tumor—nothing to biopsy—and also said that the stents did not have to be replaced! Everything flushed fine and the stents were removed altogether. A CT scan that was done in June of 2010 confirmed that the tumor had not returned in the four months since my relative had been told that he was in total remission. Once again, while we were sitting in the oncologist's office with the CT scan results on the table, the physician remarked with disbelief how unusual his case was and what an amazing response he had had to the treatment!

Rationale for the Formula

I refer to my first formula as **Orange Wunder** (no, it isn't misspelled), because the word for *miracle* in German is **Wunder**, and this drink is truly miraculous. It is like an orange burst of power and a wonderful tonic for anyone suffering from any chronic illness such as cancer, lupus, high cholesterol, CAD, high blood pressure, neuropathy, frequent colds and viruses, arthritis, migraines, Crohn's, CHF, HIV, ADD, psoriasis, MS, dry skin, senility, depression, female disorders, cystic breasts, psychosis, bipolar disorders, dementia, Alzheimer's, schizophrenia, or any number of ailments! It is the most important recipe that I developed (out of 3) during the time I was fasting and praying. It uses a modified portion of two ingredients from the Johanna Budwig Formula discussed later.

    I also added high dose liposomal C, iodine, magnesium, and other nutrients. If you have loved ones that need the Budwig Formula but don't care for the cottage cheese flax oil blend, believe me, they will drink this tasty orange formula eagerly, even children! Many people with deficiencies in omega-3, magnesium, vitamin C and iodine will benefit from this drink as well. Studies have shown that ADD, ADHD, bi-polar disorders, schizophrenia, MS, heart disease, congestive heart failure, all cancers, ulcers, irritable bowel syndrome, fibromyalgia, chronic fatigue syndrome, bowel disturbances, skin problems, migraines, and many other chronic illnesses, can be linked to omega-3, magnesium, iodine, and vitamin C deficiencies; probably many more than most of us are aware of! There are also ingredients in this formula that promote the formation of glutathione in the body, a life-saving nutrient that most cancer patients are lacking.

    Just be sure if you use the Budwig Formula by itself, without the rest of these ingredients (from the *Orange Wunder Formula*), that you have sufficient magnesium in your diet, or your body will not be able to metabolize the fatty acids in the flax oil (287).

My *Orange Wunder* recipe contains magnesium. During the time that my family member underwent two rounds of chemotherapy, he drank the *Orange Wunder* every morning. He never had a single episode of nausea, vomiting, mouth or stomach ulcers, malaise, infection, decreased appetite, feeling ill or sick, nor did he lose his hair. During his two cycles of chemo, he gained 26 pounds. And, as I said earlier, this was "good" weight. It was not edema where unhealthy fluid accumulates in the extremities. The slight edema he developed from the leg clots was at the start of the chemo and would never have amounted to 26 pounds. As noted earlier, it was subcutaneous fat and muscle mass, weight that he sorely needed. He even ate some very spicy chili at least two or three times per week while taking the chemo treatments. This was in the middle of a very cold winter, and he loves chili during cold weather. He was receiving *Cisplatin* and *Gemzar*, two commonly used chemo drugs with potentially severe side effects. At the end of the second cycle, less than 90 days after beginning this protocol, a PET scan showed that he was in **total remission!** The cancer had disappeared from the bladder and the bones! The physician gave him a 3rd cycle, just to be sure (in his words) that no malignant cells were left, and again, he had absolutely no side-effects! One day when my relative walked into his urologist's office, the physician told him that had he just walked in off the street, he would never have known that he was a chemo patient. He told him, "You don't look like my typical chemo patients."

Though I am not an advocate of chemotherapy because it is so toxic to the body's natural immunity, I believe the *Orange Wunder* drink (and the other formulas I developed, coupled with seeking God in prayer) prevented the severe toxicity that these drugs can cause to the immune system and helped in eradicating the cancer. Both his urologist and oncologist were amazed at my family member's quick recovery and kept saying so at every single visit. Without these formulas, I do not believe he would have gone into total remission with only two rounds of chemo, nor do I believe he would have escaped all the serious side effects that most people experience, and for all I know, he may have gotten well without even taking the chemo! And, just as with what happened to my four other family members before him, I believe it is possible that without taking the nutritional formulas, without the prayer of many people, he would have experienced side effects of the chemo, which might very well have killed him. One of the nurses in the oncologist's office had given him several papers right before he was to begin the chemo, outlining all the potential side effects he could expect. He was told that it was not likely that he would have all of the side effects, but to expect *at least a few of them*. He had none!

I can remember being in the oncologist's office while my relative was taking chemo and watching other patients as they came and went. Many of them, with their little caps on their heads (because of hair loss), gray-looking skin, and thin, frail, wasted bodies, appeared to be at death's door. I'm sure some of them were. One patient was even brought in on a stretcher for chemo treatment, and I heard the oncologist giving verbal instructions to one of the nurses for a patient who had developed severe mouth and throat sores and non-stop nausea and vomiting from the chemo. I recall her telling the oncologist how miserable the patient was. They were talking of hospitalizing him. I saw and heard all of this activity around us while my own family member was sitting up and watching TV, with a full head of hair, eating a full lunch with his legs propped up; no weight loss, and never missing a beat, as the chemo was infusing during his favorite TV program. During the first week of his first chemo treatment, I also gave him *Life Mel* Honey. It is a special honey that is produced from the nectar of 40 herbs (with other natural ingredients), developed in Israel (318). Two teaspoons per day (one in the morning and one in the evening) are recommended. This special honey has been shown, in **human** testing, to prevent the neutropenia (dangerously low white blood count) caused by chemotherapy and to lower the risk of severe platelet drop (thrombocytopenia), often found in chemo patients (318). You can find out more about this amazing honey at website: *http://www.lifemel israel.com* (318).

During the time he was taking chemo, my family member was also taking 1000 mg of vitamin C (ascorbic acid) by mouth twice a day (in pill form), 3000 mg of liposomal C in the orange drink, 50,000 U of vitamin D once a week (this was given to him via prescription by his physician), a multi-vitamin/multi-mineral pill once a day, 14 – 16 ounces of ***Orange Wunder*** once a day (in the am) and the 16 ounce Fruit/Vegetable Drink once a day about 2 hours after dinner, as described in the next chapter. (There were a few days that he missed the fruit/vegetable drink, but most days he drank it.) He drank the whey protein shake just occasionally during this time, about once every four days. Most of the time, he was just too full from the fruit/vegetable drink for the protein shake. When first diagnosed, he was also taking 200 mg a day of CoQ10 (something he never took before being diagnosed with cancer; he hated pills), and acidophilus PEARLS™, but had to discontinue the CoQ10 when his physician placed him on blood-thinners. CoQ10 isn't recommended when taking blood-thinners. He was also not able to take any leafy green drinks due to the blood-thinners, nor any herbs or other treatments besides the drinks mentioned below. I would like for him to have taken chlorella, barley juice, Essiac, and some other herbals, but being on blood-thinners made this impossible. Described in Chapter 2 is the simple step-by-step recipe for the **Orange Wunder** drink and the other two formulas I developed. When you have the ingredients in front of you, assembling the **Orange Wunder** takes three or four minutes to mix and drink. That formula (and the other two) is given in detail in the next chapter. The ingredients are so vital to healing, that I have devoted entire chapters to some of them later in this book, letting you know exactly why they are so powerful! I have also explained exactly where you can obtain all of the ingredients. (I would not be surprised to see *copycat* "versions" of my formulas appear not long after this book is released.)

CHAPTER 2

The Orange Wunder Formula & Others – God-Inspired Healing

****

I. Orange Wunder

If using this as part of a cancer-fighting protocol, you must prepare this drink EXACTLY as described. Use it every single morning. Do not skip days. It is best to drink it on an empty stomach before you eat or drink anything else. It incorporates a modified portion of the famous *Budwig flax oil formula* that Johanna Budwig used to cure many of her *terminal* cancer patients! Known fondly as the "Linseed Lady," her brilliant studies, research, and accomplishments won her world-wide fame as a premier German biochemist and a formidable foe for the hydrogenated fat industry! **Orange Wunder** also contains a very potent form of vitamin C known as *liposomal vitamin C*. The brand I use is made by **LivOn Labs®** and is called **LypoSpheric C™,** described by Dr. Thomas Levy in his excellent nutritional books. At the end of the recipe, I have a list of the brands I use and <u>where</u> you can find them. All but two of these ingredients can be found at your local health food store. The two that may (or may not) be found at your health food store can be found on the internet sites I have given.

Ingredients:
(Sources where you can find the items are given after this list)

1. ½ navel orange peeled and sliced in about 8 pieces. Discard peelings. If you do not use navel oranges, be sure to remove all the seeds from your orange. It is fine to leave some of the white skin (under the peeling) on the orange pieces.
2. 3000 mg of liposomal vitamin C (see below for source).
3. One small squeeze-packet of Omega 3 fish oil (see source below).

4. One teaspoon of glutamine powder.
5. 20 drops of 2% food grade iodine (Do NOT use if allergic to iodine or iodized salt). I use only ***Magnascent*©** Iodine. (Those fighting breast cancers may need more iodine than this and those with larger breasts may need more iodine.)
6. Two tablespoons of organic high-lignan, non GMO flax seed oil. (Keep this oil refrigerated and never heat it for any reason.)
7. Two tablespoons of liquid Calcium, Magnesium, and Zinc (local source below). All 3 are available in one bottle in liquid form.
8. 6 tablespoons of organic yogurt (4 to 6 ounces total).
9. Two packets of a natural herbal sweetener (I use Stevia®).
10. Orange juice (you will add fresh, organic OJ at the end of the recipe to total 16 ounces of fluid). The large size blender *(party cup),* if using a ***Magic Bullet*®** blender, will be full.
11. Maitake D-Fraction® Mushroom Extract (20 drops). You cannot use Maitake if you are taking blood-thinners or if you have M.S. Check with your physician.

How to Mix the Formula:

1. First, put the organic yogurt into a ***Magic Bullet*®** or a small individual blender (do not use a large blender.) If you have one of those hand-held, stick-type blenders, those will work too. You can also use a small, inexpensive two cup blender that you can find at *WalMart's* if you don't have a small blender or a ***Magic Bullet*®**. Add the 2 tablespoons of organic flax seed oil. Blend these 2 items well in the blender for about 20 seconds, or until the oil is **no longer visible**. You should have a very creamy consistency and the oil should not be separated from the yogurt. It is critical that you mix these TWO ingredients FIRST and get them mixed thoroughly before adding anything else. Do not short-cut by skipping this step. It is crucial. (Also, the directions on your *Magic Bullet*® blender will tell you not to ever mix anything for longer than 60 seconds at a time, so be aware of that.)
2. Next, add the 2 packets of sweetener (use 3 if you want a sweeter-tasting drink) (I use Stevia®), and add the chopped orange pieces, glutamine, iodine drops, 2 tablespoons of the Calcium, Magnesium and Zinc liquid (see brand below), the Maitake drops, and blend all of these ingredients several

seconds until the oranges are liquid and the mixture is a creamy, smooth consistency. It will take 30-40 seconds. At this point you may need to pour the contents of your small cup *Magic Bullet®* into one of the larger *party* cups provided by the *Magic Bullet®* appliance makers. Remember, your main reason for using the small cup first is to get the flax oil and yogurt easily blended before adding anything else.

3. Next, add the 3 packets of liposomal C and the one packet of Omega-3 fish-oil blend to the drink. These are little squeeze packets and the contents are very thick. Get every drop! Then, use a **fork** to mix them very gently by hand into your drink. You do NOT want to blend these in your blender or you will break up all the liposomes in the liposomal C. You want to keep the little liposomes intact as much as possible as this is how the C is absorbed so efficiently!

4. Last, add enough fresh organic orange juice to total 16 ounces or to fill your ***Magic Bullet®*** large *(party cup)* nearly to the top. Do NOT blend it again! Just use a large fork to gently mix by hand, and it is ready to drink. (If you use the smallest *Magic Bullet®* container to mix your ingredients, you will have to pour everything into one of the larger drink cups provided by *Magic Bullet®* before adding the orange juice, in order to have at least 16 ounces of fluid.) Just don't blend them again.

Sources—Where to Obtain the Ingredients:

1. Use organic, seedless oranges, such as navel oranges. A juicer will remove seeds, but a blender will not. Leaving seeds in could cause choking and will make the drink very bitter and gritty! Buy ORGANIC whenever possible. If using other than navel oranges, remove all seeds. If the oranges you use are unusually large, even using only half, you may not need to add the extra OJ at the end of the drink.

2. I use the *LypoSpheric™* brand of liposomal Vitamin C. You can obtain this at *LivOnLabs* in Henderson, Nevada. See their website at: ***livonlabs.com***. They sell 30 packets to a box. A box will last you ten days, so you will need 3 boxes to get you through one month. The more you purchase from

LivOnLabs, the bigger your discount. If you buy this product ready-made, it may seem expensive, but not compared to the thousands of dollars that drug companies charge for chemo. Also, the liposomes are actually composed of lecithin molecules and even the lecithin is very beneficial. Combining vitamin C with lecithin can help prevent and clear up atherosclerosis because it reduces harmful (LDL) cholesterol and raises good (HDL) cholesterol levels. You can also shop around for other brands, including bottles of the liquid liposomal C, rather than the small individual packets. These 3 websites have the bottled, liquid liposomal C at different prices (there are probably others):

- *http://www.letstalkhealth.com*
- *http://www.nanoliposomals.com/Liposomal_ VITAMIN_C.html*
- *http://www.lipoflow.com/index.php?main_page= productinfo&products_id=5&c Path=1_4.*

Just realize that the bottled form, though less expensive, may not have as long a shelf-life as the individually-sealed packets. I have tried the liquid from *Letstalkhealth* and it has a great taste. Always check expiration dates. Some of the bottled liposomal will last 45 days after it is opened, but it MUST be kept refrigerated. The little individual-sealed packets of liposomal C have a longer shelf-life and do not need refrigeration, but may cost more. (Note that during the time my relative was taking chemo, on the day before chemo, the day of chemo and the day after, I used FOUR of the liposomal packets, rather than three.) The rest of the time, I used 3 packets or a total of 3000 mg of liposomal C. If you absolutely cannot get the liposomal C, there is a substitute: take one teaspoon of ascorbic acid powder or crystals (which should contain 5000 mg of vitamin C per **teaspoon**) that you can get at most health food stores, and add it to 4 ounces of distilled water. Add ½ teaspoon of soda bicarb (*Arm & Hammer*® brand, for example) into the mixture. Once the fizzing stops, stir until completely dissolved and fizzing is done. Congratulations! You have just created sodium ascorbate. This removes the bitterness of the ascorbic acid crystals, and you can simply add this to the ***Orange Wunder*** drink instead of the liposomal C. It is not as potent, but is a less expensive substitute. It does add some salt to the mixture. Just be sure that you add this sodium ascorbate to the drink right before you add the orange juice. Do not **EVER** add the sodium ascorbate to the blender, put the blade on and mix it, especially when the cup is nearly full, because the sodium ascorbate could still be fizzing slightly and doing so will put pressure on the *Magic Bullet®* blender. This could damage the unit beyond repair.

3. I use ***CorOmega® 3 Squeeze*** brand of omega 3 fish oil. I find this at *Meijer's*, but some health food stores also carry these little individual packets. They come in 30 packet boxes or 90 packet boxes and are delicious! The large box will last you 3 months (using one packet per day). You can get orange or lime-flavored. I used the orange. It goes well with the orange-flavored MRM® (see below), the orange juice, and orange, vanilla, or peach-flavored yogurt.

4. **Glutamine powder**: you can obtain this powder at health food stores like ***Whole Foods Market.*** I have only seen it in large plastic jars that weigh more than a pound, but take heart. You may pay $30.00 for it, but one jar will last you more than 3 months. Use the vegetarian, gluten-free. **Don't** refrigerate after opening. Keep it dry, in a pantry or kitchen cabinet. Glutamine helps cancer patients maintain their weight and prevents the muscle-wasting that you often see in cancer patients, known as *cachexia.* It also increases valuable levels of **glutathione** that everyone needs, especially cancer patients and those with suppressed immune systems.

5. **Iodine:** I use the 2% ***Magnascent*©** Iodine brand (one small dropper bottle will last you a long time.) You can find this online at their website: ***http://www.magnascent.com.*** Lugol's iodine is not as gentle, but you can get it at 2% strength at *SwansonVitamins.com*. Go to their site and type

Lugol's in the search box in the upper left corner. You can get 7% Lugol's only by prescription. At one time, the 7% Lugol's was commonly sold in many pharmacies without requiring a prescription. The ***breastcancerchoices.org*** website recommends **50 mg of Iodoral iodine** in their protocol. That is 50 MILLIGRAMS, not MICROgrams! See Chapter 8 in this book for their full *Breast Cancer Protocol* or go to their website above. Their protocol is supported by physicians who have used it for more than 4,000 patients, and they believe that not only breast cancer patients, but others with cancer would benefit from this dosage as well.

The amount in *Orange Wunder* will give you 8 mg (if you use the 2% solution and 4 mg if you use the 1% solution). You can split the amount in divided doses during the day and take the rest (that isn't in the formula) mixed in water on an empty stomach, though I did not do so for this particular formula. I used a one-time amount of 20 drops of the *2% Magnascent©* in the **Orange Wunder Formula** once daily in the mornings. You can also use smaller amounts and gradually build up your dose once you see how you are feeling. Just realize that most cancer patients are very deficient in magnesium and iodine, and the more toxins (like chlorine, fluoride, bromide, and mercury) you are exposed to every day, the more iodine you need. Be aware that Lugol's 2% or 7% has a much higher ratio of iodine per drop than *Magnascent©*. Check the label!

6. **Flax seed oil**: I use *Barlean's®* brand or *Nature's Way®,* which most health food stores carry. Just be sure the flax oil you use is organic and **non-GMO**! Get the "high lignan" bottles. If you use the unfiltered, it has more lignans and is darker in color. If you use the filtered, it is lower in lignans and lighter and clearer in color. Not much difference in taste or price, but you want the **high lignan** product.

7. **MRM®** liquid Calcium, Magnesium, & Zinc: I find these bottles (orange-flavored) at health food stores only. You can probably order it on the internet as well. ***Whole Foods Market*** stores carry it. Note that it does use the Magnesium

Oxide form of magnesium which can have a slight laxative effect. Some cancer patients have a problem with sluggish bowels, while others have diarrhea problems. If this formula causes you diarrhea, then cut the portion in half and take only ONE tablespoon, rather than two, and use two **teaspoons** of Swanson Vitamins liquid *Magnesium Chloride* made by *Nutricology®* along with the ONE tablespoon of the MRM®. Another option is that you can switch to magnesium citrate or magnesium malate, just do not use the liquid magnesium aspartate or magnesium hydroxide! The MRM® bottle calls for one tablespoon per serving, but most people with cancer are **very magnesium deficient** and need more. You can also substitute the *Floradix®* brand of liquid magnesium which is very tasty and does not have a laxative effect, if you prefer, though I did not do this. You can get *Floradix®* at **Whole Foods** and at **Rainbow Blossom** Natural Food Markets. **Rainbow Blossom** Natural Food Markets often carry things you cannot find anywhere else. If you do not have one nearby, their website can be found at: ***http://www.rainbowblossom.com.*** (Just be sure to check the label of contents. Some of these items may contain trace amounts of apricots, or other items you could be allergic to!) *Swanson's Vitamins* also makes a liquid calcium-magnesium drink that uses the **magnesium citrate** form of magnesium. This form is more absorbable and won't usually have a laxative effect on the body, though it has no zinc. You will get more magnesium because mag citrate is more easily absorbed by the body than mag oxide. Note that *Swansons* also has a **magnesium chloride drink**. This is probably the **BEST form of magnesium you can get for absorption**, apart from the magnesium oil that you get and spray right onto the skin for absorption through the skin (available on the internet). Be sure you get your zinc in a daily multi-mineral, multi-vitamin pill, and use another source for your calcium, if not using the MRM®. The problem is that most people are getting adequate calcium in their daily diets, but not enough magnesium.

8. **Yogurt** - Use only **organic yogurt** or non-GMO organic soy yogurt. Do not use any products that contain **GMO** foods. Usually, the label will tell you that the product contains no GMO foods. Most organic products are non-GMO (not genetically-modified). I have used orange-flavored, vanilla, French-vanilla, peach-flavored yogurt, or plain. Just be sure it is **organic,** and do not use the yogurt that is full of large pieces of fruit or covered with creams, cereal, sprinkles, or other questionable substances. Use non-GMO if you choose the organic **soy** yogurt. The actual Budwig Formula uses six tablespoons of yogurt for every tablespoon of flax oil or two tablespoons of cottage cheese or quark for every tablespoon of flax oil. My *Orange Wunder* recipe does not use the same yogurt-to-oil ratio. If you prefer to use the organic cottage cheese, you will need 4 tablespoons of organic cottage cheese to the two tablespoons of flax oil—the choice is yours—but the flavor and texture will be much different. Cancer cells thrive on sugar, but this can also be a way to seal their doom. They suck not only the sugar into the cells, but the antioxidants as well, and the antioxidants clobber them!

9. *Stevia®* **sweetener**: can be found at most health food stores, *WalMart, Meijers's,* and *Kroger.* They may be available at *HEB* stores, though I have not checked there for them. (You could probably use honey or royal jelly if you wanted.) If you have lost a great deal of weight fighting cancer, the extra calories might be helpful. If you get cachexia (wasting away syndrome), or you are vomiting non-stop (from chemo), you need all the calories you can get down! Sometimes, just getting organic honey down is a blessing when you are nauseated. (Don't forget that ginger is an excellent anti-nausea herb, and is available in capsules.) You cannot use a lot of ginger if you are on blood-thinners. Do NOT use any type of aspartame sweetener **EVER** for any reason! Do NOT use desserts or drinks with aspartame (*Equal®*) sweetener in them! Don't feed them to your kids! This sweetener can be deadly. Don't be fooled by *AminoSweet®.* Avoid it! They simply changed the name of

the sweetener thinking people would be fooled into buying it under a new name! It is the same old aspartame that has been proven to cause brain cancer! NEVER use saccharin for any reason! Never give honey or honey products to children under two. Some pediatricians will allow kids over a year old to have honey. Check with your child's pediatrician first. Honey has spores in it that the immature digestive systems in babies can't handle, which can cause infant-botulism.

10. **Organic orange juice**. If using for patients taking chemo, get the **"low acid"** organic orange juice. (Unless you are eating chili twice a week! If you can tolerate chili, you don't need low acid orange juice!) Do not get the OJ with calcium or vitamin D added.

11. **Maitake D-Fraction** mushroom supplement. I use the ***Grifron*®** brand that has no alcohol. It is available on the internet and at ***Rainbow Blossom*®**. (Do not use this supplement if you are taking blood-thinning drugs.)

You can watch a video by Dr. Thomas Levy explaining liposomals at this location: ***http://www.squidoo.com/liposomal-vitamin-c,*** or at the *LivOnLabs* website ***http://www.livonlabs.com,*** which also contains a great deal of information on the product, as well as some excellent books you can order, written by Dr. Levy. I knew about liposomal C long before my relative was diagnosed with cancer.

Extras:

During the time my family member took this drink, he was also taking (every day):
- 1000 mg of vitamin C (ascorbic acid) in pill form in the am and evening (for a total of 2000 mg).
- A multi-vitamin/multi-mineral pill that contained selenium. Cancer patients need at least 100-200 mcg/day of selenium.
- CoQ10: 200 mg/day (he had to discontinue this when going on blood-thinners). It is not advisable to take CoQ10 while you are on blood-thinners.
- Vitamin D: **50,000 Units**. (This is not a typo.) This amount was

prescribed by his physician. It was a large blue-green gel capsule that he took once weekly. (If purchasing D, use only the D3. Do not ever use the D2.) Many cancer patients have severe vitamin D shortages.
- A probiotic known as *PEARLS™*, which he did not use while taking blood-thinners.

Making Homemade Liposomal Vitamin C:

I have tried this recipe. One good thing in its favor is the high level of lecithin that you will get in combination with the vitamin C, which helps lower LDL and raise HDL. I do not use this homemade recipe in my formula, though I have tried it. I use the **LivOnLabs® LypoSpheric C™**.

This do-it-yourself homemade liposomal C recipe, by Brooks Bradley, can be found at various internet sites such as: *http://alobar.livejournal.com/3346670.html*. Also, see website: *http://www.pdazzlercom/archives/62*, which says that the recipe below "will give you a product between 7.0 and 7.5 (measured with Alkaline pH Stix) or similar pH to human blood so there is no risk of over acidifying your blood should you take significant amounts of your homemade Liposomal Vitamin C Ascorbate," and that "This Vitamin C Ascorbate recipe is a compilation of several postings on forums and Pdazzler's own trials in the kitchen" (68a).

Ingredients:

- An ultra-sonic jewelry cleaner (with stainless steel interior) that will hold at least TWO CUPS of liquid. This will run about $30.00, but it is a one-time purchase and should last you a long time. Some manufacturers have a one-year warranty on the machine.
- 1 level tablespoon of pharmaceutical grade vitamin C powder. You want the powder that has **5000 mg** of ascorbic acid per **teaspoon**, not per tablespoon. [You can get pharmaceutical grade C at website: *http://www.vitamincfoundation.org/*.]
- 3 level **tablespoons** of **NON-GMO** (you do not want the genetically modified) soy lecithin granules. You can get these in one pound containers from health food stores or from internet sites like *Swanson Vitamins®*. They are usually inexpensive.
- Distilled water
- ¾ teaspoon of *Bob's Red Mill®* Bicarbonate of Soda [Bob's is guaranteed aluminum-free; however, I have checked and *Arm & Hammer®* claims that their soda bicarb is aluminum-free as well.]

How to Mix:
These instructions are given at website: *http://www.pdazzler.com/archives/62* (68a).

1. In qt mixing jar pour one cup distilled water. Add 3 level Tablespoons of granular soy lecithin [use NON GMO soy lecithin] and agitate vigorously for 3 – 5 minutes. Then place the lecithin mixture in the refrigerator for two or more hours. (You can leave in refrigerator overnight if you prefer.) This allows lecithin granules to soak up water for easy mixing into solution…After 2 hour soaking period vigorously agitate the mixture for another 3 – 5 minutes. At the conclusion there should be no lecithin granules visible. Set this smooth lecithin mixture aside.

2. Dissolve 1 level Tablespoon of **Pharmaceutical grade Vitamin C** powder in 2 oz. of distilled water. We recommend you use a 6 oz. or larger screw lid jar so you can shake vigorously. [You can obtain pharmaceutical grade C at: *http://www.vitamincfoundation.org/.*]

3. Dissolve ¾ Teaspoon of *Bob's Red Mill®* Bicarbonate of Soda (Bob's is Aluminum free) in 2 oz. of distilled water using a separate 6 oz. or larger screw lid jar. Shake or agitate the mixture 3 minutes or until soda dissolved.

   While stirring the Vitamin C/distilled water solution, very slowly pour/dribble the dissolved bicarbonate of soda/water mixture into the Vitamin C / distilled water solution. (Pour soda solution very slowly as the resulting mixture will bubble. By pouring slowly and constantly stirring you will be able to mix the two without bubbling over.)

   At the conclusion of mixing the bicarbonate of soda mixture into the Vitamin C mixture all bubbling will cease. If you have any soda settled in the jar, pour the resulting total mix together into that jar, swirl and pour the resulting Vitamin C/Bicarbonate of Soda mixture into the Ultrasonic Cleaner.

4. Pour the lecithin solution into the ultrasonic cleaner bowl with the Vitamin C / Bicarbonate of Soda mixture and stir the contents together.

5. Turn the ultrasonic cleaner on and using a plastic straw (leaving the top of the cleaner opened), gently, slowly, stir the contents.

   Note: The cleaner will, automatically, self-stop about every 2 minutes. Just push ON button to continue. Repeat for a total of 6 series (12 – 18 minutes). By that time the entire solution should be blended into a cloudy, homogenous, milk-like mixture. the LET solution is now well formed.

You can raise the level of encapsulation by continuing several more ultrasonic cycles if desired.

This protocol furnishes 12 grams (12000mg.) of Vitamin C Ascorbate. At 70% - 90% encapsulation efficiency, 8400 mg would be of the **LET** [liposomal encapsulation] type. This solution will keep, acceptably, at room temperature for 3 to 4 days. Refrigerated, it will keep much longer (68a).

If you get a more powerful ultrasonic cleaner, you can make larger amounts and also get a *higher quality liposomal or more encapsulated supplement at one time, depending on the amount you mix.* (68a).

As noted earlier, you can also buy liposomal C in ready-to-use bottles at other internet sites. I use *LivOnLabs* formula in my recipe because it is very thick, practically tasteless, easy to use, and encapsulation is said to be 100%. The Vitamin C Foundation also sells the *LivOnLabs C*. You can obtain ultrasonic cleaners on several internet sites. (Also, *Arm & Hammer®* claims that their soda bicarb is aluminum-free.)

- **The Johanna Budwig Recipe:**

    Blend 2 Tbsp. organic flax seed oil with **4** Tbsp. organic low-fat cottage cheese or quark (48) [obtain the cottage cheese or quark from a dairy farmer who makes this fresh in your area, if possible]. Blend until you can no longer see the oil (48). [ONCE mixed thoroughly (a blender works fine), you can add cinnamon to taste, or fruit of choice, such as organic raisins. Quark is a pasty type of white cheese. Some farmers make their own.]

Realize that the entire Johanna Budwig protocol involves not just this simple mix. It also involves using many other health ingredients in the diet. You can get details on her entire protocol at many internet sites and by reading my last book: ***Gentle Cures for Tough Cancers***, available at online bookstores. There is also more information in the next chapter.

II. The Fruit/Vegetable Drink

Juice the following in your juicer:
(use organic produce)

- 3 medium apples
- 8 ounces of carrots (1/2 lb.)
- ½ cup of cauliflower
- 2 stalks of celery
- 2 small pears
- A dozen grapes
(with or without seeds, black, purple, green, or a variety)

(Your juicer will remove seeds, a blender won't.)

When finished, you should have about 14 to 16 ounces of juice. If not, juice enough carrots or apples until you have 14 to 16 ounces total. Drink this once a day in the evening about 2 hours after you eat supper. Share any leftover juice (if you get more than 16 ounces) with someone else or save for the next day. You can vary this occasionally by chopping 4 ounces of blueberries, raspberries, blackberries, or strawberries in a blender (not a juicer, or you'll lose most of the berries) with 2 ounces of distilled water to keep the berries from clumping together, then pour the berry slush into the fruit/vegetable drink, or juice 2 or 3 apricots (after removing the seeds). Even if you have a juicer that will juice an entire apple without slicing, ALWAYS SLICE what you are juicing at least ONCE so you can check to be sure there are no rotten areas in the fruit or vegetable you are using! An apple can look gorgeous on the outside, but be completely rotten in the center and you don't want to be drinking mold. Drink this mix in the afternoon. You can divide it in half and drink 7 or 8 ounces in the afternoon, then drink the rest about 4 hours later. You will be using the **Orange Wunder** drink in the morning. See the article further below for the importance of apple juice in fighting cancer. If eating FRESH whole fruit, always eat it on an empty stomach, rather than with other foods, like vegetables. Fruit goes through the digestive system more rapidly. Eating it with other foods will make the entire meal acidic and it will ferment in your stomach. Juicing is different. You can mix the **juices** of vegetables and fruit together, though it is still best to drink the juices too, on an empty stomach.

III. The Whey Protein Shake

- **Ingredients:**

- 6 tablespoons of organic plain or flavored yogurt (4 to 6 ounces).
- 2 tablespoons of organic non-GMO flax seed oil (these first 2 ingredients are also found in the *Orange Wunder Formula*).
- 4 ounces of organic almond milk, or rice milk (unsweetened non GMO), or unsweetened organic coconut milk, or distilled water. Your preference. (Do not use grapefruit juice.) If you want a thinner drink, use 6 ounces, or you can add some ice cubes for a thinner and colder drink. Do not use cubes that contain chlorine or fluoride and only use cubes if your blender can handle them.
- 1 tablespoon of (non-GMO) lecithin granules or powder (you can get these at *http://www.swansonvitamins.com.*) Just go to their search box at the top left of the webpage and type in the words *lecithin granules*, and be sure to choose the **non-GMO** formula. You can also purchase them at website: *http://www.iherb.com.*
- 1 scoop of organic *whey protein powder* (check the label of contents closely). Do NOT purchase any whey protein powder that contains aspartame sweetener! The very best form of whey protein I have found that is cold-processed and contains no aspartame is called ***Miracle Whey*™** and can be found at Dr. Joseph Mercola's website: ***http://proteinpowder.mercola.com /Miracle-Whey-Protein.html;*** and for those who may have a hard time digesting protein, try his ***Whey Protein Powder with Aminogen®,*** available at: ***http://proteinpowder.mercola.com/ Whey-Protein-With-Aminogen.html.*** The container comes with a little scoop, which holds one serving. Their brand comes in chocolate, vanilla, or strawberry.
- 1 scoop of Defatted Wheat Germ Powder, Cold-pressed. You can purchase this from *www.swansomvitamins.com* and other online websites, as well as health food stores. The container you purchase should have the little scoop, which is one serving.
- 1 tablespoon of Brewer's Yeast Powder. (Available at most health food stores and some nutritional product internet sites.)
- 28 drops of Reishi mushroom liquid extract. Use the alcohol-free,

sugar-free. The brand I use is from Swanson® Health Products at *swansonvitamins.com*. (Again, you cannot use this if on blood-thinners.)
- 30 drops of Astragalus Root. Use the alcohol-free. You can also get this at *swansonvitamins.com*. GAIA Herbs makes their own brand. Do not use if you are on blood-thinners or if allergic to Astragalus.
- Feel free to add a packet of the liposomal vitamin C to this mix. It will go very well with the lecithin that is being used. I have used it both ways, with and without the C. (Or use the other half of your homemade liposomal C mix if you chose to make your own.)
- 2 or 3 packets of Stevia® to your preference – optional. (If you decide to use the coconut milk, unless you use unsweetened coconut milk, you may not want to add the Stevia®.)
- ½ tablespoon of organic dark cocoa powder or organic dark chocolate syrup (optional). This will improve the taste, especially for kids. (Check with their pediatrician.)

Remember that you cannot take herbs and mushroom extracts if they are not compatible with prescription drugs you may be taking.

How to Mix:

First, mix the yogurt and oil in your *MagicBullet*® blender until no traces of the oil are visible. (You can also use a hand-held blender or a small blender of your choice, one that holds no more than two cups). You should have a creamy mixture and the oil should not be visible. Then add the rest of the ingredients and mix in your blender until well-blended. If you want a thinner drink, add distilled water. Do not use the Astragalus or mushroom drops if on blood-thinners.

If you are having problems with constipation, or just want to increase the fiber in your diet, put the following in a large container (it should hold about six cups) that has a lid. Mix them well, keep refrigerated for freshness, and eat ¾ cup a day every day (use only organic products). You will have no trouble with keeping your colon cleaned out. This mix is full of fiber and omega-3:

- **Power Seed Mix**
  Use ½ cup of each of the following:

  - Almonds
  - Brazil nuts
  - Cashews
  - Dark raisins
  - Pecans
  - Pine nuts
  - Pistachios
  - Pumpkin seeds
  - Spanish peanuts (red-skinned)
  - Sunflower seeds
  - Walnuts

- **Apples & Unfiltered Apple Juice Help Prevent Colon Cancer**

Eating apples, which are rich in pectin, and drinking apple juice keep the colon healthy (9). A substance known as *butyrate* is found in apple juice and pectin which helps stop cancerous growths in the colon (9). A report from *sciencedaily.com* says that scientists in Germany have recommended ingesting 8 to 24 *ounces per day of cloudy apple juice (unfiltered)* for preventing colon cancer. This drink, in animal studies, decreased *small intestine* tumors by *38* and *40 percent* (112). Researchers in Poland said that the unfiltered juice has four times the antioxidants of filtered juice (112). Apples are also important in preventing osteoporosis, reducing the incidence of asthma in children, helping to prevent lung, liver, and breast cancer, and reducing the cellular need for insulin. Mix a teaspoon or two of cinnamon into each glass of apple juice you make. It is delicious and adds many health benefits! (Use a small shaker to get the cinnamon mixed well into the juice.) Caution: do not use large amounts of cinnamon if you are taking blood-thinning medications.

CHAPTER 3

An Oil of Blessing – God's Natural Cancer Killing Machine

****

Flax seed has been in use for thousands of years. Studies were done in 1986 in Canada on flax seed, showing its power at fighting cancer and harmful fats in the blood. Flax is rich in lignans, nutrients that fight cancer, especially breast cancer (278). Two other essential fatty oils that can destroy several types of cancer (in laboratory testing) without harming normal cells are *evening primrose oil* and *borage oil* (278). Many physicians also recommend flax oil (gel caps) to their patients who have problems with dry eye syndrome, psoriasis, and other skin disorders.

The wrong kinds of fat not only depress the immune system, they transport cancer-causing chemicals into and throughout the body. Avoid the use of anything that is *hydrogenated* or refined (e.g. margarines). *Hydrogenation* creates millions of free radicals that strip vitamins, especially *vitamin E* from the body (278). Obtain organic, unrefined oils from natural health food stores. Even the FDA has recognized flax seed oil as a cancer preventative (278).

Cold-pressed organic olive oil is also a good choice. (Note that most of the onion rings, french fries, fried chicken, and other fried foods that are found in today's fast food restaurants, are cooked with unhealthy oils.) Some states are finally wising up and passing laws to eliminate the use of unhealthy fats in restaurants. You will see more of these type laws go into effect as consumers become more and more aware that the unnaturally high fats that Americans consume in popular fast food dishes are a primary cause of cancer. Dietary fats are needed, but the RIGHT kinds of fat. Processed vegetable oils are contributing to the deterioration of the health of millions of people. Johanna Budwig knew this and she was determined to do something about it!

I. Budwig & the Margarine Battle

Dr. Johanna Budwig, famous for her work in isolating and identifying fatty substances in the blood, was appalled at the way margarine manufacturers took and transformed *good unrefined healthy oils* "into processed and hydrogenated health-endangering margarine," and she was very vocal about saying so (207). In *Fantastic Flax,* author Siegfried Gursche says that the government, the margarine producers, and conventional medicine basically ganged up on her to prosecute her for claiming that margarine and all such hydrogenated fats are like giving poison to the human body (207). The margarine producers were wealthy and had a lot of clout behind their lawsuits.

Johanna said the following about margarine: "[T]he process of artificially hardening liquid vegetable oils (hydrogenation) creates life-threatening fat molecules—the trans fatty acids" (207). The margarine industry brought legal action against Johanna. "She fought twenty-eight court cases," winning every single one of them (207)! We see warnings everywhere today about the dangers of trans-fatty acids (like those in margarine) that contribute to all forms of chronic illnesses, heart disease, and cancer (207), and of course, we now know that it was the margarine manufacturers who were lying and not Johanna! Recently, some margarine manufacturers have come out with products that they claim have no trans-fat in them. Always be a label reader, because even if a products says it contains 0% trans-fat, the FDA does allow a small amount of trans-fat in these "zero" products, and by the time you consume (or cook with) 3 or 4 tablespoons, you could be getting a significant amount of trans-fat, when you think you are not!

Organic butter is actually better for you than margarine. (Butter contains natural lecithin, an ingredient that lowers bad cholesterol, margarine does not.) We can thank Johanna Budwig for exposing the truth about margarine and margarine manufacturers.

One of the richest sources of *omega-3* is *flax oil*. Be careful in purchasing flax oil. On the label, you want to see the words, *cold expeller-pressed* and *unrefined,* and check the expiration date on the container (207). I discuss this in other places of my book. Combining lecithin with megadoses of vitamin C is especially helpful in fighting atherosclerosis because it raises good cholesterol and lowers bad cholesterol (232).

Perhaps this makes you wonder about other warnings that are currently being issued by natural health advocates: warnings against using homogenized, pasteurized milk; warnings against immunizations; warnings against the deadly effects of chemo and radiation to the immune system; warnings against aspartame; warnings against fluoride and chlorine in drinking water, and warnings against amalgam fillings—that are currently being ignored by conventional medicine and the AMA, the FDA, government leaders, and the FTC.

• Are the Warnings Being Heeded?

Dr. Mark Sircus, Ac., OMD tells us in his book, *Sodium Bicarbonate – Rich Man's Poor Man's Cancer Treatment* (from IMVA Books), that "The three trillion dollar medical machine in the United States is impotent against chronic diseases and is responsible itself for much of the horror that is happening" (287):

> ...oncologists just have not been able to understand that cancer patients are suffering from poisoning on a massive scale with all the chemicals scientists have already established cause cancer (288).

How much longer do you think it will take for these warnings to finally be taken seriously? How much longer will it take and how many times will history vindicate people like Dr. Johanna Budwig, Dr. Burzynski, Johanna Brandt, Dr. Simoncini, Gaston Niessens, Emanuel Revici, Dr. Linus Pauling, Dr. Robert Cathcart, Dr. Mark Sircus, Ac., OMD, Dr. Mark Levine, Dr. Thomas E. Levy, MD, JD, and Rene Caisse?

II. The Famous Budwig Flax Oil Diet

Johanna Budwig combined flax oil with cottage cheese as part of her anti-cancer program. I do not recommend cow's milk simply because many dairy products in this country are so tainted with hormones, pesticides and herbicides, and because cow's milk has been linked to juvenile or type I diabetes and sometimes carries leukemia and lymphoma cells. If you do use dairy products, such as cottage cheese, or yogurt, I would recommend that you use only organic or better yet, if you have a nearby farmer who can provide you with raw milk and dairy (providing he or she practices scrupulous farming methods and has a healthy disease-free herd), then you are quite fortunate.

There is so much controversy about soy, especially the GMO or genetically-modified soy products, you are better off without soy, unless it is fermented soy. (See Chapter Four in my last book, *Gentle Cures for Tough Cancers,* for details on the amazing fermented soy drink, *Haelan.*) In the Budwig diet, you can use yogurt, but again, see the note above about organic and raw products. Some studies indicate that giving cow's milk to babies under one-year-old causes milk allergies, and may be the culprit in Type I diabetes. Many children suffering from chronic ear infections, colds, and allergies completely recover when they are taken off all dairy products. Do you have a child who gets one ear infection (or strep) after another? Try this: take them off ALL dairy products, even powdered milk and dried products (like pancake mix) that may contain dairy in them. Take them off milk, cheeses, ice cream, cottage cheese, and yogurt – ALL DAIRY! Milk is not for children. It is for *baby cows*. I do encourage the use of the Budwig flax oil diet in anyone battling cancer, such as brain cancer or some other type of cancer, and as stated earlier, it can be done with organic, or better yet, raw dairy products if you can find them.

Many testimonials have been given of patients brought back from terminal illness to amazing health by the Johanna Budwig flax oil diet. Dr. Johanna Budwig was a premier German biochemical expert, who found that the blood of cancer patients is lacking essential fatty acids. Her diet revolves around very specific ingredients, including flax oil and cottage cheese (312). As described at *www.healingcancernaturally. com*, ingredients are combined as follows:

> For each tablespoon of flax seed oil, add 2 tablespoons of low-fat cottage cheese (or quark) or 6 tablespoons of yoghurt. The flax oil/cottage cheese or flax oil/yoghurt mixture should be fully blended until no traces of oil remain visible, proving that the highly unsaturated fatty acids have become water soluble (a hand-held mixer or a blender works well) (47). [Quark is a pasty type of white cheese.]

As you can see, the ingredients are very simple. The flax oil reacts with the sulfuric contents of the cottage cheese and dramatically increases oxygenation at the cellular level. This combination binds the fats to protein, thus making them readily available at the cellular level. The body is also supplied with natural essential fatty acids that prevent cancer cells from running rampant (312). Note that this is not all of the famous Budwig diet. There are other facets included as well. For example: the diet forbids the ingestion of margarine, any type of animal fats (e.g., including butter, and fats found in other animal products), and no sugar whatsoever, though raw juicing from vegetables is encouraged, as is *apple juice*. Herbal teas are also recommended at least three times a day (312).

It is important to realize that the Budwig diet is a complete protocol. It is a "lacto-vegetarian diet except that fish is allowed, flax seeds, fruit juices, vegetable juices, sauerkraut, sunshine, emotional and spiritual peace and stress control," as well as the ingredients above (80). More than "50% of Dr. Budwig's patients were doctors or relatives of doctors..." (47). Visit site: *www.healingcancernaturally.com* for more specifics on the Budwig diet. Dr. Budwig described her work in the following way:

> And what do I actually do? I give cancer patients simple, natural foods. That is all. I take sick people out of the hospital, when it is said that they do not have more than an hour or two left to live, that the scientifically attested diagnosis is at hand and that the patient is completely moribund. In most cases I can help even these patients quickly and conclusively (47).

There are many amazing cancer cures attributed to Dr. Budwig's flax oil diet. One example is that of Sandy A., who was diagnosed with an *inoperable brain tumor* (312). When the tumor began to bleed, he was told that there was nothing more to offer him. He started on Dr. Budwig's formula and improved so dramatically that he could partially resume normal activities. He is still being considered a medical marvel ten years later. He said that his amazing healing has been described in many prestigious health periodicals (312).

Ms. Budwig admitted that for those patients in the most severe stages (who had been told that surgery was useless), "even in these cases health can be restored, usually within a few months, I would say in 90% of cases" (47). The Budwig diet uses a natural formula that inhibits the formation of cancer. It is known throughout the world.

Many people have followed this regimen, people who were said to be *terminal*. They were cured on the Budwig diet, and are now going about their usual everyday activities without restriction (312). The substances in the Budwig diet heal the immune system, giving the body the ability to heal itself.

Dr. Johanna Budwig authored several books, including *The Oil Protein Diet Cookbook*, which contains many recipes using the Budwig protocol. Her books are available in major bookstores. Website: *www.healingcancernaturally.com*, contains a great deal of information on the Budwig diet, as does *http://www.barleans.com/budwig.html*. Be sure that you **never heat flax oil**, and that you always keep it refrigerated. Also, if you choose the Budwig diet, be sure to use only certified organic dairy products, or raw, if you can get them (as noted above).

• Oxygenation & Flax Oil

Dr. Otto Warburg won *the Nobel Prize in 1931* when he discovered that, unlike normal cells in the body, cancer cells do not use oxygen—meaning that they are *anaerobic*—and that they cannot thrive in a highly oxygenated environment (81). See website: http://*www.mnwelldir.org/docs/cancer1/budwig.html*, which explains that this resulted in the advent of many types of cancer therapies for increased tissue oxygenation, such as using *ozone* for blood oxygenation, the use of *hyperbaric oxygen*, and doing exercises (such as walking on a treadmill) while breathing in pure oxygen (*EWOT* or *Exercise With Oxygen Therapy*) (81). This is probably one reason, among many, that regular exercise lowers cancer risk; it increases oxygen levels in your cells.

It was this principle of increasing oxygen to the body at the cellular level that interested Dr. Budwig, and was part of the rationale behind her flax seed oil/cottage cheese combination. Dr. Budwig assisted many terminally ill patients in regaining their health through her simple diet of flax seed oil and low-fat cottage cheese. She was known as *Germany's premier biochemist* with "a Ph.D. in Natural Science" (312). She was also trained in *pharmaceutical science* and many other fields. Those in Germany, who were producing margarines and other solid shortening, bitterly attacked her in order to silence her and keep her from exposing the truth about their harmful hydrogenated fats (312).

Some websites vary the Budwig diet slightly by allowing the addition of fresh ground flax seed. Oncologist, Dr. Dan C. Roehm, studied the Budwig diet and said that, "this diet is far and away the most successful anti-cancer diet in the world" (312). Dr. Budwig claimed that the diet not only prevented disease, but cured disease as well. She believed that the total lack of *linol acids* in the average person's diet is the reason for the rampant epidemic of cancer and other diseases, especially in the West (312).

Apparently, Dr. Budwig cured cancer by discovering that cancer patients were always deficient in essential fats which are critical for controlling cancer cells (312). What she found in her research was a completely natural way for people to obtain the missing ingredients they needed (312).

III. Flax & Alkalinity

The importance of maintaining the body's alkalinity was noted earlier in this book and later in other chapters, devoted to that concept. It is also discussed at length in both my previous books.

As noted by Siegfried Gursche, in his book, *Good Fats and Oils,* flax can assist with sustaining a healthy state of alkalinity as it is *very alkaline* (207). It is a good preventative for *heartburn* and excellent for promotion of a correct acid-alkaline balance. When the seeds are ground into a powder and mixed with juice or water and drank, it forms thick *mucilage* in the stomach, thus providing a protective coat for those with ulcers and inflammation (207). Check with your physician first if you have bleeding ulcers or colitis. Other good natural treatments for ulcers and colon problems include: Manuka honey, bee propolis, calendula, DGL tablets, lots of WATER (but no chlorine or fluoride, use distilled or a trusted spring water source), coconut water and coconut milk, plenty of raw cabbage juice, fish oil capsules, bilberry supplements, carrot and spinach juice, organic flax seed (use a coffee-grinder to grind it up and add to water – drink before it gets too thick), probiotics (e.g. Bio-K), organic yogurt, chia seeds (mix in water and drink before it thickens too much), olive leaf extract, wild oil of oregano, organic apple cider vinegar (mixed in plenty of water), cold-pressed aloe vera juice, green tea, white tea, slippery elm, no wheat or gluten products. Use krill oil capsules, non-acidic vitamin C (8 to 10 grams per day, not milligrams, GRAMS), soda bicarb in water (check with your physician or alternative health doctor, as it is high in salt), lots of fresh fruits and vegetables (and their juices, but best to juice your own), raw broccoli, beta-sitosterol supplements, chlorophyll (as in wheat grass juice, green leafy vegetables, chlorella supplements, and spirulina), magnesium citrate supplements (or liquid), Magnascent© iodine drops, fresh grated ginger or the ginger capsules. Ginger is sometimes given to pregnant women to prevent morning sickness.

Essential fats are healthy. In normal amounts, they do not make people fat. It is all the non-essential fats that are being ingested that are causing the problem of obesity in America. Mr. Gursche described Dr. Johanna Budwig as "a pioneer in the field of health and nutrition research" (207).

IV. The Flax Cancer Killing Connection

• Flax & Cancer

If you are fighting terminal cancer, I would certainly recommend the Budwig diet. If you go with dairy, just be sure you use organic and even get raw dairy (the cottage cheese or yogurt) if you are lucky enough to live near a small dairy farmer that has healthy, disease-free herds and practices scrupulously clean farming (you don't need parasites). The very last thing you need in your diet is the addition of hormones, herbicides, pesticides, leukemia and lymphoma cells, and parasites that are often found in non-organic dairy. These are the substances that may have caused your cancer in the first place. If you cannot get raw organic, just get organic yogurt or cottage cheese and always ask God to bless the food you prepare!

• Lignans & the Cancer Link

Flax contains *lignans,* which are nothing more than natural estrogens from plants, yet these powerhouses play a vital part in fighting degenerative diseases and cancers of the "breast, prostate, uterus and colon," says Mr. Gursche. They also keep bones healthy, and because they bind with *bile acids*, they help prevent *gallstones* (207). He describes flax seeds as being so rich in lignans that they "contain 75 to

800 times more [lignans] than wheat bran, oats, millet, rye, legumes soybeans..." and many other foods (207). They are important cancer-fighters because they block the growth of cancers by causing **"excess estrogen" to be driven "from the body."** They also prevent existing fat cells from producing more estrogen (207). All of your cells have receptor sites where harmful estrogens can attach themselves and be absorbed. Lignans from flax lock onto the receptor sites blocking harmful estrogens, thus preventing them from getting into the cells. Flax is also high in fiber and protein.

When combined with cottage cheese or yogurt, as in the Budwig Formula, flax becomes a complete protein. Flax comes in brown or gold. There are several varieties, but there is little difference between the brown flax and the golden. If you buy the gold flax seed, you will get more protein and less oil than the brown flax. You may also pay more for the golden (207). Do not buy flax that has already been ground, unless it is in a sealed package and once opened, you can keep it refrigerated, but use before the expiration date. It is preferable to purchase the flax seed whole, then grind in a coffee grinder the amount you need as you use it. This will prevent the flax from going rancid (207). Once rancid, it will do you more harm than good.

Flax is rich in *vitamin F* and it provides very nutritious and healthy *mucilage*, which helps detoxify and clean the colon (170). Selene Yeager, author of *Doctors Book of FOOD REMEDIES,* says that flax is so high in lignans that you would have to eat 5 dozen "cups of fresh broccoli or 100 slices of whole-wheat bread to get the same amount of lignans that are in ¼ cup of flax seed" (314). Research showed that tumors that are estrogen-positive could be reduced to half their size in less than two months in animals given flax seed (314). As described earlier in this chapter, lignans apparently have the power to counter-attack the harmful effects of synthetic estrogen in the cells—estrogens that cause cancer (314).

Heating oil to extreme temperatures changes its molecular structure, making it unfit for human consumption. Fats that are artificially hardened, the fats that are bad for you, will be labeled *as "hydrogenated, modified, fractionated or partially hydrogenated... avoid all products that contain these dangerous fats"* (208). You will find these fats in processed foods, in fast foods, and in many items in your grocery store. Butter is actually better for you unless you burn it. Burning butter completely ruins it. Never eat anything cooked in butter that has been burned. It has become a harmful fat and will flood your body with dangerous free radicals (208).

Refined oils are considered by Siegfried Gursche, in his book, *Good Fats and Oils,* to be a *dead food*—meaning that they are completely empty of nutrients. These are the oils you will find on supermarket shelves, including the refined safflower and peanut oils. Avoid even the so-called *light olive oils.* Some oil manufacturers try to fool the public into believing that their oil is olive oil. A good example is a canola oil that is called *Olivera.* These are the high trans-fatty acid oils that are unhealthy (208). The same can be said of margarine and vegetable shortening. Some processors are now removing trans-fats from their oils, but as noted earlier, you must be a label-reader.

New studies show that eating organic foods can keep you pesticide-free, including your children! Researchers from the University of Washington in Seattle discovered that preschool kids on regular diets had "six times the level of certain pesticides in their urine" as the children who were fed an organic diet (114). Another good reason to use ORGANIC!

• Flax & Malignant Cancers

The type of GLA found in flax seed, as well as *evening primrose oil and borage oil,* in laboratory testing, was able to destroy *alpha-cell chronic lymphocytic leukemia cells.* As a matter-of-fact, their anti-tumor effects have been demonstrated against many types of cancer, including deadly brain cancers (175).

Essential fatty acids work by protecting the walls or membranes of the cells. The membranes work by allowing nutritious elements to enter, while blocking out harmful scavengers. This is why flax seed is such an important antioxidant. It works to fight inflammation and pathogens, and it contains naturally-occurring plant estrogens, also called *phyto-estrogens* (133). According to *The Healing Power of Vitamins, Minerals, and Herbs,* by the Reader's Digest Association, flax seed and flax oil have been used to treat many health disorders, including gastric problems, *shingles,* and *lupus.* It can also help the body in preventing (and dissolving) gallstones (133).

The Budwig diet works by making important oils and lipoproteins easily available to the body at the cellular level, elevating oxygenation and energy. There is one website, in particular, that describes a new omega oil product known as *Omegasentials™* that it says is already *water-soluble* and works much the same way that the Budwig diet works. You can find more information on *Omegasentials™* at website: *www.mnwelldir.org/docs/cancer1/budwig.htm,* or you can email them at: *info@integritydirectinc.com* if you want to try their product (81).

• Flax Seed Versus Flax Oil & The Colon

Animal testing has shown that ingesting ground flax seed can inhibit cancers of the colon. Ground flax meal is far better than using flax oil for this purpose, because the flax meal is much higher in disease-fighting lignans than the oil (190).

• Flax & Hodgkin's Disease

The parents of 11-year-old Timmy G were told that he had *Hodgkin's disease*. He was given just a few months to live, after failure to respond to 24 conventional *radiation treatments* (312). His mother was told of the Budwig diet, which she gave to her son. She marveled that less than one week later, he was, "for the first time in…two years," breathing normally. He eventually returned to school and is now more than 18 years of age and credits his cure and his life to Dr. Budwig's formula (312). My *Orange Wunder Formula* in Chapter 2 incorporates two of the Budwig ingredients in slightly different amounts.

Website: *www.curezone.com* documents the case of a person diagnosed with a terminal osteosarcoma using the Budwig diet; however, the patient used larger amounts of flax oil a day than the official diet calls for. He started "out with 4 tbl. [tablespoons] of flax per day," plus the cottage cheese. A few days later, he increased it to "8-10 tbl [tablespoons] of flax [oil] per day" with the cottage cheese. Three months later, all of his lab work came back negative. His cancer was cured. His physician was so incredulous that he thought there was some mistake and ordered his tests repeated **three times**. There were no errors. The patient, in his **eighties**, no longer had any traces of cancer (15). Don't give up because of age! Just remember that you are never too old to be cured of anything!

Be aware that there are other components involved with the Budwig flax oil diet, besides the oil and cottage cheese. For example: no processed sugar is allowed. *Grape juice* is used as a juicing sweetener. All processed fats and *animal fats* are forbidden. Processed and *preserved meats* are not allowed. *Fresh-squeezed* juices are encouraged, as are teas, with *honey* used as a sweetener (312). Every day, those on the diet are to drink either a glass of [organic] *sauerkraut juice...before breakfast*, or a *glass of acidophilus milk.* On the first day of the diet, nothing is taken except for "250 ml (8.5 oz) of Flax Oil with honey plus freshly squeezed fruit juices" (no sugar added) (312). Note that many people skip that 8.5 ounce flax oil dose on day one and proceed to the main diet (312). (That much oil would be in divided amounts.) As noted elsewhere in this book, you would require extra magnesium (and perhaps some pancreatic enzyme supplements) to help digest that much oil!

Just be sure (if using the Budwig diet) that you are getting two to five tablespoons of the flax seed oil daily with ½ to 1 cup of organic yogurt, or cottage cheese, thoroughly blended until no traces of the oil can be seen. If you do not care for the taste of the flax oil, you can add fresh fruit to the mix, or cinnamon and other spices, which hide the oily taste, however, don't add fruit or cinnamon until after the oil and yogurt are thoroughly mixed. You may want to eat the fruit as a side dish. See the **Orange Wunder Formula** I developed in Chapter 2 of this book for my relative, who was going through Stage IV inoperable bladder cancer. As noted earlier, the formula I gave him contains two ingredients from the Budwig diet protocol, and it is delicious! You would have no problem getting a child to drink it. Check with their pediatrician.

- **Flax Prevents Many Diseases—Helps the Heart, Kidneys & Those with Lupus Nephritis, M.S., Diabetes, Colon Problems & HIV**

Research studies have found that flax seed has an anti-cancer effect comparable to that of some chemotherapy drugs, but minus the toxic side effects. It is a well-known fact that women having the highest levels of omega-3-fatty acids (such as those found in fish and flax) are the least likely to develop breast cancer. Flax has also been very effective at treating skin disorders, and it is possible that it could extend the lives of patients with lupus who are fighting nephritis (caused when the lupus attacks their kidneys).

Flax seed and its oil can help in the prevention and treatment of many forms of cancer, including those of the female reproductive tract, intestinal tract, and prostate cancer, and offers some help for those suffering with digestive disorders, including Crohn's, colitis, and bowel irregularities (290). One physician in particular, *Dr. Roy Swank*, has shown that multiple sclerosis responds to a diet that is *low in saturated* fats, but high in *essential* fats (e.g., flax oil) (290). (If you have any of the above disorders, or are taking prescription medications, be sure to consult with your licensed health care practitioner for appropriate amounts to take, or ask for a nutritional consult.)

Essential fatty acids help to metabolize dangerous blood fats, preventing them from accumulating in blood vessels and tissues. Other sources of omega-3 oils (besides flax) are leafy greens, *cold water fish* (277), krill oil, sprouts, olive oil, Lyprinol®, chia seeds, and avocados.

Borage oil is high in omega-6. One researcher has discovered that the GLA in borage oil helps reverse some diabetic health complications, "especially retina problems" (277). Researchers have also shown repeatedly that omega-3 fish oil (the same type oil found in flax oil), in animal testing, shrank tumors and halted their spread. It helps suppress colon cancer and breast cancer in humans (196). Krill oil has omega-3 and is claimed to be much healthier and more potent than fish oil. Chia seeds also contain omega-3 and are a great fiber source. They are tasty when mixed with organic yogurt.

V. Storing & Using Flax

Always keep flax seed **oil** refrigerated. You do not need to refrigerate the seeds. Once opened, use the oil by the expiration date given, or at least "within three weeks after opening" (207). You can use the flax seeds in baking if you soak them "in water for at least an hour before using them" (207). Dr. Budwig also authored several books on flax oil. One in particular, *The Oil-Protein Diet Cookbook*, has many of her recipes for a variety of ways to incorporate flax oil into your menus.

When using flax oil or flax seed, be sure to purchase organic flax from a reputable health food store (207). I prefer flax oil in salads, juices, cold dishes (such as chopped salads or avocados), or poured over a baked potato. (Just be sure the potato is not burning hot as flax oil should never be heated.) If using fresh flax seed, take 2 or 3 tablespoons of the seeds, grind them in a coffee grinder, mix them with

8 ounces of water, shake and drink for a breakfast drink. Or you can add the crushed (or cracked) seeds to cereals (i.e. steel-cut oats), or salads. However, if adding to a drink, you must drink it quickly, because it thickens very fast! You may need to follow it with more water since it is rather gritty.

Flax seed has been called *the ideal survival food* because all the antioxidants in flax are enclosed in a small, shell-like structure that keeps the seed from spoiling for years. Once the outer shell is cracked or crushed, the oil inside begins to deteriorate as it mixes with oxygen, and will eventually spoil if not used within a short period of time. Refrigeration will retard the spoilage process, but not indefinitely (207).

In his book, *Fantastic Flax*, Siegfried Gursche lauds the many benefits of flax seed as a healing food and nutraceutical, and says that adding these seeds to the daily diet will help with all sorts of digestive disorders, including constipation. He says that it will also help those with high triglycerides, blood pressure problems, circulatory, and degenerative diseases (207).

VI. Other Healthy Oils

Fish Oil & Cancer

Studies reveal that within just a few weeks, pre-cancerous polyps in the colon could be halted by greater than half—if men would take fish oil supplements every day (196). Also, GLA and fish oil supplements were shown to greatly increase (by as much as double) the *life expectancies of* people fighting the HIV virus (196). These essential oils have been used to treat rheumatoid arthritis. GLAs work by enhancing the body's ability to increase immune cells that kill pathogens and cancer cells in the body. Good sources of GLA are *borage oil* and *evening primrose oil,* as well as *black currants* (196). (Use the fish oil capsules that are enteric-coated. This will ensure that the nutrients in them reach the colon.)

Fish Versus Flax

Though fish oil is great for the colon, and many nutrition experts will tell you that fish is the healthiest form of omega-3, studies have shown that flax and krill oil may be healthier. For one thing, many of our coastal waters are dangerously polluted. There is much documentation available on mercury poisoning in fish, and we still don't know what lasting effect the disastrous BP Gulf oil leak will have on the oceans and their food supply! Even if you are able to get untainted fish, while some fish may be good, eating it more often may not be best. When researchers completed a **human** study that lasted 30 years and involved 2000 male participants, they discovered that those eating more than "8 ounces of fish a week," had greater risk of *stroke*. My advice, when eating fish, don't consume more than 4 ounces at any one time and stick to healthy varieties, such as arctic cod, herring, Atlantic salmon, mackerel, and sardines. Do not use the farm-raised salmon.

While the Japanese do eat a large amount of fish in their diet, it is also true that they have high statistics for stroke (314) in their population. During research studies, when mice received fish oil, flax oil, or corn oil, and were then injected with cancerous breast cells, the only oil that successfully retarded the growth of the cancerous tumors and their spread was the flax oil (256).

Krill Oil

A high antioxidant marine oil (perhaps one of the best new sources), that also provides omega-3 fatty acids, proteins, phospholipids, and astaxanthin carotenoids, is the oil from the tiny shrimp-like creature known as the *Antarctic Krill*. This oil can also help alleviate arthritic pain, PMS, seasonal allergies, autoimmune disorders, and high cholesterol levels (278a). The amazing health properties of the oil of this little sea creature are described in *The Healing Power of Neptune Krill Oil,* by Tina Sampalis, M.D., Ph.D. Be certain if you obtain supplements, that you get the Neptune Krill Oil (NKO™) patented formula that uses a proprietary process to keep the oil potent. For PMS, they recommend 600 mg/day; to lower high cholesterol 1000 mg/day; to maintain good cholesterol 500 mg/daily; and for "joint pain and inflammation 300 mg krill oil" daily (278a). Of course, consult with your physician about new supplements.

Oil of the Green-Lipped Mussel

Another form of oil that should be considered for those fighting diseases, such as cancer and arthritis, is the oil from the green-lipped mussel from the country of New Zealand, known as *Lyprinol®,* an anti-inflammatory that some say is equivalent in potency to **Celebrex**, but without the side effects associated with Celebrex. This is a rare type of omega-3 that has an anti-inflammatory affect on the body. It is described at website *http://www.primohealth.com,* and is said to have hundreds of times the potency of salmon oil, evening primrose oil, or flax oil. The damaging gastric side effects of NSAIDS, over-the-counter, and some prescription drugs, are well known, yet Lyprinol® is without toxic side effects and exerts a protective effect on the GI system. As a matter-of-fact, when Lyprinol® was given at the rate of *50 capsules* a day to those who were very ill, no toxic effects were experienced (87). It has been used for everything from arthritis to asthma, and even given for CFS or *Chronic Fatigue Syndrome* (87). This supplement is marketed at the above website. Even those with severe *rheumatoid arthritis* have had tremendous results using Lyprinol®.

Another supplement made from the oil of the green-lipped mussel is a *concentrated superfood* from New Zealand known as *Moxxor* (158). Many people are using Moxxor to rid themselves of the painful inflammation caused by arthritis, without the side effects of NSAIDS and other drugs. Many researchers believe cancer is an inflammatory process. This oil fights inflammation (158). Testing on this supplement is currently underway. You can purchase it at: *http://www.mymoxxor .com/productListPage.aspx?ID=consumerwellness* (158).

Olive Oil

Organic, cold-pressed, extra virgin olive oil (unrefined) can be purchased at your local health food store and some retail grocers. Research continues to point to the heart-healthy benefits of extra virgin olive oil (EVOO). Apparently, the extra virgin oil benefits exceed other types of olive oil for helping lower harmful blood fats and for its antioxidant properties. For best results, the *unrefined,* organic EVOO is considered best (303).

Perilla Oil & Salba

Perilla oil and salba are other healthy sources of plant-based oils. See Life Extension's website: *http://www.lef.org/magazine/mag98/nov98_*

perilla.html and *healthtrends.com* at: *http://www.allhealthtrends.com/salba-information.html.*

Pumpkinseed Oil

Another good oil (if organic, unrefined) is pumpkinseed oil (which has been shown to prevent prostate enlargement), but beware, some oils are watered down (208). Mr. Siegfried Gursche in his book, *Fantastic Flax*, says "one drop of genuine pumpkinseed oil on a lettuce leaf will remain a solid drop..." (208). If it has been *mixed* with another oil, it will run (208). Pumpkinseed oil is famous for boosting the health of the *urinary tract* as well as the prostate (208). Make it a habit to be a label reader.

Walnut, Coconut, Almond Oil & Blackseed Oil

Look for other good oils (unrefined, cold-pressed) such as natural organic *coconut oil, walnut,* and *almond* oil (208). Organic perilla oil, krill oil, and black seed (*nigela sativa*) are also good healthy oil sources.

CHAPTER 4

Vitamin C – Premier Cancer Killer & Health Sustainer

****

I. Vitamin C – Unique Protector

I had a nephew remark to me one time that he only takes a certain amount of vitamin C a day (a small dose); because he had read that anything beyond that small amount is just lost out through the urine. His comment made me realize how truly uneducated most people are about vitamin C and why it is so important for staying healthy.

Vitamin C neutralizes free radicals in the body. Free radicals are generated with exercise, stress, and toxic chemicals in our environment that we breathe in or ingest every day, even toxins in shampoo, detergent, toothpaste, and food. The more free radicals and stress you are exposed to on a daily basis, the more likely you are to suffer disease and illness, and vitamin C helps to neutralize free radicals! Every time you inhale things like air pollution and cigarette smoke (even second-hand smoke) your body needs vitamin C to neutralize the toxins in the smoke. Every time you get stuck in traffic and you sit for an hour stressing out and inhaling toxic fumes from other cars' exhaust pipes, your body burns up thousands of milligrams of vitamin C. Any sort of stress, such as stress on your job, surgery, lack of sleep, lack of proper exercise and fresh air, being angry, depressed, sick, losing a loved one, hearing bad news, losing a job, going through a new marriage, separation or divorce, or moving to a new city, will burn up vitamin C in your body. No one can survive long in a healthy state with inadequate levels of vitamin C in the body, and the amount you need will vary from day-to-day depending on where you live and the toxins, life stressors, and free radicals that constantly bombard you. You inhale them through your lungs and they are absorbed through your skin. You also ingest them through all the chemicals, preservatives, and dyes that are put into our food supply every day. These include pesticides and herbicides sprayed on foods, toxic chemicals that the FDA allows added to the food supply, and hormones in the meat and dairy industry. Our planet is an increasing mess of dangerous chemicals and there is no escaping them. We have managed to nearly drown ourselves in a toxic soup of our own making, mostly while no one was really looking.

My nephew knew nothing of the research by Linus Pauling, who was the only person who ever won "two unshared Nobel Prizes," and "probably generated more attention in advocating high doses of vitamin C for the common cold than for anything else he did" (230). Dr. Robert Cathcart treated what he considered a "mild cold" with "30,000 to 60,000 mg of vitamin C to reach bowel tolerance," noting that a more "severe cold could require from 60,000 to more than 100,000 mg of vitamin C [per day] to reach bowel tolerance," and usually gave these large amounts in "six to 15 divided doses daily" (230). (Bowel tolerance is the highest dose of vitamin C you can ingest before getting diarrhea.)

• Liver Protector

There are many different forms of vitamin C, but only one was discovered to actually have the ability to protect the liver from damage caused by acetaminophen (Tylenol®) in test animals. The type vitamin C used was **ascorbyl palmitate** and the mice in the study received "600 mg/kg body weight dose of ascorbyl palmitate, a vitamin C derivative" (230).

• Poison Detoxifier

Vitamin C is protective against many toxic substances, not only acetaminophen, but cyclosporine, cyanides, Cisplatin, benzene, nicotine, methanol, ozone, phenol, PCP, selenium poisoning, sulfa drugs, pesticides, deadly mushrooms, strychnine, mercury, radiation, arsenic, lead, cadmium, aluminum, vanadium, fluoride, and toxic venoms, to name a few (230). Dr. Thomas Levy, M.D., J.D., reports that "in Australia alone, some 100 physicians have administered [intravenously] as much as 300,000 mg of vitamin C per day to their patients...in most cases the results have been spectacular, the only side effect is 'chronic good health'" (230), and if you are concerned about SIDS and vaccination safety, you might consider "generous doses of vitamin C before and after" any type of vaccination exposure (230)!

The US RDA for vitamin C is 45/60 mg. Can you see how ABSURD this amount of vitamin C is in relation to keeping you healthy? This amount of vitamin C is just enough to keep you in a state of borderline scurvy and may not even prevent scurvy if you are not consuming a lot of vitamin C rich foods in your daily diet.

Studies have shown that animals that can produce their own levels of vitamin C will produce as much as 60,000 mg a day when exposed to a disease. Humans cannot produce their own vitamin C. They must ingest what they need. If an animal automatically manufactures 60,000 mg a day when they are sick, why in the world would the Committee on Dietary Allowance Food and Nutrition Board get the idea that a human being can survive on less than 100 mg a day, especially with all the stress, toxins, and free radicals we are exposed to on a daily basis!?

• Chronic Diseases & Vitamin C

When it came to hemorrhagic diseases, Dr. Frederick Klenner believed that the presence of hemorrhage meant that vitamin C had been totally burned up in the body, producing a rapid hemorrhagic scurvy, and that the best way to battle the disease was with immediate intervention using massive doses of vitamin C (230). Klenner gave IM injections of "2,000 to 3,000" mgs "of vitamin C" to eight shingles patients "every 12 hours, and 1,000 mg was given orally every two hours. "…within two hours of the first vitamin C injection, 7 out of 8 of the patients were totally and permanently pain-free of the disease and "within 72 hours," 7 of the patients had no "skin lesions" (230).

As noted by Dr Thomas Levy, "published results show complete resolution of 327 of 327 shingle cases within 72 hours after administering vitamin C injections," with similar results noted in children with chicken pox, and a remarkable case of mono clearing up. In another mono case, a woman was well after just one week of receiving "Only three daily 2,000 mg injections of vitamin C" (230). If you are a person who is always getting fever blisters and colds, pay attention. What you may need is to increase your vitamin C by about 10,000 mg (or more) per day!

II. Cancer & Vitamin C

I consider vitamin C a ***premier nutrient*** simply because every single cell in the body uses vitamin C and re-uses vitamin C, and desperately needs this nutrient for proper cell functioning and total health, yet most people are severely deficient in C. They are totally unaware of the important place this vitamin plays in the role of overall health, believing, erroneously, that drinking a glass of orange juice once a day will give you all the vitamin C that you need for optimal health. Nothing could be further from the truth!

The RDA daily recommendation of vitamin C is so dismally low that what they have done is to allow just enough to keep people from developing full-blown scurvy, yet not allowing for adequate amounts to help the body neutralize the millions of free radicals that constantly bombard us on a daily basis causing disease. Ewan Cameron, M.B., Ch.B, C.S., F.R.C.S., and Linus Pauling, Ph.D., lamented this fact in their book: *Cancer and Vitamin C* (362c). For all cancer patients, they recommended Dr. Abram Hoffer's daily nutritional regimen which included: "about 12,000 mg of vitamin C, 800 IU of vitamin E, 1500 mg of niacin (vitamin B3, either nicotinic acid or nicotinamide) 25 or 50 times the RDA of other B vitamins, 0.200 mg of selenium, and for some patients...zinc or calcium" (362c).

If you check the *Orange Wunder Formula* I discuss in Chapters 1 and 2 of this book, it does contain calcium and zinc. This is a drink that I developed for a family member fighting Stage IV inoperable bladder cancer. It also contains 3000 mg of liposomal vitamin C, believed to be a much more potent form of C than any other oral form available. Dr. Thomas Levy, a staunch advocate of vitamin C therapy, discusses it in his excellent books on vitamin C: *Curing the Incurable*, and *Stop America's #1 Killer!* If you read these books, as I have, you will never think the same about vitamin C again!

- ### New Research Shows Vitamin C Can Shrink Stage IV Bladder Tumors, Lymphoma & Kidney Cancers

During the 60's and 70's, urologists from Tulane University discovered that megadosing with Vitamin C on a regular basis had the ability to wipe out chemicals that cause bladder cancers and prevent the chances that bladder tumors would return and progress (181).

As described by writer J. Laurance at *The Independent News,* when three cancer victims "were given large intravenous doses" [of vitamin C] for "several months," and "their tumours shrunk," this got the attention of some in the medical profession. One of the recipients of the intravenous vitamin C was a man with stage 4 "terminal bladder cancer" in his late forties, who survived and is still living a normal, disease-free life "nine years later", after refusing chemo and radiation and opting only for the vitamin C (229). The second patient was a woman in her mid-sixties with a "dismal prognosis," due to a particularly "aggressive lymphoma," treated only with the I.V. vitamin C. Ten years have passed and she is still alive and cancer-free (229). The third patient, a woman in her early fifties, had "kidney cancer that spread to her lungs" (229). The cancer was discovered in 1995. She received the intravenous vitamin C, and "had a normal chest x-ray two years later" (229).

Linus Pauling, "Nobel prize winner, 30 years ago," first began expounding the benefits of vitamin C, which is harmless to normal cells and toxic to cancer cells (229), though there is controversy about dosing levels. Pauling used oral doses, but scientists say that when given intravenously, a person can maintain "blood levels 25 times higher that persist for longer" than oral doses, and at these higher doses, vitamin C will kill cancer (229).

Does vitamin C kill cancer? If still in doubt, read the rest of this chapter and please go back and read Chapters 1 and 2 again. There is a new form of vitamin C called *liposomal C* that you take by mouth, and it is believed to be just as potent, if not more so, than receiving intravenous vitamin C, and it is only a fraction of the cost of chemotherapy! I used this liposomal vitamin C in my nutritional formula that I gave to a close relative who had a very aggressive stage IV inoperable bladder cancer, which I discuss at length in Chapters 1 and 2 of this book.

When someone I know tells me that they are fighting a cold, flu, virus, high blood pressure, high cholesterol, heart disease of any kind, a chronic illness, COPD, CHF, MS, high blood pressure, diabetes, CAD, infection, asthma, sore throat, strep, nagging allergies, or cancer, the very first thing I ask them is how much vitamin C they are taking daily. Why is this? After years of research and reading the materials of Linus Pauling, Dr. Matthias Rath, Ewan Cameron, Frederick Klenner, Dr. Robert Cathcart, Bernard Rimland, Dr. Thomas Levy, Irwin Stone,

Abram Hoffer, and many others, I am convinced that most people get ill primarily because they are not getting high enough levels of this miraculous vitamin in their bodies on a daily basis. I'm not speaking of 300 mg or 500 mg or 1000 mg a day! I am talking 10,000 mg a day or more in divided doses throughout the day. This is TEN GRAMS a day (10,000 milligrams). If you go to your local health food store and get a bottle of vitamin C with 1000 mg capsules, you would take TEN of them every day in divided doses.

If you are not willing to increase your vitamin C intake and the vitamin C intake of your children in this world we live in, where we are constantly being bombarded with billions of free radicals on a daily basis, you and they will have to suffer your share of colds, flu viruses, chronic illnesses, bacterial infections, strep, chronic ear infections, tonsillitis, and other diseases that might very well have been prevented. Though I believe glutathione to also be one of the most vital nutrients in protecting the health of the body, unless you replenish daily stores of lost vitamin C (which helps protect glutathione levels), all the glutathione in the world isn't going to help.

• Proof that Vitamin C Cures Myelogenous Leukemia & CSS

As discussed by Irwin Stone, a "case history published in the *Medical Times* 22 years ago…" showed that *ascorbate* [vitamin C] could be used to bring about a total *remission* in "myelogenous leukemia" (291). The patient was given "24,500 mg to 42,000 mg of ascorbate…" and enjoyed a total "remission" (291). Whenever the ascorbate was deliberately stopped (twice) *as an experiment,* all symptoms returned. As soon as the vitamin "was resumed, the temperature returned to normal within six hours…and the remission reoccurred." For some reason this research was mysteriously discontinued (291). Dr. Stone believed that the puny 45 mg of ascorbate that is recommended daily, known as the RDA, is terribly inadequate at preventing lifelong CSS [chronic subclinical scurvy], which brings with it all manner of chronic disease, leukemia, "heart disease, cancer, the collagen diseases, kidney diseases, and the many infirmities found in the senior citizens" (291).

• Vitamin C & Other Cancers

The National Institute of Diabetes and Digestive and Kidney Diseases in Bethesda, Maryland, discovered recently, that giving large amounts of vitamin C intravenously to mice with ovarian cancers, glioblastoma, and cancers of the pancreas, restricted the cancer *growth by up to 53%* (160). The study was headed up by Dr. Mark Levine, who said that the vitamin C worked by forming *hydrogen peroxide,* which destroyed the *cancer cells* (160). Cancer Treatment Centers of America *(CTCA)* in Zion, Illinois, has been testing intravenous Vitamin C on patients with advanced cancer (160).

• Vitamin C & Cancer Research – Recent Studies

There was a lot of publicity in the news in the latter part of 2008 that vitamins such as C, E, and selenium, in human studies, were not shown to prevent cancer. When you read about these studies, many factors need to be taken into consideration:

1. In the study on vitamin C, only 500 mg a day was given. You will read throughout this entire book that not a single advocate of vitamin C therapy ever proposed such a ridiculously LOW amount of vitamin C for fighting cancer! You can probably burn that much vitamin C in five minutes stressing out in a traffic jam! It has also been proven that vitamin C given in huge doses intravenously is much more effective at fighting cancer than C taken orally. Also, some forms of vitamin C are better than others (e.g., the whole form of C that includes all the bioflavanoids, not just the ascorbic acid). See Chapters 1 and 2 and later in this chapter for a discussion on liposomal C, which may be just as important for fighting cancer as intravenous C, even though it is taken by mouth!

2. In the study using vitamin E, only 400 IU were given every OTHER day, not every day. Why was it not given daily? Also, what KIND of vitamin E was given? The synthetic dl-alpha? The natural d-alpha, mixed tocotrieols? This would make a HUGE difference. Even synthetic beta carotene is so far inferior to natural beta carotene, prior human studies showed that the

SYNTHETIC variety can actually increase the risk for lung cancer in smokers – not so with the natural!

3. There are numerous other human studies that have been done using vitamin therapy that contradict the findings of these studies. What about the control group? How healthy were they? Did they eat normally? If so, how do they know that the group not receiving the vitamin or mineral supplements did not get the SAME amounts in their daily diets—via food intake—as those given the supplements, making the entire study flawed?

4. Whenever I have read research studies on the importance of minerals like selenium and vitamin C antioxidants for cancer prevention, then along comes another study that tries to contradict 30 that were done before it, a red flag goes up. WHO sponsored these studies? How many drug companies were involved in these studies? Pharmaceutical companies are ALWAYS trying to discredit natural substances like vitamins and minerals. They would like to see every man, woman, and child in the country taking their prescription medications for things like high cholesterol, rather than natural foods and nutrients that lower cholesterol levels without drugs. Most of them test 200 mg of vitamin C against a disorder, and then pitch it as useless when it does not work. (What they need to be testing is 100-500 GRAMS of vitamin C intravenously at a time! Or using the new *liposome-encapsulated Vitamin C* that is taken orally (233). They should try using 5 mg of an antibiotic, that usually requires 2 grams, and see where it gets them in fighting disease!

5. Two new studies by German scientists showed that selenium boosts the body's natural immunity. Of significance was the fact that all the men in the study with prostate cancer already had low levels of selenium in their body. What about the other recent study that claimed that selenium did nothing to prevent prostate cancer? Were blood levels of selenium taken BEFORE the study began to determine if some of the men were already deficient in selenium before even beginning the study? While it was shown that those men taking selenium alone (rather than

with vitamin E) had increased incidence for diabetes, this should come as no surprise, because minerals and vitamins need each other for best performance. Also, one has to wonder what FORM of selenium was used in this study. Was it a natural form of the mineral, such as organic selenomethionine, selenocysteine, methylselenocysteine, or the inorganic selenite, selenate, or selenide, which are poorly absorbed by the body?

6. While one large study said that selenium did not affect melanoma, the same study revealed that it decreases the risk for all other cancers. Those giving the results of the study said that natural foods are a better source of vitamins and minerals than supplements. Of course, this has always been true; however, there are some nutrients that you simply cannot get enough of in your daily diet without supplementing (such as with vitamin C, alpha lipoic acid, and CoQ10), and there are many areas of the country, for example, where you can eat foods that SHOULD be rich in selenium, but they are not because the soil has been stripped of selenium, so you need to supplement. Brazil nuts are a great source of selenium, but only if the soil they are grown in is selenium-rich.

7. Individual situations will also determine vitamin and nutrient needs. If you have just had a devastating illness or major stressor in your life (e.g., death of a loved one in your family, major surgery, newly married, divorced, moving to a new location, changing jobs), you are going to require more vitamin C to offset the stress in your life than someone dealing with no stress.

Be VERY suspicious of people who tell you that you don't need vitamin and mineral supplements, but it's fine to take multiple prescription drugs, and that your only CHOICE for cancer is chemo or radiation.

Perhaps health advocate, Mike Adams, said it best in his website article *http://www.naturalnews.com/027705_chemotherapy_fraud.html*, when he explained the reason that most people take chemo:

> The answer: *Because they're desperate*. They're dying, and they're willing to pay anything for hope, even if it's a false

hope thrust upon them by their oncologist. It is in this context that these cancer drug companies charge $10,000 a month, $20,000 a month or even now **$30,000 a month** to treat you with their 'breakthrough' cancer drugs. The purpose of all this isn't to cure your cancer: It's to *drain your bank account before you die*, extracting every last dollar of your savings and retirement money before you expire. No one out-quacks the cancer industry in terms of exploiting the fears of dying <u>elderly patients</u> (156).

• Vitamin C Cures a "Fatal" Hodgkin's Disease

Have you or someone you love been diagnosed with leukemia? Be sure that what you (or they) have really **is leukemia** and not a vitamin C deficiency, or even a *folic acid* or *B12 deficiency* (278). Those words of warning from Maureen Kennedy Salaman, author of *Nutrition: The Cancer Answer II* (278). A *vitamin C* deficiency (scurvy) can resemble leukemia, as can *folic acid* and *B12* deficiencies (278).

In a report by Irwin Stone, he describes what happened when Dr. Bernard Rimland (their Program Chairman) had a daughter who was diagnosed with terminal *Hodgkin's disease* (291). She was admitted to the hospital with serious *renal failure*, and graded as "the most severe Stage IV-B, with" spread into "the kidneys and liver" (291). Dr. Rimland began her on a high dose vitamin C regimen. Her physicians "gave her less than one year to live" (278). She received chemo, which made her much sicker, and she became severely depressed. Once back home, her father immediately started her on a regimen that included *1000 mg/day* of *niacinamide* and *40 grams* per day of *vitamin C*. (That's GRAMS, not milligrams.) He divided the dose throughout the day (278) (291).

Dr. Rimland believed in high-dose vitamin C for leukemia. He noted that Irwin Stone had documented many cases of people who recovered from leukemia using this treatment. The high dose nutritional program saved his daughter's life and he feels might have spared other children, but he could not convince the oncologists (278) (291). See this internet site: *http://www.seanet.com/~alexs/ascorbate/197x/stone-i-ort homol_psych-1976-v5-n3-p183.htm,* for reports on other cancer cases treated successfully with vitamin C (291).

Not only did Rimland give his daughter megadoses of vitamin C throughout the day in divided doses, but he himself takes these megadoses. They also included vitamins E, A, and the minerals selenium and calcium (278).

(Note: Since vitamin A can be toxic when taken in large doses and natural beta carotene is not, I would recommend taking the vitamin A in beta carotene form by juicing fresh carrot juice daily. It is believed that the body converts natural beta carotene into vitamin A.) For those who are concerned about stomach upset from high dose (oral) vitamin C (ascorbic acid), get the buffered C powder or crystals in health food stores, use the sodium ascorbate (rather than the ascorbic acid form), or purchase *Ester-C®*, which is buffered vitamin C with calcium ascorbate. High dose vitamin C is also given intravenously (sodium ascorbate form) by many alternative health physicians. It is a non-acidic form and bypasses the stomach, so does not cause gastric upset.

You can make your own sodium ascorbate by mixing one teaspoon of the ascorbic acid C crystals (which contain either 1000 mg or 5000 mg of vitamin C per teaspoon, depending on the brand you buy) with ½ teaspoon of soda bicarb, as described in Chapter 2, and dilute in ½ cup of distilled water or orange juice to remove the tartness and make it gentler on the stomach. Be sure you wait until it stops fizzing before you mix it with a spoon, or it may foam over the top of your glass. *Ester C®* may have more calcium than you need. (Most people get too much calcium and not enough magnesium in their diets.) If you love lemonade, but not the tartness, you can reduce the acidity of lemonade much the same way. Just put a teaspoon of soda bicarb in 2 quarts of lemonade and the tartness and acidity will be greatly reduced. Drink after it stops fizzing. This does add sodium to the lemonade.

• Vitamin C - Research
Multiple Human Studies Reveal it Cures Cancer

When 59-year-old Arlindo O. was told that his advanced lung cancer had gone into his brain, physicians sent him home to die (64), yet today he is *cancer-free* (64), and he credits his survival to vitamin C. Recent studies *from* the *National Institutes of Health* showed that vitamin C given *intravenously* could halt the growth of "aggressive brain, ovarian and pancreatic tumors…" in mice (64).

The treatment is non-toxic to healthy cells, with none of the adverse, damaging side effects associated with standard *chemotherapy and radiation*. According to Dr. Scott Greenberg, who treated Arlindo with high intravenous doses of vitamin C, "it is a valuable option for those who don't respond to other treatments," and is safe to combine with most standard "chemo and radiation" (64). He said that the vitamin C creates "hydrogen peroxide," which kills the cancer cells much "like chemotherapy does" (64), except that vitamin C is non-toxic to healthy cells. He even talked about a woman he treated with massive intravenous vitamin C, who had "a large breast mass protruding out of her chest" (64). Within just "a few months of treatment," the mass disappeared. It has been five years and she has had no further "sign of cancer whatsoever," says Dr. Greenberg (64).

• Vitamin C & Lymphoma

Human scientific data written up by the National Institutes of Health has shown that giving vitamin C intravenously could "have unexpected implications for treatment of infections where" hydrogen peroxide "may be beneficial," and showed that **lymphoma cells**, which are very sensitive to vitamin C, were killed because the vitamin C generated **hydrogen peroxide** within the cells, as noted above, which killed the cancer (185). The research proved that giving intravenous vitamin C does kill cancer cells. Why? Because as stated earlier, it forms peroxide and peroxide kills the cancer (185). This is exactly what the pioneers of vitamin C therapy for killing cancer have been saying for more than 60 years—that vitamin C given intravenously in large amounts will KILL CANCER! No one has listened to them. Why? Because vitamin C is cheap and the pharmaceutical industry runs the medical system in America. Most chemo costs thousands of dollars per round. Drug companies can't make a profit on vitamin C, a natural substance, because it cannot be patented! I can vouch for this. See Chapter 1. After only two rounds of chemo, my relative's oncologist sent his insurance carrier a bill for $30,000! (I told him that this is why his oncologist was smiling every time he saw him coming!)

Racing for a cure? Running for a cure? Pink ribbons for a cure? Who's really interested in a cure at those profits? If the "cure" is out there, do you really think the current medical-pharmaceutical monopoly in the U.S. is going to acknowledge it? They would all have to close up shop. They would all be out of business! All these new billion-dollar cancer centers being built? What would they do with them if a "cure" were found? There are countless entire institutional medical complexes dedicated to treating cancer with their chemo drugs and radiation and surgical procedures, not to mention the billions that the diagnostic tests generate in profits. What would happen to all of them and their employees? Would the U.S. government consider the current cancer industry in this nation too big to fail and bail them out like they did the banks and the car companies if a cure were suddenly announced? The National Cancer Institute and American Cancer Society rakes in millions of dollars a year in donations. Do you think THEY want to turn those dollars away? Do you think they want their jobs terminated? What will become of all those massive programs, government grants, and cancer-dedicated building programs? What will they do with them? Turn them into massage parlors and nail salons? No. As stated in my first book, The SEARCH for a cure is extremely profitable, finding one isn't!

For those who think that socialized medicine is simply terrific, don't bet on getting the breast cancer drug Tykerb (Lapatinib) in the UK anymore. Their National Institute for Health and Clinical Excellence (?) decided recently that the drug was not "cost-effective" for people with advanced breast cancer. Why? Because it costs "$2,300 per treatment course in Britain" (142a), and under socialized medicine, guess what, you simply are not worth it! The government will no longer pay for it. But this could be a plus, because some of the chemo drugs are killing more people than they are curing and some are simply killing them faster than their cancer does! It won't be long, under socialized medicine, before health care will be denied to anyone sixty or over. In the U.S. Medicare and Medicaid are going broke. All those dollars you paid out over a lifetime to social security have already been stolen from you! Why do you think that they are changing the retirement age to 70? They are hoping that you will drop dead on the job so you won't LIVE long enough to collect the retirement you've paid into for 50 years that the government has already squandered! It won't take the sociopathic beaurocrats long to legislate that there isn't enough to go around and the younger, more fit populace, who are more valuable contributors to society deserve the funding. Think it can't possibly happen? There are already countries in this world where elderly patients are being euthanized (permanently "put to sleep") like household pets, without having any say in the matter whatsoever! Your best insurance? Stay healthy as long as possible so that you can avoid the death grip of conventional medicine's "health" treatments.

• Those Who Were Cured

In their book, *Cancer and Vitamin C,* Ewan Cameron and Linus Pauling discuss several cases of people who halted the progression of their cancer, or cured it completely by taking megadoses of vitamin C every day (usually in divided doses), including the following:

- Two women with **breast cancer**, both of them having breast removal and radiation, but in the first woman the cancer returned in her spine. Her cancer disappeared completely after she began taking 10 grams of vitamin C by mouth per day. The other woman (who had *adenocarcinoma* of the breast) had a return of her cancer within two years and no improvement after trying androgen hormones. After another bout of Stage IV cancer and ovarian removal, she began taking 10 grams of vitamin C every day and went into total remission. At last check, more than SEVEN years later, she was still cancer-free and healthy (362c).
- Two men with **prostate cancer,** one with *adenocarcinoma* of the prostate that had gone into his left lung. He was not offered any type of treatment, considered "incurable," but began taking 10 grams of vitamin C a day. Within 60 days, the lung tumor was totally gone. Three-and-a-half years later, he was still healthy and enjoying a normal life. The second patient began taking 8 grams of vitamin C daily, increased it to 10 grams per day along with Laetrile that he also took by mouth. He became symptom-free, and then the cancer went into his pelvis. The only treatment he would take was to increase the vitamin C to 12 grams, then 20 grams per day, and he started taking vitamin A in large doses and a vegetarian diet. His cancer disappeared completely (362c).
- Three patients with **lung cancer**, one of whom halted the growth for nearly a year by taking 10 grams of vitamin C daily, then had surgical removal; the other with malignant tumors in both lungs, given up as untreatable, who began taking 15 grams of vitamin C daily, putting herself into total remission lasting for years. The third patient also used 10 grams of vitamin C daily, which resulted in total remission (362c).

- Two **carcinoma** patients, one who failed conventional medicine, then made a remarkable recovery taking 10 grams of vitamin C daily. The other patient, after having surgery to remove three malignant tumors, began taking 10 to 12 grams of vitamin C per day. She too remained cancer-free for several years (362c).
- A **colon cancer** patient who was cured taking 8-10 grams of vitamin C daily (362c).
- A **reticulum cell sarcoma** patient, who accomplished the same thing taking 10 grams of vitamin C daily (362c).
- A **bladder cancer** patient who went into regression taking 3 grams per day of vitamin C (362c).
- A **cerebral brain tumor** patient whose tumor disappeared after 3 months of taking 10 grams a day of vitamin C (362c).
- A young woman with extensive **Hodgkin's disease** who refused conventional treatment, and cured her cancer by taking 10 grams of vitamin C daily (362c).
- An 80-year-old woman with **Stage III lymphosarcoma** who underwent radiation and began taking 10 grams of vitamin C a day on her own, resulting in a cure (362c).
- A middle-aged woman with **ovarian cancer** who underwent surgery and radiation, then colon surgery when the cancer returned. When it was found that the cancer had gone into multiple areas of the peritoneum, she was given six months to live. She ended up living long enough to take Leukeran and 3 to 12 grams of vitamin C a day, resulting in a complete cure. At last check, six years after her ordeal, she was still cancer-free (362c). These are people, not mice.

Note that most of the above patients managed to put their disease into remission taking only small amounts of C, about 10 grams or so per day. There were also cases noted by Cameron and Pauling where much larger doses of vitamin C (in divided doses) were taken to successfully eradicate cancer, including the following few examples out of many:

- A patient with **chronic myeloid leukemia** (and *alcoholic cirrhosis*) who went into remission for two years taking 42 grams a day of vitamin C orally. He took 500 mg tablets in divided doses several times a day to get this amount (362c).

- A woman with **cancer of the pancreas** who took 16 grams of vitamin C a day, then gradually increased to 30 grams of sodium ascorbate (Vitamin C). She was in total remission in less than a year, but continued to take 30 grams a day of the vitamin C (362c).
- A 77-year-old patient with **mesothelioma** who underwent once-a-week 5-Fluorouracil, causing him severe skin reactions. He began taking 10 grams of vitamin C a day, then increased to 25 grams over a two-week period. All diagnostic tests came back clear. He had no trace of cancer (362c).
- A patient with **"hairy cell" CLL** (chronic lymphocytic leukemia) who opted out of conventional therapy, ingesting 35 grams of vitamin C daily. He did undergo spleen removal, but continued on the same dose of vitamin C resulting in a total cure (362c).
- A **mycosis fungoides** patient who went into remission taking only 4 grams of vitamin C daily, reducing his dose to 3 grams after his recovery (362c).
- A young man with **pheochromocytoma** who failed surgery and was considered untreatable, with the cancer spreading into his abdominal region. He began taking vitamin C at 30 grams per day, slowly increasing to 80 grams per day (in divided doses) over a 14 month period. He became pain-free and returned to a normal and very active lifestyle (362c).
- A 67-year-old man with **carcinoma of the stomach** that had gone into his pancreas. He had partial removal of the tumor, but the pancreas was left intact. He received no other treatment except he began to take 12 grams of sodium ascorbate [vitamin C] daily. He worsened, was hospitalized, then his relatives insisted he be discharged when he was not improving. After getting back home, he began taking 20 grams of the vitamin C daily and then 28 grams per day. He had a remarkable improvement, then had gallstones removed. During that surgery, it was noted that his cancer was totally gone. He continued to take the large daily doses of vitamin C and went on to enjoy a normal, active life (362c).

Note that if you are hospitalized for any reason, you will NOT be given megadoses of vitamin C unless you ask for them, and even if you ask for them, your doctor may still refuse to give it to you. They will tell you that it is not on the "hospital formulary," so it isn't available and your insurance won't cover it. This was one enigma that used to puzzle me as a nurse, and other nurses I worked with. On our medical floors, we often had people with huge, gaping wounds that we were doing daily dressing changes on, yet none of their physicians ever put extra vitamin C on their medication sheets, the main vitamin that the body needs for HEALING! When we asked them about it, the physicians simply told us that their patients were eating a regular diet, so they should be getting plenty of vitamin C.

• Vitamin C & Pancreatic Cancer

I have an email friend of mine who was totally cured of "terminal" pancreatic cancer with megadoses of **intravenous** vitamin C. This was more than FIVE years ago. She worked the entire time she was receiving the treatment, had no adverse effects, felt healthy and well, and her cancer totally disappeared, in spite of the fact that her oncologist told her that she was dying. She obtained the megadose intravenous vitamin C from a Naturopathic physician. When she returned to her conventional doctor, he told her that this was impossible and that he must have made an error in diagnosing her!

III. Chronic Diseases, Illness & Vitamin C

Vitamin C is essential in nearly all cellular functions in the body. It is found in our blood vessels, joints, bones, muscles, and ligaments. It is found in the brain and is important in nerve transmission and in behavior and mood. It also helps the body convert fat into energy and is vital in the process that keeps cholesterol levels healthy. It is one of the most important antioxidants found in nature. It protects the strength of our cells and the integrity of blood vessel walls.

A lack of vitamin C brings on a disease known as scurvy. When scurvy occurs, your teeth begin to fall out, the walls of your blood vessels actually begin leaking blood and you will hemorrhage or bleed to death. Vitamin C protects against free radicals, fights the effects of deadly heavy metals, neutralizes toxins, venoms, and pollutants, and protects other antioxidants in the body from being oxidized—essential nutrients like GSH (glutathione) and vitamin E. Simply put, deprive yourself of vitamin C and you will die a miserable death. Many sailors who spent months on long ocean voyages succumbed to scurvy, until it was discovered that eating citrus fruit could protect them (though they did not know exactly why, since vitamin C hadn't been discovered yet). This is where the word "limey" comes from. They began carrying crates of limes on board vessels bound for long voyages for the sailors to ingest. They referred to the sailors (or soldiers) as *limeys* from their ingestion of limes to prevent scurvy.

Vitamin C is not only important in disease prevention, but in treating disease. Nearly every major disease known to mankind has responded favorably to megadoses of vitamin C. This has been shown repeatedly in the studies and writings of Linus Pauling, Dr. Abram Hoffer, Dr. Matthias Rath, Dr. Robert Cathcart, Irwin Stone, Dr. Frederick Klenner, Ewan Cameron, Dr. Thomas Levy, and many others who recognize how valuable this vitamin truly is!

Of Vitamin C and cancer, Irwin Stone said:

> In one case where complete remission was achieved in myelogenous leukemia...the patient took 24—42 gms vitamin C per day...it is inconceivable that no one appears to have followed this up...without the scurvy, leukemia may be a relatively benign, non fatal condition. I wrote a paper...in an attempt to have the therapy clinically tested...I sent it to 3 cancer journals and 3 blood journals...it was refused by all...Two without even reading it (136).

Do you realize that 24—42 grams is 24,000 to 42,000 mg a day? He also advised parents how to avoid SIDS or *cot death*, as it is sometimes called, by telling them to be sure their babies had sufficient levels of vitamin C in their blood:

> Cot-death is no longer a problem of clinical medicine, but is one of medical politics. We have long had the knowledge and experience as to how these unnecessary deaths can be avoided. In the meantime...to prevent your offspring from becoming a SIDS statistic just make sure that its daily intake of ascorbate [vitamin C] from conception on is sufficient. Under this regime the neonate is so robust and healthy that there has never been a case of SIDS among these ascorbate-corrected infants, not even a case of respiratory distress during birth (136).

Dr. Ewan Cameron and Linus Pauling also agreed that "a properly large intake of vitamin C may well be found to be the most important of all dietary factors in the prevention of cancer" (181). How much vitamin C have YOU had today? Your children?

Want to prevent your child from getting colds, flu, viruses, SIDS, RDS (respiratory distress syndrome), ear infections? Make sure they keep sufficient blood levels of vitamin C. A good way to do this is through the **timed-release** vitamin C supplements.

In his book on vitamin C, *Curing the Incurable,* Thomas E. Levy, M.D., J.D., proved that vitamin C can be effective in preventing and successfully treating many diseases including, but not limited to:

African hemorrhagic fever
Argentine hemorrhagic fever
Bolivian hemorrhagic fever
Botulism
Brazilian hemorrhagic fever
Brucellosis
Cancer
Chicken pox
Hemorrhagic diseases
Herpes
HIV
Kyasanur Forest Disease
Lassa fever
Leprosy
Malaria
Measles
Mononucleosis
MRSA
Mumps
Omsk hemorrhagic fever
Parainfluenzavirus type 2
Pertussis
Plasmodium falciparum parasite
Pneumonia (viral)
Polio
Rabies
Radiation poisoning

Crimean-Congo hemorrhagic fever
Cytomegalovirus
Dengue Fever
Diphtheria
Dysentery
Ebola virus
Encephalitis (viral)
Hantavirus
Respiratory syncytial virus
Rheumatic fever
Rift Valley fever
Rocky Mountain spotted fever
Scarlet fever
Scurvy
Shingles
Staph infections
Strep
Tetanus
The common cold
Trichinosis
Trypanosomal infections
Tuberculosis
Typhoid
Urinary tract infections
Venezuelan hemorrhagic fever
West Nile fever
Yellow fever

Dr. Levy used 12 packets of liposomal C to **cure** a woman of **dengue fever** (though the news media is telling people in Florida there is no cure for this disease)! He does caution against the use of megadoses of vitamin C in people having the rare genetic disorder, *G6PD deficiency,* especially if they also have **sickle cell disease** (230). According to his research, HIV and AIDS could also be "controlled quite effectively if a high enough chronic dosing of vitamin C is maintained" (230).

• Infectious Diseases & Vitamin C

Dr. Robert Cathcart, Dr. Thomas Levy, Linus Pauling, Dr. Frederick Klenner, Ewan Cameron, Dr. Matthias Rath, and many others also studied the effects of vitamin C in fighting infection and disease. Dr. Frederick Klenner was giving his polio patients megadoses of vitamin C and they were walking home, while other physicians (using conventional medicine) were sticking their polio victims in iron lungs, and more often than not, sending them to the morgue!

I discussed the new liposomal vitamin C in my last book *Gentle Cures for Tough Cancers,* and talked about its use in fighting infectious diseases like dengue fever. I used it to help my own family member recover from a Stage IV inoperable bladder cancer (see Chapters 1 and 2 of this book). Dr. Robert Cathcart believes that the toxins created by infectious diseases eat up vitamin C so rapidly that what really happens is a widespread fulminating SCURVY occurs. This is why you have the profuse bleeding and hemorrhage found in diseases like Ebola and others, and the quick deterioration of health found in diseases like the West Nile Virus, polio, Epstein-Barr virus, HIV and others; however, even the World Health Organization has refused to follow Dr. Cathcart's suggestions and treat these patients with high doses of intravenous vitamin C. Is it because vitamin C is so much cheaper than some of the state-of-the-art antibiotics and other premier drugs that are being developed by the big pharmaceutical companies?

Sometimes you have no choice but to use antibiotics, depending on the circumstances, but remember this: vitamin C in the right dosage at the right time will rapidly kill just about any infection and prevent them from occurring in the first place.

How many people would have taken the chance of being vaccinated with the H1N1 vaccine had they known that megadosing with vitamin C might have protected them just as well, if not better? How many moms would have given their newborns extra vitamin C drops had they known it might have helped in the prevention of SIDS or autism in their babies?

• Diabetes, High Cholesterol & Vitamin C

Board Certified Cardiologist, Dr. Thomas Levy, M.D., J.D., has written many incomparable books on health. I believe that his book *"STOP AMERICA's #1 KILLER – Reversible Vitamin Deficiency Found to be Origin of ALL Coronary Heart Disease,* should be mandatory reading for all nurses and physicians, regardless of their specialty, and anyone else concerned about heart disease. He is one of the most informed health leaders in the world when it comes to expertise on the use of vitamin C for optimal health. Not only does he discuss the role that low levels of vitamin C cause in promoting the current scourge of heart disease in this country (and others), he also shows the important link between deficient C levels in the body and diabetes. In his book he reports that "…diabetics have depressed, scurvy-like plasma levels of vitamin C," the very same problem that is found in coronary heart disease (232). He says that there is competition in the cells between their uptake of vitamin C and glucose and because of this, high levels of glucose (sugar) in the blood will always drive down vitamin C amounts (232). Insulin actually removes "vitamin C out of the blood," and the kidneys also work against vitamin C levels because high levels of sugar in the blood will cause the kidneys to excrete this valuable vitamin before the body can use it (232).

These high sugar levels in the blood will strip the immune cells (white blood cells) from their much-needed vitamin C, rendering them incapable of fighting off infection (232). Perhaps this is why diabetics are so prone to inflammation, infections, and diseases that do not affect non-diabetics as easily. Vitamin C is important in telling the pancreas how much insulin to release and also helps in keeping harmful blood clots at bay by actually dissolving them (232). Not only are these dangerously low blood levels of vitamin C found in diabetics, they are found in patients with coronary heart disease. Since diabetes drives out vitamin C and the coronary arteries desperately need vitamin C, is it any wonder that diabetics develop heart disease much earlier in life than the non-diabetic population (232)? Take non-GMO lecithin with your vitamin C for reducing harmful cholesterol and atherosclerosis and for elevating good cholesterol (232).

• Hepatitis, Encephalitis & Vitamin C

Frederick Klenner (1974) used mainly vitamin C for the treatment of viral hepatitis. He gave "500 to 700 mg per kilogram of body weight...every eight to 12 hours by vein..." and "at least another 10,000 mg daily by mouth in divided doses," and his hepatitis patients usually recovered within "two to four days" (230). In one particular case, where his patient was needle-phobic, he gave the patient 5000 mg of vitamin C mixed in either "water or juice every four hours," with a complete recovery from the disease within 96 hours. The total amount the patient received in that four-day period was 120,000 mg taken by mouth (230). This is like buying a bottle of 120 pills of 1000 mg each of vitamin C at your local health food store and taking the entire bottle in 4 days at the rate of 30 pills every day in divided doses.

Another clinical study reported by Dr. Thomas Levy, M.D., J.D., was that of 63 children who all "markedly improved" from acute hepatitis after taking "10,000 mg of vitamin C daily for only five days". It was given either rectally or by I.V. infusion, and he reported "similar excellent clinical responses in 245 children with acute hepatitis" (230). Children, not mice.

Dr. Robert Cathcart admitted that he never lost "a single case of acute viral hepatitis...to properly dosed intravenous vitamin C," and Dr. Frederick Klenner "repeatedly used vitamin C to cure patients who were already comatose with viral encephalitis" (184).

• Osteoporosis & Vitamin C

In his book on *STOP AMERICA'S #1 KILLER!*, Dr. Thomas Levy, MD, JD, noted that having adequate levels of vitamin C in the body causes "greater bone mineral density" for women after menopause. Starve your body of vitamin C and risk the disease of osteoporosis (232).

• Vitamin C Deficiency & CSS Syndrome

Irwin Stone presented much of his work on the connection between *CSS Syndrome* (*Chronic Subclinical Scurvy*) and ascorbate deficiency in his book, *The Healing Factor*, 1972 (291). He believed that the disease we refer to as "scurvy," is actually the result of "...a potentially fatal genetic liver-enzyme disease called 'hypoascorbemia,'" and that this disease "affects 100 percent of the population," due to a genetic abnormality that we carry (291). He says that taking the very small amounts of vitamin C we humans take each day will simply "avoid the terminal signs" of CSS, but if you want to actually "correct this human genetic defect," you must be concerned about taking much larger daily doses of ascorbate (vitamin C).

Most animals are able to produce thousands of milligrams of their own ascorbate daily, something we humans are not capable of doing. Leukemia is caused by CSS (291). If you wish to get a test strip that can check your urine (or saliva) to determine if you have sufficient vitamin C in your body, you can order them at website: *http://www.nutri.com/strips/index.html*. This is for informational purposes only. I am not affiliated with them. I cannot vouch for the integrity of their products and have not used them.

• Viral Pneumonia, HIV, Chediak-Higashi Disease & Vitamin C

Klenner also noted that viral pneumonia could be prevented and cured with vitamin C. He even used it for infants and small children, giving them "500 mg of vitamin C intramuscularly every six to twelve hours," and in every instance, he had "complete clinical and x-ray response after only three to seven vitamin C injections" (230). The vitamin has been given to dogs and cats to treat distemper successfully (230). Dr. Robert Cathcart reported great success giving huge doses of vitamin C (180,000 mg) "per day until" he was able to get the patient stable enough to "switch to oral" doses in AIDS patients with "herpes or cytomegalovirus" (230). Some of the patients Dr. Levy discusses received as much as **3,000,000 milligrams** of vitamin C, yet there was never any "toxicity or side effect" from the massive amounts given

(230). Try this with some of your new and improved state-of-the-art antibiotic drugs with all their potentially toxic side effects!

Chediak-Higashi Disease is a genetic disease from birth that causes severe infections because of a defect in the leukocytes, also making these victims especially vulnerable to diseases like cancer (181). Though vitamin C cannot reverse this genetic defect, megadosing with vitamin C has been shown to help restore the potency of the leukocytes, decreasing the severity and occurrence of these infections (181). If vitamin C can help such a sick immune system in these patients, how much more **protective** can it be in those with a well-functioning immunity?

- ## Vitamin C & Heart Disease

In his book on vitamin C: *STOP AMERICA'S #1 KILLER! Reversible Vitamin Deficiency Found to be Origin of ALL Coronary Heart Disease,* Dr. Thomas E. Levy, M.D., J.D., sets forth research-backed data pointing out the importance of adequate vitamin C in preventing a type of arterial scurvy that is the actual cause of all coronary heart disease. Many times, problems originate with root canal treated teeth (232). In **human** studies, even small amounts of vitamin C (as low as 300 mg to 3000 mg a day), proved that vitamin C lowers harmful cholesterol levels and triglyceride levels, even in diabetics, and raises healthy cholesterol (232). His entire book brings the message that current conventional medicine's treatment of heart disease is taking the wrong approach. They really don't even know how it begins!

Reams of research material have shown that adequate amounts of vitamin C can prevent and even help reverse atherosclerotic heart disease. The best way that vitamin C works at reducing harmful cholesterol and raising healthy cholesterol is in conjunction with lecithin (232). Dr. Levy found that it is of utmost importance to take vitamin C with non-GMO soy-based lecithin in order to raise HDL cholesterol and lower LDL cholesterol (232). You can get this lecithin at *http://www.swansonvitamins.com.* Just go to their search box at the top left of the webpage and type in the words *lecithin granules*, and be sure to choose the **non-GMO** formula. You can also purchase them at website: *http://www.iherb.com.* Lecithin in gel tabs is available at most health food stores and pharmacies.

We are subjecting millions of people to a method of treating heart disease by vilifying the wrong culprit. High cholesterol in the body neutralizes toxins. You can lower cholesterol, but this also lowers the body's ability to fight off infections because cholesterol binds with toxins and neutralizes them. Is this why people with low cholesterol levels are more likely to get cancer and die from it (232)? Not only that, but those with low cholesterol also suffer from more depression and suicidal tendencies.

Many animals can manufacture their own vitamin C, something we humans are incapable of. When these animals are fed a high cholesterol diet, they respond by manufacturing MORE vitamin C, which then LOWERS their cholesterol levels (232). Apparently, these animals have a built-in mechanism that "recognizes" exactly when they have too much cholesterol, and their bodies respond by making more vitamin C to lower the excess cholesterol (232). Severe vitamin C deficiencies also appear to elevate levels of histamine in the body, which contributes to atherosclerosis (232), not to mention problems for asthma and allergy sufferers. Antihistamines appear to lower cholesterol. This could be a reason that niacin works so well at lowering harmful cholesterol. It helps remove histamine from the body.

Heart disease increases the inflammatory process in the body. Being deficient in magnesium, glutathione, vitamin C, and increased stress and depression all lead to inflammation in the body, increasing the risks for CAD, cancer, stroke, chronic illness, and death. Stress also suppresses the immune system and allows viruses to take an opportunity during a weakened immunity to attack us with cancer, colds, flu, shingles, CFS, CMV, HIV, Epstein-Barr, sub acute endocarditis and all other types of chronic illness and disease.

According to Dr. Levy, the leading cause of coronary disease is the continuous load of toxins produced non-stop by anaerobic bacteria "generated in root canal teeth," which he compares to being bombarded by botulism (232). These toxins rapidly use up all the vitamin C in the body. A cancer physician discovered that "98% of his patients had between two and ten 'dead teeth,' most of which were root canal-treated teeth" (232). Also, most people develop a type of arterial scurvy in the vessels around the heart caused by insufficient levels of vitamin C, which leads to weak and damaged blood vessels, an inflammatory response by white blood cells, and the build-up of dangerous plaque in the body. (232).

The most amazing thing of all about vitamin C is that it will help lower unhealthy cholesterol, but elevate healthy cholesterol. Dr. Levy pointed out that vitamin C therapy can help bring about total remission in cardiomyopathy and edema sufferers who also had scurvy (232). Are you aware that if you are scheduled to have your blood drawn for labs, they will tell you NOT to take vitamin C beforehand? It's because vitamin C lowers harmful LDL and raises HDL levels!

Remember, if using vitamin C for heart health, use non GMO soy-based lecithin as well, which helps reduce the harmful form of cholesterol (232). Dr. Levy also recommends taking the amino acids proline and lysine with vitamin C for those who are fighting heart disease or simply want to help prevent it from occurring in the first place (232). He recommends at least "3,000 to 9,000 mg" per day of ascorbic acid, the same amount of L-lysine; "500 to 1,500 mg" daily of L-proline and L-arginine, and at least "200 to 1,000" mg daily of a "magnesium-amino acid chelate" such as "Magnesium glycinate" (232). He also recommends daily supplements of vitamin D3, vitamin K2, vitamin E, beta carotene, L-carnosine, Omega-3 fatty acids, thiamine, niacin, the rest of the B vitamins, CoQ10 ("50-250 mg" per day), SOD, MSM, glutathione, NAC, selenium, boron, and other minerals: the complete list and doses, which you can find in his book, *STOP AMERICA'S #1 KILLER*, on pp. 253-254. He does not recommend dental implants any more than he does root canals or amalgam fillings and says that you can find a healthcare dentist who will do a "Total Dental Revision" for you by calling Scientific Health Solutions, Inc. at 800-331-2303 or 719-548-1600, or you can email them at: *dentists @bestdentalmaterials.com* (232).

Human studies have proven that sufficient levels of vitamin C will help prevent many of the complications commonly experienced by diabetics: gum infections, decayed teeth, high blood sugar levels, kidney damage, inflammation, infection, eye problems, and atherosclerotic heart disease, and prevent the dangerous effects of high homocysteine in the blood (232). Also, you can greatly minimize your chances of death from cancer and heart disease by cutting out foods from your diet that are high in copper, and greatly decrease your risk for *dangerous* clots by keeping high levels of vitamin C in your blood (232). Are you aware that vitamin C will even "help dissolve dangerous blood clots after they have already been formed" (232)?

- **Chondroitin Versus Heparin & No Unwanted Side Effects**

I discussed the importance of chondroitin sulfate in preventing dangerous blood clots in my first book that came out in 2005 and my second book, which was released in late 2009. Dr. Levy says that because of this ability of chondroitin sulfate to prevent dangerous clots, it helps fight coronary artery disease (CAD) and atherosclerosis (232). Chondroitin sulfate has long been combined with glucosamine to prevent cartilage degeneration in joints, but most people do not realize that it works much like Heparin at keeping the blood thin, without the dangerous side effects often accompanied with Heparin (232).

Realize too, that while most of the media keeps ramming calcium down our throats as a way to prevent osteoporosis, it isn't calcium that prevents osteoporosis, it's MAGNESIUM, vitamin D, boron, selenium, iodine, strontium,* zinc, and sufficient levels of vitamin C in the blood, as well as the proper ratio of hormones, especially natural progesterone in women. (*Not to be confused with strontium-90.)

- **Vitamin C — Universal God-Designed Disease Fighter**

Fighting high cholesterol, high blood pressure, diabetes, heart disease, CHF, asthma, infections, viruses, and colds? I have a challenge for you. Begin taking 10,000 mg of vitamin C (either in ascorbic acid form or a timed-release form if the higher doses give you diarrhea) in divided doses throughout the day. Do not give babies and toddlers doses this high. Check with their pediatricians about increasing their vitamin C levels. Check with your doctor, but also keep in mind if you mention this to most conventional medicine doctors the "pat" reply you will get is – "OH don't worry about vitamin C! As long as you eat a well-rounded diet, you'll get plenty of vitamin C." This common belief is a fable, and one reason why many people get one cold after another, many children get one ear infection after another, and disease is so rampant in this country!

Until conventional doctors understand that the current toxic-load of chemicals that we are constantly bombarded with every day in the air we breathe and the foods we eat, keep destroying the

vitamin C in our bodies at a rate much faster than we are replacing it, they will never recommend vitamin C as a disease preventative, and the fight to regain our health will continue to be a losing battle for most people who do NOT recognize this fact! Do not depend upon your physician to keep you well. You must take charge of your own health.

IV. Vitamin C – The Controversy

There is a lot of erroneous information out there on vitamin C. Some physicians are so adamantly against anything alternative, that they will tell you that vitamin C causes kidney stones. This is not true. In most cases, vitamin C will dissolve kidney stones. If you get adequate water in your diet, as well as magnesium, B vitamins, and vitamin C, and cut the sugary soda pop from your diet (which is high in phosphorus), and the excess calcium and acid-forming foods, your chances of kidney stones are next to nothing. Of course, if you are going to take large amounts of vitamin C and go all day long without drinking water, you may get stones even without the C. If you are deficient in magnesium and B vitamins, you are more likely to get stones. A high fat diet makes you more prone to stones and so do high oxalate foods and high protein meals. If you are prone to develop stones and are able to obtain one of them, have it analyzed to find out the stone's composition. Depending on what the stone consists of, will tell you how to prevent a reoccurrence. For example, if you have stones that consist mostly of calcium phosphate or magnesium ammonium phosphate (sometimes called *struvite stones*), keeping your urine acidic with things like cranberry juice and/or ascorbic acid (vitamin C) will help prevent, and in some cases, even dissolve these type stones. If you have cystine stones or calcium oxalate stones, keeping your urine acidic will not help dissolve them, nor if you have uric acid stones. Even though vitamin C may increase oxalate formation, it won't cause you to form these type stones.

If you have a problem with gout caused by uric acid and purines, try eating sour cherries, increasing your intake of vitamin C, and decreasing meat, sugar, and coffee intake. It is also important to maintain good water hydration, restrict sugar consumption, and avoid carbonated sodas to prevent stones. Be sure to get adequate B vitamins and alkalize your body.

If you would like to keep your vitamin C levels up and consistent throughout the day, consider taking the timed-release tablets of vitamin C. Large doses are not as likely to cause diarrhea.

• Media Bias Against Vitamins

In an article by *Orthomolecular Medicine News Service*, April 3, 2010, a group of doctors spoke out against a recent article in *Reader's Digest* that attacked the usage of supplemental vitamins (46). One does not have to look very far to figure out why *Reader's Digest* attacks natural substances like vitamins. James A. Jackson, Ph.D. from Wichita, KS says:

> This is not the first time Reader's Digest has written about 'bad' vitamins, and they always seem to manage to put it on the front page but look at their advertising: so much of it is for pharmaceutical drugs. No wonder the article states virtually nothing of the thousands of positive results with vitamins.

Did you catch that line about the ***pharmaceutical drugs***? This is nothing new! When you look at many current trade publications and magazines such as this one, you will find that they are getting literally thousands and thousands of dollars from pharmaceutical companies for paid advertisements for prescription drugs in their pages.

Readers, remember this, anytime you find material written AGAINST natural substances, such as herbs, minerals, and vitamins, just **follow the MONEY TRAIL!** MOST of the time, you will see that it ends at the doorstep of some drug company. Though I am acutely aware of the many life-saving medications that have been developed by pharmaceutical companies (things like insulin and antibiotics and other drugs to extend lives), for the most part drug companies stay in business because people stay sick. Vitamins and natural substances help people to GET WELL and STAY WELL! Companies that make a living off of selling prescription drugs to a population that gets sicker and sicker are not interested in natural, inexpensive, God-given substances that can prevent sickness in the first place and effectively treat it when it does occur.

Allan N. Spreen, M.D. of Mesa, Arizona, said this of the article:

> From start to finish, the Reader's Digest article, '5 Vitamin Truths and Lies' was one of the worst bits of propaganda I ever saw. There was not one word in it discussing the benefits of multivitamins, vitamin C, and studies supporting the use of vitamins for preventing cancer and heart disease... (46).

And when comparing the safety of vitamins (even in large doses) to prescription drugs, Dr. Erik Paterson, M.D., from Vancouver, BC had this to say:

> Vitamins are among the safest substances known. They have the most minimal side effects, even in large doses, compared with the death rate **due to conventional drugs** taken according to the manufacturer's advice. **Vitamin C is among the most powerful immune modulators if given in large doses.** Scare stories against the use of vitamins do the public no good (46). [Emphasis mine.]

Cardiologist, Dr. Thomas Levy from Colorado Springs, Colorado, said that "The material was not well-researched, and a bias was clearly in play. 15 pages of drug advertisements in that issue of Reader's Digest are very telling indeed" (46).

Steve Hickey, Ph.D. from Manchester, UK, pointed out that the magazine referred to the 2007 "Cochrane report", but that report has been updated often and the most recent update was 02/02/2010, which was totally ignored by the writer of the Reader's Digest article. The review was about low vitamin intakes (46). Even Linus Pauling "recommended at least 5,000 mg of vitamin C daily for reversing heart disease" (46). The article did not account for all the amazing health benefits researchers have been able to obtain from high vitamin doses, such as with vitamin C.

- ## Vitamin C – Ignored for 40 Years

The forgotten fact is that Dean Burk of the NCI (National Cancer Institute) knew nearly 40 years ago that ascorbate (vitamin C) could destroy cancer cells and leave normal cells unharmed, and he shared this information with his peers. They even published the results in the *Oncology* paper, revealing their *findings*:

> 'In our view, the future of effective cancer chemotherapy will not rest on the use of host-toxic compounds now so widely employed, but upon virtually host non-toxic compounds that are lethal to cancer cells of which ascorbate…represents an excellent prototype.' They also point out that ascorbate **was never tested for its anticancer effects by the Cancer Chemotherapy National Service Center, because it was too non-toxic to fit into their screening program. They don't want to test anything unless it helps kill the cancer patient.** [Emphasis mine] (291).

If you scanned that very last paragraph briefly, you should read it again, because this is exactly what has happened in the last **40 - 60 years**. The Cancer Industry, historically, has NOT been interested in promoting non-toxic drugs. They are only interested in drugs (and treatments) that are so toxic, that they often kill the patient before the cancer does!

You will find that just recently, some pharmaceutical companies (probably due to public outcry, competition with European drug makers, and perhaps all the new competition from alternative therapies), are beginning to develop drugs and treatments for fighting cancer that are less toxic to the body, many of which are described in my last book, *Gentle Cures for Tough Cancers.*

Cameron and Campbell did, in fact, conduct a clinical trial in 1974, giving "50 advanced cancer patients…10,000 mg of ascorbate a day either intravenously or orally." They discovered that the "large doses of ascorbic acid" were able to "enhance natural resistance to cancer" (291).

• How Those Who Promote the Cancer Drugs Are Often the Ones Causing the Cancer

In an article entitled "Eli Lilly (Satan's Chemist)", the writer points out the fact that some drug makers (such as this one) have a "perfect cancer profit cycle," because Eli Lilly makes the drug Evista, "which might help reduce the risk of breast cancer, may lower IGF-1 (according to one small study)." Well in effect, the company is marketing a "milk drug that might increase cancer, and on the other, it comes to the rescue with drugs to treat or 'prevent' cancer" (50).

If it's possible to breach the pinnacle of hypocrisy, they've done it, but so have many other drug makers. There are many drug makers who produce drugs that increase the risk for cancer, and also produce drugs that they say help prevent or treat cancer too! (There is something terribly WRONG with this picture! It is pure GREED, pure EVIL!)

• Pharmaceutical Madness

Dr. Matthias Rath says that "It is the multinational pharmaceutical companies that control the world," and according to website: *http://www4.dr-rathfoundation.org/publication_library/interview/dsalud_interview.html*, Dr. Rath's research work "on the positive effects of lysine and vitamin C as alternatives to pharmacological treatments for some of the most serious diseases faced by mankind, including cancer, has brought him into open confrontation with the guardians of conventional medicine and with the pharmaceutical industry" (271). He says that high cholesterol is not the main reason humans have coronary heart disease. It is a lack of sufficient vitamin C, and the reason most animals do not get heart disease is because most of them can self-manufacture this vitamin within their own bodies and humans cannot (271).

This is a belief that is shared by many other prominent physicians in our society, but ignored by mainstream medicine, which is controlled by pharmaceutical drug companies. Dr. Rath wrote about his findings in his book: *Why Animals Don't Get Heart Attacks...But People Do.* Want to keep your blood vessels healthy and clear and prevent cancer and strokes? Be sure you are megadosing with vitamin C and getting plenty of lysine, CoQ10, beta carotene, B-vitamins, magnesium, iodine, selenium, vitamin D, E, zinc, glutathione, boron, niacin, and heart-healthy omega-3s on a daily basis.

• Vitamin C Intentional Cover-Up

An article from the National Institutes of Health (08/04/2008) says that three decades ago, interest in vitamin C for fighting cancer and other diseases was at its height (148). That is, until other researchers [who did not know what they were doing], stated that taking megadoses of vitamin C by mouth did not produce *benefits* for cancer patients enrolled in their "two double-blind, placebo-controlled clinical trials" (148).

There was one gross problem with this study. Had it not been so flawed, multitudes of people possibly could have been saved from cancer and other diseases by the thousands before now. The reason I say it was "flawed" (which was not just my personal opinion, but the opinion of many others in the health industry), and the reason I say that the researchers did not know what they were doing, is because for many years, Dr. Virginia Livingston, Dr. William J. Saccoman, Dr. Frederick Klenner, Dr. Abram Hoffer, Dr. Thomas Levy, Dr. Bernard Rimland, Linus Pauling, Dr. Matthias Rath, Irwin Stone, Dr. Robert Cathcart, and many others (who checked their research), told the public that vitamin C given in the form of sodium ascorbate INTRAVENOUSLY, which bypasses the GI tract, is absorbed directly into the circulatory system, into the cellular level and patients can tolerate 100—300 GRAMS a day (that is not a typo either—it is GRAMS, not milligrams) sometimes more, depending on if doses are spread out over the day, and the condition of the patient. You can also tolerate larger doses if you take the timed-release form of vitamin C by mouth or the new **liposomal C** that you mix with water or juice (see chapter 2).

Some physicians will start out giving megadoses of C, the patient begins to improve, and then they lower the dose, and the patient gets worse. This is typical, because all vitamin C proponents agree that you cannot suddenly reduce vitamin C megadosing, or the patient may regress. You MUST keep the megadoses going continuously until there is full recovery!

Researchers are just now [after 40 - 60 years of ignoring men smarter than them], figuring out that these early pioneers of Vitamin C intravenous megadosing knew exactly what they were doing (148). Also, there are no toxic side effects to intravenous vitamin C in the form of sodium ascorbate or calcium ascorbate (the ascorbic acid is too acidic to be given intravenously) (148). Oral doses will eventually cause diarrhea. Chemo can cost thousands of dollars per dose. Intravenous vitamin C therapy usually runs about $125.00 per dose (64), depending where you live, and even though Vitamin C doses are so much cheaper than chemo, insurance companies will pay for the chemo, but not the Vitamin C (64). (Of course not—that would make too much sense—and the current health system in the U.S. operates with absolutely no common sense whatsoever!)

More studies (using intravenous vitamin C) are planned in human trials. These are studies that should have been done decades ago, had anyone taken Linus Pauling, Ewan Cameron, Irwin Stone, Dr. Thomas Levy, Dr. Matthias Rath, Frederick Klenner, and Dr. Robert Cathcart seriously, instead of dragging their feet, while people who could have been saved by megadoses of C died prematurely. Not only did researchers discover that high levels of ascorbate could kill cancer in lab studies (without harming normal cells), but they found "that these high ascorbate concentrations could be achieved in people" (148), something that Linus Pauling and Irwin Stone already knew (when the current researchers were mere babes), had anyone just listened to them and taken them seriously!

Scientists have proven that vitamin C, in laboratory testing, at "3 mgms per 100 mls" can effectively wipe out cancer and without any adverse side effects (71). This was discovered by scientists from the Bio-Communications Research Institute in Wichita, USA. The article is available from website: *http://www.alternative-doctor.com/cancer/ca_ advanced.htm* (71). The blood level of vitamin C needed to achieve this amount would be available if 50 grams of vitamin C (50,000 mg) were given intravenously to a patient (71). This amount of sodium ascorbate given intravenously is usually well-tolerated by the patient, as stated earlier. As noted by Dr. Irwin Stone in *The Genetics of Scurvy and the Cancer Problem,* "Dr. Frederick Klenner uses up to 300,000 mg of sodium ascorbate, intravenously, each day in his successful therapy of the viral diseases" (291).

How many people are aware that as levels of vitamin C fall in the body, pancreatic insulin levels drop? This was proven when guinea pigs were allowed to develop scurvy and they also had a drastically reduced output of insulin from their pancreas, **indicating a clear connection between low levels of vitamin C and the development of diabetes** (232). It is interesting in the experiment with the guinea pigs that as soon as their vitamin C levels were restored, the pancreas began producing insulin again (232). (Do you know someone with diabetes? How much vitamin C do they take on a daily basis?)

V. Vitamins for Breast Cancer Prevention & Treatment

Vitamins A, C, D, and E are important in the prevention and treatment of breast cancer. Studies have shown that deficiencies in these vitamins can contribute toward, not only breast cancer, but many other types of cancer, including colon cancers. Megadosing with vitamin C has been used to treat some cancers, including breast cancer and pancreatic cancer. This is also known as *Orthomolecular Medicine* and requires intravenous dosing in high amounts, from 80-120 grams or more per day. When given intravenously, sodium ascorbate is commonly used. Ascorbic acid is too acidic.

Sodium ascorbate is simply a mixture of soda bicarb and "powdered ascorbic acid crystals" (310). If you purchase the C crystals, check the label. It will tell you how much vitamin C is in each teaspoon. Under their Candida article, website *nourishedmagazine.com* recommends mixing "equal amounts of ascorbic acid and baking soda, and then add filtered water," to take "4,000 mgs or more daily in divided doses" (310). They are mixing it this way because if you take vitamin C crystals and mix them in water or juice, you will have a very BITTER-tasting drink that is acidic and hard to swallow; however, the soda bicarb removes the bitterness and instead of ascorbic acid, you now have sodium ascorbate! Here is the exact recipe that I use:

> Add 1 teaspoon (containing 5000 mg of ascorbic acid powder or crystals), and ½ teaspoon of soda bicarb to ½ glass of distilled water. Still until well dissolved and drink.

It is recommend that if the 4000 mg of vitamin C causes diarrhea, cut back to a lower dosage, and increase the dosage gradually over a period of time, "every 5 days" (310). This website (above) also warns people that you should not take cod liver oil for your vitamin A and D supply until you know for sure that the company has not removed "all the [natural] vitamin A and D" and replaced them with "synthetic vitamins A and D," which "can be toxic" (310). For the best cod liver oil brand, they recommend **Blue Ice™** cod liver oil, which you can find at these websites:

http://www.greenpasture.org/retail/?t=products&a=line&i=royal and
http://www.drrons.com/blue-ice-high-vitamin-cod-liver-oil.htm

For those with **Candida** yeast, *nourishedmagazine.com* recommends *20,000 to 30,000 IUs* a day of vitamin A; *800 to 1200 IUs* of vitamin D each day and *2000 to 3000 mgs* of Omega-3 each day (310). They recommend that people with lighter skin get at least 10-20 minutes per day of sun exposure, while darker-skinned individuals need from 90–120 minutes of sunshine each day, and since the natural oils in the body are required to assist in this vitamin D manufacture in the skin, don't bathe, shower, or swim "in a chlorinated pool for one hour after [sun] exposure" (310).

Your "best fish oils are from 'wild-caught cold-water fish,' i.e. anchovy, arctic cod, herring, krill, mackerel, salmon, and sardine" (310). Remember the warning about avoiding a shower or bath (or swimming) for at least one hour after sun exposure? If you lay out in the sun for 20 minutes, then immediately go jump in a shower, you may completely cancel out any of the vitamin D that your skin is still in the process of forming.

VI. Testing Your Vitamin C Levels

If you would like to keep track of your urine vitamin C content, you can get vitamin C test strips at this website: *http://www.nutri.com/strips*. The website itself has a great deal of information on how you can tell if you have sufficient levels of vitamin C in your body by the results of their urine testing strips. If you have healthy levels of vitamin C in your body, you should have some C in your urine; however, if you have cancer, or are severely deficient in vitamin C, you will have no vitamin C in your urine. (It simply means that all the free radicals in your body are neutralizing the vitamin C and you have basically run out of C.)

This website tells you how to do an ascorbate "flush" to help you determine your vitamin C needs: *http://www.vitamins-today.com/c_flush.html*. Always check with your physician.

VII. Final Evidence for Vitamin C

Linus Pauling was an early advocate for high dose vitamin C therapy. He won the Nobel Prize twice, once in 1954 for chemistry, and then in 1962, the Nobel Peace Prize. He authored several books on chemistry, quantum mechanics, vitamin C, and cancer. He has been followed by others, mentioned earlier in this chapter, who have taken up the banner in favor of megadosing with vitamin C. Dr. Robert Cathcart's website at *www.orthomed.com* gives startling revelations about diseases, such as "Ebola...and West Nile," as well as many others that he says could possibly be "cured or ameliorated by massive doses of vitamin C" (184).

I spoke at length with Dr. Cathcart by phone on July 5, 2005, regarding many of these issues. He was greatly concerned about the low levels of vitamin C in the entire population. If you look at a table of the U.S. RDA (Recommended Daily Allowance, sometimes referred to as the Recommended Dietary Allowance) for vitamin C, currently it is between 45/60 milligrams. (Most people could probably burn this much up during two minutes of stress.) Others recommend what is known as the DOI or Daily Optimal Intake for vitamin C at 1000 to 5000 mg daily. This amount is for optimal health, not just to prevent you from getting full-blown scurvy. And in this world of toxins we are inundated with, I believe the DOI should be closer to 10,000 mg daily in divided doses or timed-release capsules.

Did you know that scientists are very concerned about the health of their laboratory monkeys? They have to keep them on healthy diets so that they stay well (213). It is amazing that monkeys, used in animal experiments, require many times the vitamin C that is recommended for humans, yet studies show that their nutritional requirements are very similar to that of humans (213).

If you still have doubts about the way that natural cancer cures are being suppressed, consider the scientific findings on vitamin C, which show it is lethal to certain cancer cells (213). Thousands of grams of vitamin C per day have been ingested by humans, as well as given intravenously, without noxious side effects. Just be sure to use the buffered form of vitamin C if you are taking large amounts, or are concerned about stomach upset or diarrhea, or simply do as described earlier. Change your ascorbic acid into sodium ascorbate by simply taking half a glass of distilled water and adding 1 teaspoon of ascorbic acid (powder or crystals) and ½ teaspoon of soda bicarb. Wait until the fizzing stops, stir, and add to orange juice or another type of juice like grape juice, if you want, or just drink as is.

VIII. Vitamin C Dosing & Forms

When taken by mouth, vitamin C is usually taken in the form of ascorbic acid. The best NEW form of vitamin C is liposomal C, which I discussed in other areas of this book, including use in my *Orange Wunder Formula* in Chapters 1 and 2.

Huge vitamin C doses (ascorbic acid) usually cannot be tolerated by mouth because they cause diarrhea (211). Other forms of vitamin C (besides the liposomal C) may not cause diarrhea. I also use the timed-released vitamin C. It's released slowly into the body, so does not usually cause diarrhea. When given intravenously in the form of sodium ascorbate (see below article), there is normally excellent tolerance. The human body can tolerate vitamin C (ascorbic acid) by mouth in large enough doses until diarrhea occurs. Once diarrhea occurs, this tells you your *bowel tolerance level* (212). For example, if you take 3500 mg of vitamin C and have no problems with it, then take 4000 mg of vitamin C four hours later and it gives you diarrhea, then your bowel tolerance level would be below 4000 mg. Your body is tolerating less than 4000 mg doses and will not tolerate doses higher than that. If you have stomach irritation from vitamin C, take it with food and in divided doses, or use the non-acidic *Ester-C®* (calcium ascorbate), or the sodium ascorbate non-acidic form, rather than the ascorbic acid form of vitamin C. You may also wish to try the liposomal C, which is so rapidly absorbed, it is not likely to cause diarrhea. You may also wish to try the recipe given earlier in this chapter for mixing ascorbic acid crystals with soda bicarb in distilled water, which creates sodium ascorbate and removes the bitter taste, though it does add sodium to the vitamin C. Usually, the larger amount of vitamin C you can tolerate without getting diarrhea, the sicker you are. Over time this will change, however, because once you start taking it, your body will build up a higher tolerance for it as it gets used to it. Some people use the higher doses just for the bowel cleaning effect.

IX. Starting Early - How to Prevent Leukemia in Your Children Before They Are Born

Seven studies by researchers at the University of Toronto from 1960-2005, looking at how a mother's vitamin intake could affect her child's later development of cancer, had some surprising results (202). As noted by *CancerConsultants.com* website, all vitamins were studied, including *folic acid*. Mothers who took vitamin supplements (that included folic acid) had children with *36% fewer cases of pediatric leukemia; 18% reduction in pediatric brain tumors*, and *47% reduction in neuroblastoma* in their children. Authors of the study theorized that folic acid might have been the most important of the vitamins (202), and it is already a well-known fact that women who take folic acid can prevent neural tube birth defects in their babies.

This study is described in the Journal *Clinical Pharmacology and Therapeutics* from the website article: "Vitamins During Pregnancy Decrease Childhood Cancer Risk" at:

> *http://patient.cancerconsultants.com/CancerNews_Neuroblastoma. aspx?DocumentId=393773* (202).

More proof that nutrition plays a critical role in disease prevention, even in the womb!

X. Resurgence of Dengue Fever & Vitamin C Cure

Dengue Fever is rearing its ugly head in the U.S. in Florida. Though uncertain about how the disease came into this country, the national news media is already insisting that there is *no cure*. I have already reported that Dr. Thomas Levy has been successful at curing this disease by giving 12 packets of liposomal C to a patient with the disease. This is another disease that rapidly depletes vitamin C from the body, so rapidly in fact, that it is only a short matter of time before the victims start having early signs of hemorrhagic scurvy (e.g. bleeding gums). You Floridians, stock up on vitamin C. It's a better weapon than mosquito spray, and if you get the disease, consider Dr. Levy's protocol above, or at least 10,000 mg or more of vitamin C daily in divided doses for adults. (See pp. 79-80 and 167.)

CHAPTER 5

God's Healing Sunshine Gift – Vitamin D

****

I. Vitamin D Prevents All Forms of Cancer & Even Shrinks Existing Cancers

In my first book written five years ago, I discussed the importance of using vitamin D to prevent and treat cancer. Well, a few days ago there was a report on national news about discoveries with test animals showing that vitamin D not only shrank tumors in some of the animals, but totally cured others! (Where were THEY five years ago?)

When my own family member was fighting an aggressive bladder cancer last winter, his physician checked his vitamin D levels, found them to be low, and placed him on 50,000 units of vitamin D a week until his levels were more normal. (See Chapters 1 and 2.) That equates to a little more than 7,000 units per day. Most people try to get by with taking about 400 units (or less) a day, and let's face it, most multi-vitamin formulas on the market only contain about 400 units in them, and much of that vitamin D is D2, the synthetic D, not the natural D3 form of D. Taking synthetic D2 is a waste. (See below for more information on the difference between D2 and D3.)

If you really want to prevent and fight cancer, you must be sure you are not vitamin D deficient and you must make sure your kids also have sufficient vitamin D. Never take D2, the synthetic D that is put into milk and dairy products. Always use D3, the natural form of vitamin D, and don't forget that one of your best sources of vitamin D is natural sunlight. These same tests (noted above) showed that when animals had their cancerous tumors injected directly with vitamin D, the vitamin shrank the tumors or totally eliminated them in a short amount of time! Will the same results work for humans, they wanted to know? Well, I don't think it should take a rocket scientist to figure out that perhaps the reason why so many people are getting cancer to BEGIN WITH is because they are so deficient in this vital nutrient!

Recent studies have shown that insufficient amounts of natural sunshine (resulting in vitamin D deficiency) increases the risk for nearly all types of cancer, including cancer of the breast, and may even promote other chronic illnesses, such as MS, *Type I diabetes* (152), and lupus. Nutritional experts are now concluding that most people need *1,000 to 2,000 IU* per *day* of vitamin D for maintaining health and preventing disease. This is a much higher amount than the RDA of *200 to 600 IU* (152). Adequate amounts of this vitamin are crucial for preventing colon, breast, and gastric cancers. The best natural source is sunshine. A nutritious diet and *supplements* can also help keep vitamin D levels normal (152). A research study that spanned eight years and involved more than 3000 people, showed that those people having the lowest vitamin D levels were twice as likely to die from all causes. They concluded that insufficient levels of vitamin D greatly increase the risk for early death (293). Caucasians need ten to twenty minutes a day of natural sunshine (without sunscreen) for vitamin D synthesis and darker-skinned individuals need more. Recent studies also show that increased levels of vitamin D can help prevent heart attacks, and many human studies have already proven that a lack of vitamin D will raise your risk for nearly all types of cancer.

Adequate amounts of this vitamin are especially crucial to preventing colon, breast, and gastric cancers. A nutritious diet and *supplements* can also provide vitamin D (152) for those unable to get out in the sun. Use caution and have your levels checked, because vitamin D is fat soluble, so it is stored in the body. Too much can be toxic, however, people usually get too much D from taking excess in supplements, not from daily sunshine exposure.

Professor Holick and his colleagues discovered that there is an essential substance within our colon which helps in the "processing of vitamin D," which also fights colon cancer, thus the reason why vitamin D deficiencies will lead to colon cancer (275).

• Vitamin D Reduces Risk of Pancreatic Cancer 43%

A human study, described in the September 2006 issue of *Cancer Epidemiology Biomarkers & Prevention,* found that taking as little as *400 IU*/day of this vitamin could cut the risk for pancreatic cancer by 43%. Those taking under *150 IU*/day cut their risk by 22%. Individuals taking more than the *400 IU*/day did not seem to have an advantage, at least not for preventing pancreatic cancer. This study reaffirms other research, which shows that populations getting adequate sunshine (which triggers the natural production of vitamin D in the skin) have much lower incidence for not only pancreatic cancers, but also breast and colon cancers (149).

• Sufficient Sunlight = Vitamin D = Cancer Prevention

Everyone has been so brain-washed by the health community and news media that sunlight is so bad for you, that there are even new cases arising of children with rickets, a disease where the bones are soft and malformed from vitamin D deficiencies. This is a disease that we thought had long ago vanished in America. What is happening? Parents are over-reacting to the hype about skin cancers and the sun, bundling their children up against **all sunshine exposure**, or slathering them with globs of sunscreen and sending them outside to play. Since the best source of **natural vitamin D is sunshine,** children are sometimes suffering from vitamin D deficiencies from not getting adequate sun exposure. Some parents go to the other extreme and let their kids play for hours outside in the sun with no protection, only to come indoors with dangerous, painful sunburns!

Scientists showed that African-American children were at more risk for developing rickets. Most of the children studied were of Muslim descent with mothers who wore heavy covering over their skin, neither did the moms or their babies ingest dairy products. Even the children *were covered by blankets much of the time.* This information was from Nutrition Research Newsletter, Sept. 1994 (151). This is what I find interesting: "none of the parents had received advice from the children's physicians on how to prevent the deficiency disease," and all the babies had been breast fed, but no vitamin supplements had been given to them or the moms (151).

When sunshine hits the skin, a chemical reaction occurs that creates natural vitamin D in our bodies. People who live in northern states often have problems with vitamin D deficiencies (more so than those living in the south) because of less sun exposure in colder climates.

Many health writers and physicians (e.g., Dr. Joseph Mercola, author of the *Total Health Programs*—website: *www.mercola.com),* are reporting that inadequate sunlight is putting us at increased risk for cancer (245). A study in the journal, *Cancer,* supports this belief. Researchers found that those suffering from low levels of ultraviolet B-light were more likely to die from cancer (245). It is believed that the body needs ultraviolet B-light in order to produce vitamin D (245). The author of the study, Dr. William Grant, is concerned that people in northern climates (who experience longer winters) may have no opportunity at all for *vitamin D synthesis* (245). The study also found that people with darker skin require as much as "10-20 times" more sunlight for adequate amounts of vitamin D synthesis as those with lighter skin (245). There were 13 different malignant cancers that were affected by this sunlight phenomenon, but the ones most affected were: "breast, colon, and ovarian cancer" (245). Others included: "tumors of the bladder, uterus, esophagus, rectum, and stomach" (245).

Dr. Mercola believes that skin cancers could be linked to an excessive consumption of the "omega-6 fats", which increase cancer risk during excess sun exposure. He says that we can stay out of the sun to cut skin cancer, but in so doing, we run a greater risk for other lethal cancers (245).

Another thing to consider: just because you or your children get outdoors in the summer and do a lot of yard work, or swim in a pool every day and get very tanned, do not assume you have adequate levels of vitamin D. This is no guarantee. (The chlorine in swimming pools is one of the worst chemicals for your skin or your body.) I would have thought that my own family member (see Chapters 1 and 2) fighting bladder cancer had plenty of vitamin D reserves because he keeps a dark tan in the summer from yard work. This was not the case. He was found to be severely deficient in vitamin D levels. The best insurance? Have your physician check your vitamin D levels at least once or twice a year.

• How & Why Vitamin D Works at Preventing & Killing Cancer

A recent study from Denmark shows exactly how and why vitamin D is so important in fighting cancer. They discovered that the **T** cells of the body's immune system are activated by the presence of vitamin D (299). When levels of this vitamin are low, the T cells do not have the capacity to *mobilize* and fight invading diseases. This same study says that half the people in the world are deficient in vitamin D (299). An Ezine article also says that vitamin D helps ward off "diabetes because it regulates blood sugar" (173). It also maintains a healthy thyroid, fights high blood pressure, autoimmune diseases, viruses, and relieves arthritis, fibromyalgia and other health disorders (173).

Dr. Joseph Mercola even wonders if vitamin D could be the "New Silver Bullet for Cancer," in an article at his website (244). Scientists studying the effect of the vitamin on the elderly found that high enough levels of this vitamin could slash their risk for "heart disease or diabetes by 43 percent" (244). It is believed that increasing the intake of calcium and vitamin D3 may prevent as many as "58,000 new cases of breast cancer and 49,000 new cases of colorectal cancer" every year in Canada and the US, preventing 75% of the deaths that these cancers cause (244). If you are Caucasian, what you need is enough sunshine each day "to turn your skin the lightest shade of pink," and this means you will have made "about 20,000 units of vitamin D (244). Also, never take synthetic vitamin A at the same time you are taking vitamin D because it can neutralize the vitamin D (244). In the same article, it is recommended for children below 5 to get at least 5 units of vitamin D3 "per pound per day"; 5-10 year olds need "2500 Units" of vitamin D3 per day; 18-30 year olds need "5000 units" per day, and those who are pregnant need "5000 units" per day (244).

Ask your physician to check your vitamin D levels using the "25-hydroxyvitamin D" test, and if you are fighting cancer, you want your levels from this test to be "65-90 ng/ml" in order to help your immune system overcome the cancer (244). I have also read other sources that say that adults 60 and over should get 10,000 units per day of vitamin D3. See my last book: *Gentle Cures for Tough Cancers*, for more information on using vitamin D3 for specific cancers.

II. Vitamin D & Chronic Illnesses

• Vitamin D & Skin Disorders

Many people suffering from psoriasis and eczema find, to their delight, that simply increasing their vitamin D3 levels to 5000 U or 6000 U/day totally eradicates their skin disorders. Others have also been helped with flax oil, milk thistle supplements, the Johanna Budwig Formula (see Chapters 1 through 3), magnesium, vitamin C, beta carotene, and iodine supplements, and/or increasing their water intake. Turmeric, used topically, has also been helpful for psoriasis sufferers.

Always check with your doctor, especially if you have a history (or family history) of skin cancer. Human studies have shown that the majority of Type I diabetics have deficient levels of vitamin D.

• Vitamin D, Asthma, Depression & Autoimmunity

Just within the last month, new studies have come out showing that insufficient levels of vitamin D are linked to asthma in children, depression, and autoimmune diseases (98). In one human study that was done, "86% of the children in the study with asthma had insufficient levels of vitamin D" in their system (98). And don't think breast-feeding will prevent this! As a matter-of-fact, most babies do not get enough vitamin D in breast milk (98). Those conducting the studies are now recommending that "most babies" get supplemental vitamin D in their diets (98). Just be sure it is D3 they get and not D2. Be a label reader.

• Vitamin D & the Lupus Connection

Human studies have shown that lupus patients have abnormally low levels of vitamin D, indicating that supplementation may be needed (150), and that they may also be low in magnesium, vitamin C, and CoQ10. Lupus is an autoimmune disorder. You should know that autoimmune disorders are symptoms of a sick immune system. Your body is being attacked, not because of an immune system that is too strong, but one that is very ill. When the immune system is ill, it becomes confused, attacking indiscriminately, causing debilitating diseases. Many of the items in this book can help heal your immune system.

• Vitamin D, MS & Type I Diabetes

Being deficient in this vitamin may promote other chronic illnesses such as multiple sclerosis (MS) and *Type I diabetes* (152). Nutritional experts are now concluding that most people need *1,000 to 2,000 IU per day* of vitamin D, a much higher amount than the RDA of *200 to 600 IU* for maintaining health and preventing disease (152), and some of them are insisting that if you are over 60, you may need 10,000 units per day.

Scotland has more MS sufferers than any other country. These alarming statistics promoted a study at Oxford (headed up by Professor of Neurology, George Ebers), which found that not only is vitamin D important in prevention of cancer and autoimmune disorders, but in prevention of MS as well. It was revealed that the disease rarely afflicts those in warmer countries, where people get more vitamin D from sunlight exposure. It was also found that children who develop MS all seem to have one thing in common – they are seriously deficient in vitamin D (272)! Recommending supplementation to children and pregnant moms is on the horizon (272), just as it finally took thousands of babies born with neural tube birth defects to convince the FDA that pregnant moms should supplement with folic acid (even though vitamin manufacturers were warning of the problem years before the FDA would allow them to put the advice on their folic acid supplements)! Another great example of FDA incompetence!

III. Having Vitamin D Levels Checked

Always have your MD check your vitamin D levels as part of your physical. Consider supplementing with vitamin D3. I use 3000 - 5000 Units of D3 daily, except on days that I manage to get plenty of sunshine exposure. Too much vitamin D can be toxic as it is stored in the liver, but most people don't have to worry about excess vitamin D, because studies show that MOST people are deficient in this vitamin! Overdosing usually happens in people who take large amounts of cod liver oil or overdose on supplements.

Why is it that the mainstream media and conventional medicine is always about FIVE years behind those who advocate nutritional healing via alternative medicine? I wonder how many items I am writing in this book TODAY will not make it into mainstream medicine or media for FIVE more years!? They are always, ALWAYS years behind alternative nutritional recommendations! I and other alternative health writers advocated vitamin C, D, E, beta carotene, resveratrol, selenium, and CoQ10 to prevent cancer FIVE years ago. Now, the news media is announcing this fact as though they just thought of it and it was their big discovery! How long will it take conventional medicine to figure out that humans cannot stay healthy on a paltry 400 units a day of vitamin D, when in reality most of us need 2000-10,000 units a day or more? How long will it take them to realize that 60 mg a day of vitamin C won't keep anyone well or prevent cancer, when in reality, most of us need at least 5,000 - 10,000 mg a day of vitamin C, or more? We are fighting toxins (e.g. mercury, cadmium, aluminum, lead, stress, deadly chemicals added to our food supply) that we didn't have to worry about 50 or 100 years ago. 100 years ago we were not being bombarded with the intensity and frequency of free radicals that are attacking our cells today! And every year, thousands of tons of NEW chemicals are surreptitiously added to our food supply (and our environment that we are never told about), that increase our risks for all forms of disease.

IV. Synthetic Versus Natural Vitamin D

Perhaps you are thinking you will just get your vitamin D from milk and supplements. After all, we see commercials about milk and its vitamin D content plastered everywhere to make us **think** that milk is actually good for us, right? As described in H. Winter Griffith's, *Vitamins, Herbs, Minerals & Supplements,* the vitamin D you find in milk and most vitamin supplements is "synthetic...D2...also called *ergocalciferol,"* and it's a poor substitute for the one that comes from natural sunlight "or natural food sources... vitamin D3 or *calciferol"* (205). Other sources of vitamin D (besides sunlight) are: "...Egg substitutes...Herring, Mackerel, Salmon, Sardines... [and] Tuna..." (205). Cod liver oil and mushrooms also contain vitamin D.

There is no way that mankind, hard as he tries, can improve on what our great Creator God has given us in its natural state. Vitamin D from natural sunshine is one of God's many gifts to us, intended for our well-being. As with any good thing, over-exposure can be harmful.

As described at *www.mercola.com*, vitamin D is critical in promoting supplies of minerals like phosphorus and calcium (245). One reason for the rampant osteoporosis in this country is because people are not getting adequate vitamin D from sunshine (and inadequate magnesium, iodine and zinc). Magnesium and vitamin D regulate our body's absorption of calcium, assisting with the maintenance of a strong skeletal system. Taking all the expensive calcium supplements in the world will not help you if you are deficient in vitamin D, magnesium, iodine, boron or zinc. Vitamin D is fat soluble, meaning it can be stored in the body, so over-dosing, especially with synthetic forms, can be dangerous. This is another reason why getting vitamin D through sunlight is best (245); however, this won't always be possible, especially if you have an indoor job and you go to work when the sun is just rising and come home when it is getting ready to set! (Just be sure to take precautions if you have a family history of melanoma. Check with your physician about sun exposure.)

V. The Excess Calcium Disaster

The dairy industry has largely contributed to the excess calcium intake disaster in this nation. You should not drink lots of milk and ingest lots of dairy products and other calcium sources without also taking in magnesium. It takes magnesium for the calcium to be properly absorbed and used, and that is what you are not being told! It is sad but true that the nations of the world that consume the most dairy products have the **highest** statistics for osteoporosis (287)! These two minerals, calcium and magnesium, are competitive; take in too much calcium and it will block your body's ability to absorb magnesium (287). What does THAT tell you about all the calcium you are taking and all the calcium that the dairy industry keeps pushing on people? It has been well-established in **human** research that high consumption of dairy products increases the risk for prostate, breast, ovarian, and uterine cancers. Currently, the RDA for calcium is 1500 mg for women and 1000 mg for men, but any calcium intake should always be accompanied with magnesium, boron, selenium, glutathione, zinc, vitamin E, iodine, and other nutrients, as you will read in other chapters of this book.

There is a new form of easily absorbable calcium known as *calcium lactate gluconate* that can be found in a new insomnia drink known as *Sleep Minerals*. It also contains magnesium chloride (287). You can find this product at many websites including: *http://www.naturalsleepminerals.com.*

A study revealed that 23,000 people die from preventable cancers every year—preventable by adequate amounts of vitamin D—and this statistic may be much higher (275)! One physician in particular, estimated that (in the UK) at least a fourth of those who die from cancer of the breast, do so because they had insufficient amounts of vitamin D, which caused the breast cancer (275). This is so unnecessary, but much of it can be attributed to the fact that we are no longer an agrarian society.

My grandparents and parents were farmers and spent many hours outdoors in the sun (as I did as a child), as did many millions of others in their generation, yet cancer was rare in those days. In our industrialized, mechanized society today, consider how many people work long hours INDOORS every day without ever setting foot out in the natural sunlight until after 5 or 6 pm when the sun is ready to set, especially in the winter months! How many people work long hours at INDOOR jobs where they are constantly exposed to radiation, molds, harmful chemicals (industrial workers, chemists, computer techs, beauticians, nail technicians?), or bacteria, viruses, radiation, and other pathogens (physicians, nurses, lab workers?)

Just consider someone you know that may be elderly, or live in a northern climate with very short summers. How much sunshine are they exposed to every day? Could this be one reason that the elderly have higher cancer statistics than their younger counterparts? Some office complexes are trying to compensate by using higher spectrum lighting.

What about those who spend their time in nursing homes, hospitals, rehab and assisted-living centers? How much natural sunshine do you think they get every day—if any—or fresh air?

Sunshine has been proven to boost the immune system, lower blood pressure, and relax the body. Have you had **your** dose of sunshine today? What about fresh air (oxygen) and exercise?

VI. Suncreens - Which Are Safe to Use?

Some health advocates are warning against the use of commercial sunscreens. One such website warns that "...sunscreen...is one of the last things you want to put on your body. Sunscreen is a toxic chemical that can cause problems in your liver and blood" (201). They suggest that you cover up with clothing or use a "natural sunblock of which there are only a few acceptable brands," and agree that natural sunlight may help protect against "MS and breast cancer" (201). For a list that describes ten of the best organic sunscreens, see this website:

http://www.associatedcontent.com/article/803893/10_of_the_best_organic_natural_sunscreens.html?cat=69

This includes *Jason Natural Sun block SPF 30* and *Burts Bees* products, and see the entire line of toxin-free sunscreen and tanning oil products available from Dr. Joseph Mercola at website: *http://products.mercola.com/summer-survival-kit/?source=nl.* From what I have studied, you will find no toxins in his sunscreen products; instead, you will find antioxidants, like GREEN TEA, that are good for your skin!

CHAPTER 6

Magnesium & Zinc – Mineral Mania

****

I. Magnesium – Forgotten Miracle

Thanks to the multi-million dollar dairy industry, we are constantly being bombarded with ads about how desperately we need calcium for our bones and for the prevention of osteoporosis. For those of you who read my first and second books (and Chapter 4 of THIS book), you know by now that it isn't calcium that prevents osteoporosis. As a matter-of-fact, it is excess calcium that CAUSES osteoporosis. It is natural progesterone (especially in post-menopausal women), **magnesium**, boron, iodine, GSH (glutathione), selenium, zinc, vitamins C, D, and E that protect the bones and prevent osteoporosis.

In his book on *STOP AMERICA'S #1 KILLER!* Thomas Levy, MD, JD, noted that having adequate levels of vitamin C in the body = "greater bone mineral density" for women after menopause. Starve your body of vitamin C and risk having osteoporosis (232)!

The problem is that most people get too much calcium in their diets and they get their calcium from the wrong sources. Carrot juice and green barley juice actually have more calcium than milk, and are much better for you. Magnesium in the body directs the calcium where to go, making sure it gets deposited in the bones, not in joints where it causes inflammation, in the eyes where it causes cataracts, in the kidneys or gallbladder where it can cause stone formation, or the skin where it causes premature aging.

II. Magnesium – When to Use it - Where to Find it

• Deficiency Symptoms for Magnesium

As noted at: *http://www.ithyroid.com/magnesium.htm*, symptoms of not having enough magnesium in your body include:

> …gastrointestinal disorders, irregular heart rhythm, lack of coordination, muscle twitch, tremors, weakness, apprehensiveness, personality changes, disorientation, confusion, depression, and irritability. A deficiency interferes with nerve and muscle impulses. Long-term deficiency can lead to tetany as in a calcium deficiency, alcoholic hallucinations, unusual face and eye movement, alopecia (baldness), swollen gums, and lesions of the gums (89)…[and seizures].

• Dietary Sources of Magnesium

According to Dr. Carolyn Dean in her book, *The Magnesium Miracle*, some of your best food sources of magnesium are almonds, kelp, molasses, cashews, wheat germ, peanuts, pecans, brewer's yeast, English walnuts, leafy greens like spinach, whole grains, egg yolks, parsley and apples (192), but not unless the plant sources are grown in magnesium-rich soil. Eating "…beans, nuts and vegetables" will increase your magnesium levels (69), but only if they are grown in magnesium-rich soil. Other sources are green drinks, "vegetable juices, kelp, seawater, seafood, green leaves, molasses, soaked nuts, oily seeds and sprouted seeds" (228). See other sources later in this chapter.

• Best Supplemental Forms of Magnesium

There are good types of magnesium and types you want to avoid! For best absorption, use magnesium citrate, magnesium malate, magnesium orotate, magnesium taurate (192), or magnesium chloride that you take by mouth, or the kind that you spray directly onto your skin that is absorbed right through the skin. You can obtain this great form of magnesium at website: ***http://www.magneticclay.com***, as well as Swanson Health Products (***http://www.swansonvitamins.com***)**,** and a good deal of information on magnesium, including books on transdermal magnesium at **IMVA** website: *http://magnesiumforlife.com*. **Magnetic Clay** website and **Swanson Health Products** also have a crystal form of magnesium chloride that you can pour into your bathwater for soaking or for foot soaks. It is not for oral use. It can be helpful for those with diabetic neuropathy.

Take magnesium supplements between meals in divided doses during the day, not all at once, and take it with B6. If it gives you diarrhea, lower the dosage, use the transdermal spray, or try another oral supplemental form. Getting diarrhea from your magnesium usually means your body is not absorbing it (192). This is what happens when MOM (Milk of Magnesium) is taken as a laxative. It uses magnesium hydroxide for its laxative effect. The transdermal spray is magnesium chloride. It is the same form of magnesium that is found in the Dead Sea in the Middle East. That entire ocean is made up of magnesium chloride.

Bathers go to the Dead Sea to soak in the healing waters. Scientists have done experiments to prove that the Dead Sea water enhances the skin and "reduces inflammation in atopic dry skin" (269a). Bathers in the Dead Sea find that they automatically float due to the high magnesium salt content.

• Other Sources for Magnesium Supplements

You can also find food-grade liquid magnesium chloride at *http://www.iherb.com* website, one of the most easily absorbed forms of magnesium.

There are many other websites that have magnesium chloride, including some that sell it in a liquid drinkable form, such as: *NutriCology®* brand, available at their website: *http://www.nutricology.com/Mineral-Products-p-1-c-256.html*, along with many other mineral and vitamin supplements, and from **Swanson Vitamins** in 8 ounce bottles with 66.5 mg of mag chloride per ½ teaspoon. Their website is at: *http://www.swansonvitamins.com*. They offer the *NutriCology®* brand. You can also get a form of liquid magnesium known as **Floradix®** at *http://www.florahealth.com/flora/home/USA/Products/64728.htm*. They use magnesium citrate and magnesium gluconate in their formula, and it is often more expensive than NutriCology® brand.

The NutriCology® magnesium is magnesium chloride; the same form of magnesium that is sprayed onto the skin, except this form is drinkable. Do NOT take the spray magnesium chloride by mouth. It is only for applying to the skin.

Realize that if you are low on magnesium, you might need to start out at higher doses, and then gradually reduce the dosage over time. The RDA for magnesium is 400 mg, but most people will find that they need 500 to 1000 mg per day for staying healthy and most Americans do not get enough magnesium in diet alone. Always read the instructions on the label for the type you purchase.

Did you know that you can also get a dose of magnesium by taking *Milk of Magnesia* (MOM)? This form of magnesium is magnesium hydroxide. Instead of taking the recommended two to four tablespoons (adult dosage), which will cause bowel movements, you simply take ONE teaspoon and you will get a small dose of magnesium that usually won't have a laxative effect (192). Do NOT use any form of magnesium aspartate. I **never** recommend this form of magnesium. Do not use any milk of magnesium that contains aluminum! If you want to make your own magnesium drink using milk of magnesium, there is a recipe here: *http://www.earthclinic.com/Supplements/magnesium2.html.*

In his excellent e-books on Magnesium: *Magnesium Medicine, Magnesium The Lamp of Life* and *Magnesium The Ultimate Heart Medicine*, among others, Dr. Mark Sircus, Ac., O.M.D., discusses the acute shortage that most Americans have of magnesium in their systems and recommends as the best form of magnesium, the transdermal form that you can get in a spray bottle and spray directly onto the skin for direct absorption (magnesium chloride). You can find this wonderful form of magnesium chloride at website: *http://www.ancient-minerals.com,* and *http://magneticclay.com.* The brand known as *Ancient Minerals* is available at: *L.L. Magnetic Clay* as well. Their website is: *http://www.magneticclay.com/store/Departments/Ancient-Minerals-Magnesium-Oil.aspx.* They also have a form of bentonite clay that will absorb poison from your mouth. You can either sprinkle the calcium bentonite clay (or sodium bentonite clay) on your toothbrush to let it absorb poisons or "pack the gums" with the clay, "which will absorb poisons from deeper in the oral tissues" (287). This type of clay is said to be pure enough that you can swallow small amounts to help absorb toxins in the G.I. tract and move them out of your body (287).

L.L. Magnetic Clay has **Ancient Minerals** Magnesium Oil, the Bentonite Clay, and Magnascent© Iodine (discussed elsewhere in this book). You can also get magnesium chloride spray from **Swanson vitamins.com** website. Their brand is referred to as: *Dr. Barbara Hendel's Magnesium Oil, Magnesium Chloride Brine* from the **Ancient Zechstein Sea.** They also have the bath crystals for soaking your feet, or for pouring in your bathwater.

Many people pour Epsom salts into their bathwater. It is not an easily absorbed form of magnesium, but it does contain sulfur, and as noted elsewhere in this book, parents of autistic children sometimes use this type magnesium in their children's bathwater for the sulfur supply (51). The magnesium found in Epsom salts is mag sulfate and is inferior to magnesium chloride for absorption and use by the body, but it is better than nothing.

If you are using magnesium in your bath soaks or foot soaks and experience "redness in local areas...diarrhea or even muscle spasms," these are indications that you need to reduce the amount being used (287).

When you buy table salt, do not use sodium chloride; use sun-dried (not kiln-dried) SEA SALT or use Himalayan crystal salt. Sea salt and Himalayan crystal salt are full of vital trace minerals and are actually more healthy for you—store bought table salt is not—the ONLY thing it contains is sodium chloride and nothing else.

Other recommended salts are *Dead Sea Salt, Himalayan Salts, Real Salt* and *Celtic Salts* (287), which can be found on the internet and some health food stores. Use only reputable suppliers.

Many magnesium liquids or pills you pick up will have magnesium oxide. This form is not as easily absorbed as magnesium chloride and magnesium citrate, and it sometimes causes diarrhea. I did use it in the **Orange Wunder** drink (see Chapters 1 and 2), because it keeps the bowels regular, like clockwork, and it worked well for my relative who was using the formula. If you are going to use it, you might consider a second supplement such as magnesium taurate, or the oral form of liquid magnesium chloride (from *NutriCology®*), or magnesium citrate (in liquid or pill form) that you know will give you good absorption, especially if you are fighting a disease like cancer, heart disease, lupus, Crohn's, diabetic neuropathy, or any other type of chronic illness or disease.

Many people who are severely deficient in magnesium will need much higher doses than those suggested in the RDA, usually about 500 mg for every 100 lbs of body weight. This means if you weigh 200 lbs, you may very well need as much as 1000 mg of magnesium per day. If you are fighting a deadly disease like cancer, you may also need these higher amounts, especially if you are severely deficient in magnesium, which most cancer patients are. Since taking 1000 milligrams may not mean that your body absorbs the entire amount, you may need even more.

It is better to take magnesium in small doses several times a day, rather than a large dose once or twice a day. If you get the *NutriCology®* liquid magnesium chloride, which has 66.5 mg in a ½ teaspoon (to mix in a glass of water or juice), you may need much more if you are a cancer patient or severely magnesium deficient - as much as a full teaspoon taken 6 or 7 times a day to get the magnesium you need. Take the magnesium chloride with food or meals. (Check with your physician too, because as noted later in this chapter, there are times when you cannot use supplemental magnesium.) To avoid taking this much by mouth, you could alternate by using the transdermal spray magnesium as described earlier. When you use the spray, you are also getting immediate absorption through the skin, bypassing the digestive system and eliminating any problems with gastric irritation. (The magnesium crystals for foot soaks are great!) See Appendix II for sources.

In an article by Dr. C. Norman Shealy, he notes that using the topical magnesium raises beneficial levels of DHEA hormone in the body. Website: *http://www.yourlifesource.com/cwr-dhea.htm* markets a topical magnesium solution that you can apply directly to the skin or put into your bath water for soaking. It is called: *Aim Cell Wellness Restorer* (43).

• Extra Magnesium – When You Need It

If you or a loved one has any type of gastrointestinal problems, diarrhea, Crohn's, magnesium wasting (as found in renal problems), diabetes, or are taking diuretics, suffer from chronic alcoholism, or may be elderly, these will all increase your need for magnesium (42). Those with heart disease, diabetes, depression, cancer, bowel problems, autoimmune disorders, COPD, CHF, MS, insomnia, autism, asthma, liver problems, allergies, and migraines are very often deficient in this mineral, especially children and the elderly. Just be aware that you must check with your doctor about taking magnesium if you have renal problems or other health issues.

III. Magnesium & Disease

• Alcohol & Stress Decrease Magnesium Levels

Women are warned against drinking alcohol due to the increased risk for breast cancer; however, alcohol consumption uses up magnesium in the body, so is it possible that the magnesium deficiency, thus created, is the real culprit in causing the cancer (284)? Stressors in the body also decrease magnesium levels (284). Why is it that, according to Mark Sircus Ac., OMD, a whopping *78%* of children diagnosed with leukemia have a past record of *anorexia*, and these same children are also very deficient in magnesium (284)?

Human studies have shown that high magnesium amounts in the body can help prevent stomach cancer (284). Many chronic illnesses are linked to magnesium deficiencies, including: migraine headaches, chronic fatigue syndrome, autoimmune diseases, arrhythmias, asthma, COPD, heart disease, fibromyalgia, and others.

• Atrial Fib & Other Cardiac Arrhythmias & Magnesium

In an article by Dr. Ray Sahelian, he describes the importance of magnesium for treating atrial fib and other arrhythmias (276). Atrial fib can be caused by an "overactive thyroid... vigorous exercise... obesity" and certain prescription drugs such as *Fosamax and Novartis AG,* and drinking alcohol (276). Dr. Sahelian also discusses the importance of using fish oil containing *n-3 fatty acids*, and vitamin C for arrhythmia prevention (276).

• Cerebral Palsy in Premies & Mag Sulfate Use

Recent studies have shown that moms who are at a greater risk for having premies can help prevent cerebral palsy in their child by having sufficient amounts of magnesium sulfate. There were *five trials* involving more than 6,000 babies which showed that giving magnesium sulfate to women "at risk of very preterm birth" can help prevent cerebral palsy in infants (116). The full story is here:

http://www.washingtonpost.com/wp-dyn/content /article/2008/08/27/AR20080882702634.html (195).

• Chronic Fatigue Syndrome & Magnesium

Chronic fatigue patients are often suffering from a critical shortage of magnesium (287). This type of magnesium wasting is also seen in a kidney disorder where magnesium is lost, known *as Bartter's Syndrome* (287). Research scientists from Britain have found that being deficient in magnesium may contribute to chronic fatigue syndrome (33). In a trial with 32 CFS patients, 15 were given magnesium sulfate injections (33). Of those 15, 12 improved. Scientists were not sure as to why these particular patients had such low magnesium levels to begin with, but it was apparent that bringing their levels up to normal brought significant improvement in their symptoms (33).

Another disorder linked to magnesium deficiency is fibromyalgia. Many specialists recommend that those with CFS and fibromyalgia use "a combination of Mg plus malic acid, an extract of tart apples," which seems to work well for these patients (93). If you use malic acid as your magnesium source, the tablets are usually very large.

• Chronic Health Disorders & Magnesium

Magnesium is also important in fighting high blood pressure, arrhythmias, insomnia, muscle aches and pains, Raynaud's Syndrome, Tourette's Syndrome, prevention of blood clots, muscle spasms, stroke prevention, restless leg syndrome, senility, dementia, slow healing of wounds, migraines, Alzheimer's, depression, bi-polar disorders, Bell's palsy, chronic fatigue syndrome, high cholesterol, ADD, angina, MS,

COPD, CHF, coronary artery disease, asthma, anxiety, kidney stones, eye tics, ADHD, SIDS, cerebral palsy risk, atherosclerosis, osteoporosis, arthritis, cancer, seizure prevention, preterm delivery prevention, fibromyalgia, Parkinsonism, and the treatment of polio victims, as well as many other chronic disorders (192). Many people are loading up on calcium when their real problem is a severe magnesium deficiency. Don't depend solely on your physician to find a magnesium deficiency. It is often overlooked.

Magnesium, in combination with vitamin B6, has also been used with tremendous success in treating autistic children (11), and topical magnesium works wonders for some people in clearing up their psoriasis, eczema, acne, and dermatitis (85).

Many of the prescription drugs that physicians are giving their patients are responsible for stripping magnesium out of the body! Medical schools continue to churn out new doctors who are trained that it is better to prescribe noxious drugs with an entire burden of dangerous side effects to the general populace than to recommend safe, nutritional vitamins, minerals, and whole foods for restoring health and vitality. The pharmaceutical companies will continue to see to it that this deplorable situation continues for as long as people remain indifferent enough to tolerate it. For emergency situations (e.g. hurricane, power outage), be sure that you are well-stocked in vitamins (especially vitamin C, D, E), iodine and other essential minerals, magnesium chloride, soda bicarbonate, peroxide, and water. Remember that soda bicarb makes one of the best non-toxic cleaners AND toothpastes you can use. It will instantly alkalize your entire mouth. Peroxide will purify water and clean out wounds. So will iodine, which is non-poisonous.

If you know someone who has suffered a stroke or needs healing after brain surgery, ask their physician about using the RELOX procedure described at:

http://odeo.com/episodes/23983188-The-Relox-Procedure, or see this website: *http://www.nihadc.com/therapies/relox.html.*

• Colon Cancer & Magnesium

While it is already known that magnesium can help prevent high blood pressure, heart disease, *Type 2 diabetes, migraines and osteoporosis,* animal studies and human studies in Japan showed that a diet high in magnesium ("at least 327 milligrams of magnesium" per day) could cut in half a man's risk for developing colon cancer (194).

• Colorectal Cancer & Magnesium

In a research article from the U.S. National Library of Medicine and NIH, the dietary habits of more than 40,000 Japanese men and 46,000 Japanese women showed that a "higher dietary intake of magnesium may decrease the risk of CRC [colorectal cancer] in Japanese men" (239). The cancer risk for women in the study did not show a significant correlation between their magnesium intake and this type cancer (239); however, in another study that involved more than 35,000 women, it was clearly shown that "a diet high in magnesium may reduce the occurrence of colon cancer among women" (93). Human studies have also shown that most Americans simply do not get enough magnesium in their diets, which, among other problems, can cause an *elevated CRP (C-reactive protein), a marker of inflammation,* and this can increase the risk for heart disease (93).

• Diabetes & Magnesium Deficiency

Jerry L. Nadler, M.D., tells us that not only does magnesium play a critical role in a healthy heart, but taking magnesium enhances "insulin sensitivity," and that making sure you have sufficient magnesium on a daily basis can help prevent you (and your children) from developing type 2 diabetes and the multiple problems that accompany it – "cardiovascular disease, retinopathy, and nephropathy" (260). He admits that at least "50% to 85% of the population of the United States is receiving an inadequate" amount of magnesium, and it is also true that African-Americans have unusually low levels of this vital mineral, increasing their risks for heart disease, diabetes, stroke, and high blood pressure (260).

The reason that most diabetics have deficient magnesium is because they do not ingest enough in their diet, they lose magnesium in their urine, and many of them take diuretics that strip magnesium from their body, not to mention the problems they have with insulin resistance (260). (Did you know that many prescription medications actually strip magnesium out of your body?)

- **Headaches, Strokes, Autism & Magnesium**

1. Headaches:

An article from PubMed's website, testing the use of 1 gram of mag sulfate infusion for 40 people with various types of headaches (23 with migraines) resulted in the "complete elimination of pain...within 15 minutes of infusion of MgSO4 [mag sulfate]...in 80% of the patients," and there was also total elimination of light [sensitivity], noise sensitivity, and nausea (240). This study also suggests that migraines could be caused when people become deficient in magnesium levels. Magnesium appears to protect the brain, the heart, and can even help people recover from injuries caused by strokes.

2. Strokes:

Magnesium relaxes blood vessels. Excess calcium constricts vessels. This is why a deficiency in magnesium can constrict blood vessels and also cause not only high blood pressure and heart attacks, but strokes as well. This is exactly what 3 hospitals in New York discovered when they studied *98 stroke patients* (125). The victims all had low magnesium levels and high calcium levels. This was also proven in another four year study involving more than 17,000 people in Taiwan. It was discovered that "the higher the magnesium levels in drinking water used by Taiwan residents, the lower the incedence (sic) of stroke" (125).

3. Autism:

Similar research has been done using magnesium and vitamin B6 for treating autistic children with amazing results (147). Researchers used "as much as a gram a day of vitamin B6 and half a gram of magnesium," however; a multiple B-vitamin tablet was also given to the children to prevent them from getting too low in the other B vitamins (147). One of the researchers remarked that autism is "in many cases a vitamin B6 dependency syndrome" (147).

• Heart Disease & Magnesium

Magnesium is critical for a healthy heart. Most people who die from heart attacks are found with "very low magnesium but high calcium levels in their heart muscles" (228), and it has been proven that countries with "high calcium and low magnesium levels in soil and water have the highest" statistics for "cardiovascular disease. At the top of the list is Australia" (228). Here in the West (and other countries) that has an excessive dairy consumption, "average calcium intake is about 1000 mg. The higher the calcium intake, especially in the form of cows' milk products (except butter) the higher the incidence of osteoporosis", and countries with low levels of magnesium in their water supply and soil have much higher statistics for cancer (228). When 4,000 men were followed for an 18 year period, those with "high levels of magnesium" had "a 50 percent decrease in cancer mortality, and a 40 percent decrease in cardiovascular and all-cause mortality" (228).

Another human study involving more than 2300 people found that injecting magnesium during acute heart attacks "reduced deaths by a fourth," and the magnesium was just as effective as *aspirin* and clot-dissolving drugs and it was noted to be "simple and safe" (161). How many physicians give their acute heart attack patients intravenous magnesium immediately afterwards? Very few, but it can save patient's lives and reduce their chances of death by greater than half (192). Are you thinking that a mineral like magnesium can't possibly be a healing miracle? Well, if you or a loved one suffers an acute MI and your physician fails to give you magnesium immediately afterwards, you could be dead in less than seven minutes!

• Heart Rescue in Seaweed

Many people suffer sudden death from heart attacks brought on by a deficiency in magnesium (192). Seaweed (which is high in iodine), magnesium, and trace minerals, has been processed into a wonderful new product by Israeli scientists that may save the lives of thousands of people suffering from heart disease. The product is known as ***Biogel (BL-1040)*** and is described in at article at *www.canadaisrael.ca* by

Karen Kloosterman (225). The studies by Professors Smadar Cohen and Jonathan Leor from Ben Gurion University, have been "licensed by BioLineRx," a pharmaceutical company. The product which is processed from "common brown seaweed" can "dramatically strengthen weakened heart tissues," and "90 percent of animals treated with the gel survived a heart attack" (225). In the group not treated with the gel, "40 percent survived" (225). Trials have been done on humans in several countries and the gel product may soon be available to Americans and Canadians (225). The formula works when it is injected into a catheter that has been placed in the groin. Once "contact with damaged heart tissue" occurs, the formula "gels" acting as "mechanical support for heart tissue, allowing damaged heart muscles to regrow...lessening the risk of future heart attacks" (225). This seaweed "prevents... enlargement of the left ventricle after the MI," and "It is excreted naturally from the body within six weeks...leaving behind a stronger, more stable heart muscle" (225).

• Inflammation & Magnesium

In his blog on magnesium and inflammation, Dr. Michael R. Eades, M.D., notes that many in the medical field are beginning to believe that metabolic syndrome in itself "is nothing but a manifestation of a magnesium deficiency," because all the problems in this syndrome, "'diabetes, high blood pressure, obesity and lipid disorders are associated with low magnesium'" (91) levels. He says that he takes 300 mg of mag citrate at bedtime. When it comes to all the data on elevated cholesterol, the problem of risk involves inflammation. Having high cholesterol (LDL) along with an "elevated C-reactive protein (a measure of inflammation) is a better gauge of heart disease risk," and he says one way to fight inflammation is to keep magnesium levels elevated (91). Of even greater concern, he says, is the fact that, according to the *Journal of the American College of Nutrition,* "as consumption of magnesium fell, the levels of C-reactive protein went up" (91). This shows that deficient levels of magnesium in the body actually causes much of the inflammatory process that is being blamed solely on high cholesterol (91) as the culprit for heart disease in this country. Just think of all the millions of people taking cholesterol-lowering drugs that may simply need to increase their magnesium levels (as well as selenium, boron, zinc, CoQ10, vitamin D3, and vitamin C).

• Inflammation, Oil of Oregano, Turmeric & Pepper

There are many things you can do to reduce inflammation naturally, besides the need for magnesium. According to Bob Condor, a writer at Insiders Health, an Alternative Health Blog, using wild oil of oregano, fresh ground black pepper and turmeric (which I have discussed at great length in my last two books) are excellent ways to reduce inflammation in the body (189). Of wild oil of oregano, he says that it can be used for those with inflammatory Crohn's Disease and for warding off osteoporosis, and may be important in fighting autoimmune disorders. He adds that "5 drops in a bit of water, then gargle with it, stops a sore throat in its tracts" (sic) (189). The problem with using wild oil of oregano as a gargle with kids is that it is very bitter and smelly and most kids (and some adults like me!) won't get anywhere near it! Here is a great tip if you want to ingest wild oil of oregano and can't stand the taste or the smell. Get some empty vegetarian capsules at any health food store, put 5 – 10 liquid DROPS of the wild oil of oregano into an empty gel capsule, close it back up, then simply swallow it with water, and you will not taste it. Take with food. Oil of wild oregano has also been known to help asthma and allergy sufferers, as has olive leaf supplements.

If kids are not allergic to iodine, or iodized salt, *Magnascent©* iodine drops in a little water as a gargle will do the same thing, but beware, because iodine can stain the teeth. (Using a bit of soda bicarb to brush the teeth will help eliminate stains.) 3,000—4,000 mg of liposomal vitamin C mixed in a little orange juice and swallowed down will also help ward off oncoming colds, but keeping your vitamin C and magnesium levels elevated at all times will help prevent colds and flu in the first place.

• Killing Disease with Magnesium

Professor Pierre Delbet, MD, discovered in 1915 that magnesium chloride was the best antiseptic for wounds and a "powerful immune-stimulant" when taken internally (228). He also found it to be "beneficial in a wide range of diseases," including:

> ...diseases of the digestive tract such as colitis and gall bladder problems, Parkinson's disease, tremors and muscle cramps; acne, eczema, psoriasis, warts and itching skin; impotence, prostatic hypertrophy, cerebral and circulatory problems; asthma, hay fever, urticaria and anaphylactic reactions. Hair and nails become stronger and healthier and patients had more energy. Prof. Delbet also found a very good preventative effect [in magnesium chloride] on cancer and cured precancerous conditions such as leukoplasia, hyperkeratosis and chronic mastitis (228).

Dr. Mark Sircus, Ac, OMD, agrees and says that "Magnesium chloride is the only form of magnesium known to have anti-infectious properties" (285).

A French physician, A. Neveu, used magnesium chloride to cure "several diphtheria patients...within two days," and he also cured poliomyelitis patients (228). Magnesium chloride has also been successfully used in high doses for "symptoms of Parkinson's disease," and for treating the following illnesses:

> Bronchitis, pneumonia... tonsillitis... Influenza, whooping cough, measles, rubella, mumps, scarlet fever...boils... infected wounds...osteomyelitis...acute asthma attacks, shock, tetanus, herpes zoster, acute and chronic conjunctivitis, optic neuritis, rheumatic diseases, many allergic diseases [and] Chronic Fatigue Syndrome (228).

On tests with guinea pigs and rabbits, both survived snake venom when they were given a solution of magnesium chloride (228).

Many researchers believe that Alzheimer's could be caused by excess levels of aluminum that accumulate in the brain, and indeed, autopsies of Alzheimer's victims bears this out, but is it possible that the disease itself begins with a severe magnesium deficiency? The brain requires magnesium and if it is deficient, it will settle for "the next available mineral that will work which is aluminum" (90). If the brain can't find adequate magnesium, the receptors will search for aluminum instead (90). The problem is aluminum is toxic!

As described at website: *www.health-science-spirit.com*, it has been noted that areas with low magnesium in their soil or water, have higher suicide statistics (228). Many epileptic patients have been helped with daily magnesium supplementation, with studies showing "that the lower the magnesium blood levels the more severe was the epilepsy" (228). Magnesium should be used "in combination with vitamin B6 and zinc" (228).

- ## Leukemia Seen in Many Children with Magnesium Deficiency

Many people, women and teens especially, are aggressively encouraged to take calcium for their bones as they grow and as they age, but health care professionals do not always emphasize the importance of magnesium, without which the cells cannot use calcium efficiently. Many of the most important nutrients in our cells must have magnesium to perform their antioxidant properties (284). Studies with animals have shown that keeping them magnesium-deficient will cause malignant cancers. **Human** studies have also shown that high magnesium amounts in the body can help prevent stomach cancer (284).

Natural sources of magnesium include: sunflower seeds, pumpkin seeds, almonds, walnuts, cashews, Brazil nuts, green leafy vegetables, the green grasses, peanuts, and whole grains. Remember that green foods contain chlorophyll, and chlorophyll contains magnesium!

Other good food sources for magnesium are kelp, molasses, wheat germ, pecans, brewer's yeast, egg yolks, parsley, and apples, "oily seeds and sprouted seeds" (228).

To find out more, including information about a way of delivering magnesium chloride directly into the skin in an easily absorbable form, see website: *http://www.ancient-minerals.com* (287).

- ## Leukemia & Lymphoma, Magnesium & Zinc

A human study has shown that magnesium and zinc are so important in "cell growth, division and differentiation," that a deficiency in these minerals can cause malignant cancers (289). When children with acute lymphoblastic leukemia and malignant lymphoma, were tested, it was found that "chronic magnesium and zinc deficiency seems to be associated with the development of ALL [acute lymphoblastic leukemia] and malignant lymphoma" in children (289). Being deficient in magnesium causes cancer—all types of cancer—not just lymphoma and leukemia. Colon cancers and breast cancers are also higher in people who have low magnesium levels. One reason could be that high levels of magnesium have a protective effect on the cells against toxic heavy metals. Magnesium levels drop in alcoholics. This could be one reason why women who drink alcoholic beverages have an increased risk of developing breast cancer.

Chemo strips magnesium out of the body and many oncologists do not use magnesium in their cancer regimens. One of the best ways to get a rapid dose of magnesium into the body (besides intravenously) is to apply an ounce of the magnesium oil spray all over the body. Magnesium given in this way helps relieve pain and is also used as a prevention and treatment for diabetic neuropathy and migraine remedy. Sources for the spray are given earlier in this chapter and in Appendix II at the end of the book.

• Magnesium Prevents Stones

Many studies have shown that adequate magnesium, either through dietary means or supplementation, may be all you need to prevent kidney stones and even gallstones (96). If you are going to use it as a prevention for gallstones, combine it with lecithin (228).

A physician at the Army's Fitzsimons General Hospital in Denver was able to prevent his kidney stone patients from getting any further stones by having them take 250 mg/day of magnesium oxide. There were no side effects and the patients were followed for two years, during which time they remained stone-free (96).

• Peripheral Vascular Disease (PVD), Peripheral Artery Disease (PAD) & Magnesium

J.M.H. Howard in the *Journal of Nutritional Medicine*, described some amazing **human** studies that proved magnesium deficiencies cause the circulatory problems linked to peripheral vascular disease or PVD. The results of the study showed that magnesium deficiency is a "highly significant factor in peripheral vascular disease" (216). People who suffer with this disease often develop such severe circulatory disorders that they end up with leg ulcers, gangrene, and sometimes require limb amputation. Later, in Chapter 12, I talked about Ann Wigmore, who healed gangrene in both her legs by eating and juicing greens like wheat grass. Her physicians wanted to amputate her legs. She wrote several books about the wonderful benefits of juicing fresh wheat grass and sprouts and even went on to win a runner's marathon years after she was told she needed to have both legs amputated! This is miraculous, but not surprising, because green foods (chlorella, wheat grass juice, barley grass juice, leafy green vegetables) contain chlorophyll and chlorophyll contains MAGNESIUM and oxygen! Ms. Wigmore even claimed that the wheat grass juice restored her natural hair color. It is a known fact that a deficiency in magnesium, B12, folic acid, and zinc can cause premature gray hair.

There are many helpful things you can do for your legs if you are fighting PVD (peripheral vascular disease) or PAD (peripheral artery disease). Use niacin (the type that causes flushing, but not the timed-release), green drinks like wheat grass, barley grass, the ***Orange Wunder Formula*** I developed (see Chapters 1 and 2 of this book), ginger, ginkgo biloba, green tea, magnesium, Magnascent© iodine (see Appendix II at the back of this book for suppliers), liposomal vitamin C, a good vitamin B complex supplement daily, garlic, plenty of fresh water (no chlorine and no fluoride), daily exercise, fresh air, prayer and worship (see the last chapter in this book). Also, see my book on *Gentle Cures for Tough Cancers,* which has many recommendations for circulatory disorders. It is available at online websites and some local bookstores like *Barnes & Noble,* and can be ordered at most other local bookstores in the U.S., United Kingdom, Asia, Australia, Europe, Canada, and many other countries for arrival (usually) within a few days.

• A Bonus for You - A Great Skin Treatment Discovered by Accident

If you want a great skin treatment, one I discovered quite by accident one day: while all your pores are open from the niacin flush, take a cotton ball and soak it with 3% hydrogen peroxide that you get at any pharmacy or grocers (squeeze out any excess peroxide) and use the cotton ball to cleanse your face and other areas of your body with skin breakouts. It works great, cleans out all your pores while they are open, and will help clear up acne breakouts. Be sure to keep the peroxide away from your eyes! Also, if you have the transdermal magnesium spray on hand, this is a good time to use it, while all your pores are opened up during the niacin flush! Just remember not to eat anything until the flush wears off, because it can dry out the throat. Usually, this flushing effect only lasts a few minutes, but your throat can remain rather dry for 20 minutes or more, and of course, it will depend on the dosage of niacin you take. Larger doses will have a more dramatic effect. This is why I always caution people to begin with a smaller dose and work up as you see how it will affect you. If you take the niacin on an empty stomach, you are likely to get a more rapid, dramatic flush. It can quickly turn your entire body a beet red. For those who do not like the effect, purchase the flush-free niacin, or take a baby aspirin or two about 20 to 30 minutes before you take the niacin, but it will not open up your pores as dramatically. Do not **ever** get the timed-release niacin. Check the label carefully.

One drug company has decided to cash in on niacin's cholesterol-lowering effect by producing a PRESCRIPTION form of niacin known as *Niaspan*. Besides niacin, this product also contains synthetic dyes, including *FCF Aluminum Lake*, which is a food coloring made from coal tar. It is the same artificial coloring that is used in some of the blue mouthwashes. Is this going to be the next step for the pharmaceutical companies? When they find that people are getting well without their expensive prescription drugs, start blending their own vitamin versions and selling them in prescription form only? Then the FDA simply removes all the natural products off the shelves and makes it ILLEGAL for you and me to purchase them without a prescription, so you have to go to a doctor, pay a $75.00+ office visit charge, then pay four times the price for the prescription "vitamin blend" that was once available in your local health food store in its NATURAL form! Don't be surprised to see this happening! It already has in the past! The pharmaceutical industry and FDA will stop at NOTHING to drain your pocketbook and keep you dependent on THEM for your "health" needs! You can see more proof of this in my last book in the chapter on synthetic hormone replacement therapy. Millions of women were placed on synthetic HRT which is known to increase the risk of breast cancer, blood clots, strokes and death. Their physicians never told them that estrogen and progesterone are available in their NATURAL forms that you can get by walking into any health food store and purchasing as a cream that you simply apply to your skin, without the toxic side effects that the synthetic forms cause! The drug companies could not patent the natural forms. So what did they do? Change a molecule or two in the natural forms, create their own synthetic versions (that are foreign to the body) with a whole list of undesirable side effects, as the price an unwary public would have to pay, then pressure the physicians to prescribe their new deadly, synthetic versions! What was their answer to the toxic side effects? Well their usual answer, of course! "The benefits far outweigh the risks!"

IV. Reliable Magnesium Testing

If you are concerned about magnesium levels, do not rely on a simple blood test to give you an accurate measurement. As noted by the University of Wisconsin School of Medicine and Public Health: "Serum (extra-cellular) blood tests of magnesium are not sensitive enough to check for deficiency since magnesium is the second most prevalent intracellular ion (Potassium being the first). **Checking red blood cell magnesium is better"** (128), though a Magnesium Loading Test is the most accurate (130). Usual blood testing for *magnesium deficiency* is *irrelevant and unusable* (88).

If your doctor relies on a blood test to check to see if you are magnesium-deficient, only about 1% of the total magnesium in your body is going to show up, because most of it is found in the cells and bones of the body, so there is no way to tell if you are deficient or not. Insist on a **red blood cell magnesium level or one of the THREE tests described below to** get an accurate level of your magnesium (128). Blood levels will not *reflect total body magnesium* or *TBM* (88). Your blood levels or "serum magnesium," the "standard test used by medical doctors, means nothing until you are about to die" (94). They can appear "normal" when your body is seriously lacking in magnesium (94). [This is important and can make a big difference in whether you recover or not!] According to *www.diagnose-me.com/treat/T347488.html*, you should request one of the following magnesium tests:

- **Intracellular Free Magnesium** test, which is a "nuclear magnetic resonance (NMR) spectroscopy," a "noninvasive measure of the active magnesium ion in blood cells or tissues" though this test is not always available (130).
- **Sublingual Magnesium Assay.** Also known as the "Exatest," is a "safe, non-invasive test [that] measures the minerals inside cells." The physician simply takes a sample "from under your tongue and affixes it to a slide" which is sent to "IntraCellular Diagnostics, Inc." (130).
- **Magnesium Loading Test.** This is a test that will measure how much magnesium is excreted in your urine based on "a loading dose of magnesium." It is a test that can even find "individuals with…mild degrees of magnesium deficiency," and as long as your kidneys are functioning normally, this is "**the most accurate test**" (130). [Emphasis mine.]

There are other tests, such as the *Serum Ionized* magnesium test, and the *Total Red Cell* magnesium test (discussed earlier), but the above three bulleted items are probably the most accurate tests in the list (130). If your test results are less than *1.7 meq/L*, you have insufficient levels of magnesium (130).

It is interesting that the U.S. National Academy of Sciences "has estimated that a nationwide initiative to add calcium and magnesium to soft water might reduce the annual cardiovascular death rate by 150,000 in the United States" (95), but does anyone seriously think this will ever be done? We have an FDA in this country that believes MERCURY in vaccines and dental amalgams is SAFE for its citizens and thinks nothing of allowing alloxan in bread and chlorine and fluoride in the water supply, when there are safer alternatives for purifying water. Why should they suddenly care about actually putting stuff into the water that might promote health?

V. Magnesium - Youth & Vitality Mineral

Magnesium can help "reverse the age-related degenerative calcification of our body structure," rejuvenating us (228). One gynecologist noted that, in women, the ovaries are the first to "calcify," which causes "premenstrual tension." After putting his "patients on a high magnesium intake their PMT vanished..." (228) It is also helpful for men to improve symptoms of prostate enlargement, and remember this, in taking magnesium, the body will only absorb "as much as it needs" (228). If you have high blood pressure, you should be ingesting about twice as much magnesium per day as you do calcium (228). Many people who ingest a lot of dairy and calcium-rich foods (e.g. leafy greens or carrot juice), do not need extra calcium supplements.

Only recently did scientists discover exactly why magnesium plays such a critical antioxidant role in the human body. In an article by Carey Rossi at website *www.stopagingnow.com,* she points out that the Nutrition and Metabolism Center at Children's Hospital Oakland Research Institute discovered that when cells are deprived of magnesium they age faster (273). This rapid aging causes DNA damage and eventual cellular death (273). This is why a lack of magnesium will pre-dispose you to all manner of chronic diseases, including high blood pressure, high cholesterol, autoimmune disorders, viruses, cancer, COPD, CHF, asthma, diabetes, MS, MD, osteoporosis, and many other ailments. Being sure that your magnesium levels are normal (see above lab tests for determining this) can literally make the difference in life, longevity, health, illness, or even death for you and your loved ones.

VI. Calcium & Magnesium

You must have magnesium for your body to properly use the calcium that you take. Without magnesium, you will end up with too much calcium in the blood which gets deposited in all the wrong places. This is a primary reason for so much heart disease in this country. Deprive your body of magnesium and your heart and brain will both suffer. Both organs need large amounts of magnesium to work properly (192). According to Dr. Carolyn Dean in *The Magnesium Miracle,* if you take in too much calcium without sufficient magnesium, you will end up with "twitches, spasms, convulsions...asthma, HTN" and "painful periods," due to uterine cramps, and don't forget that drinking water with chlorine and fluoride in it will strip magnesium from your body (192). For those with heart problems, Dr. Dean recommends using magnesium taurate. Magnesium malate is often used for those with fibromyalgia and chronic fatigue syndrome (192). Be sure to include sufficient vitamin D3, B vitamins, and selenium in order for your body to efficiently use the magnesium you take (192), as well as boron and zinc.

Studies involving more than 47,000 men showed that a high daily calcium intake (*1500 and 1,999 mg of calcium per day*) could double the occurrence of advanced cancer of the prostate. Using 2000 mg or more quadrupled the risk (as compared to men ingesting *less than 500 mg* daily), and another study involving over 20,000 men, revealed that those who ingested greater amounts of *dairy products* in their diet increased their risk for this type cancer by *32%* (284).

Many people, women especially, are aggressively encouraged to take calcium for their bones as they age, but some health care professionals do not emphasize the importance of magnesium, without which the cells cannot use calcium efficiently. Many of the most important nutrients in our cells must have magnesium to perform their antioxidant properties (284). Studies with animals prove that keeping them magnesium-deficient raises free radical activity and will result in malignant cancers (284).

There are some medications that you should not take with magnesium because it may keep them from being absorbed. Always check with your physician or pharmacist to be sure your medications are compatible with your supplements.

For those of you concerned about taking iodine, magnesium, selenium, CoQ10, vitamin C, and other nutrients for your health, they are much safer than some of the pharmaceutical drugs that have killed THOUSANDS of American citizens without conscience, some that were deliberately NOT taken off the market even when the drug makers KNEW they were deadly, all in the name of profiteering! And don't depend on your doctor to protect you from the harm that prescription drugs may cause. Studies show that many times when patients complain about various symptoms while taking prescription drugs, their own physicians will tell them that their symptoms are not related to the drugs they are taking! How many U.S. citizens are aware that drug side effects kill more than 100,000 people every year in this country? (How many people do you know that have been hospitalized recently from complications taking vitamins?)

There are a lot of complaints about the new grab by government to gain control of the health care of the U.S. I am against socialized medicine, but a shortage of doctors could result in a new wave of dependence on natural substances for healing, rather than toxic drugs dispensed by prescription pads, which would be a positive outcome (except for those pushing pharmaceuticals), especially when you consider those 100,000 people that die in this country every year because of lethal side effects of their prescription drugs. But, a little poison is fine, right? As long as the patient doesn't die, at least not right away (so no connection can be made)! We are fast becoming a generation of people who are dependent on pharmaceutical drugs for every aspect of our lives, and if there is no disease to "fit" a new drug, the drug makers will simply invent one, something they are already doing! Do you have twitchy legs at night? Well, then you must have "restless legs syndrome," and you need a drug for it. Are your kids ingesting too much sugar during the day and bouncing off the walls? Well, then they must have ADHD and they need drugs to calm them down. Have you lost your energy and drive? Well maybe you have a problem called *Low T*. Are you disorganized and forgetful lately? Well, not to worry, you probably have early onset of adult ADD and a new drug will take care of that for you (but please notice the fact that some of the side effects are much WORSE than your original problem was)! See how it's done?

VII. When NOT to Take Magnesium

Do not take magnesium supplements if you have myasthenia gravis, adrenal weakness, kidney problems, are on dialysis, or have low blood pressure. If you do find that you experience muscle tiredness or weakness after taking magnesium, taking calcium will reverse the problem (228). Do not use extra magnesium if you are suffering with diarrhea, bowel obstruction or an abnormally slow pulse, since magnesium can worsen these conditions (192). Also, realize that calcium "is a magnesium antagonist," meaning that ingesting "too much milk or…too many other calcium rich foods" and not enough magnesium foods "may lower magnesium levels." Research has shown that "older women who took calcium supplements had an increased risk of heart attack" (69). The more calcium you take in, the more magnesium you need! If you are seriously low in magnesium, the calcium in your body can end up being toxic to you.

In an article at: *http://www.naturalnews.com/023279_magnesium_cancer_calcium.html* (Natural News) by Dr. Mark Sircus, Ac., O.M.D., we are advised that:

> There is no substitute for magnesium in human physiology; nothing comes even close to it in terms of its effect on overall cell physiology. Without sufficient magnesium, the body accumulates toxins and acid residues, degenerates rapidly, and ages prematurely. It goes against a gale wind of medical science to ignore magnesium chloride used transdermally in the treatment of any chronic or acute disorder, especially cancer (284).

In an Ezine article, Dr. Randolph Meresmaa notes that as far back as 1915:

> Prof. Delbet...found magnesium to be a powerful immune-stimulant...He found out that white blood cells destroyed up to three times more microbes than before, after the intake of **magnesium chloride**...Magnesium chloride was found to be beneficial in a wide range of diseases by Prof. Delbet. He found an excellent **preventative effect on cancer and cured precancerous conditions such as hyperkeratosis, leukoplasia and chronic mastitis.** He was surprised by many of these patients experiencing bursts of energy and euphoria (247) [emphasis, mine].

That isn't all. In animal testing, researchers in India discovered that they could shrink "tumors of the breast in rats...from 100% to between 46-57% by single applications of magnesium chloride, Vitamin C, Vitamin A or selenium," and even greater when at least two of these nutrients were given, "And finally tumor incidence was reduced to only 12%, when all four nutrients were given" (247).

In his excellent e-books on Magnesium: *Magnesium Medicine Magnesium The Lamp of Life* and *Magnesium The Ultimate Heart Medicine*, Dr. Mark Sircus, Ac., O.M.D., tells how iodine and selenium both help remove dangerous mercury from the body, but it is not necessary to take both of them together. Iodine also removes harmful fluoride, bromide, and percolate out of the body as well (287). He also discusses the acute shortage that most Americans have of magnesium in their systems and recommends as the best form of magnesium, the transdermal form that you can get in a spray bottle and spray directly onto the skin for direct absorption. You can find this transdermal form of magnesium chloride at: *http://www.ancient-minerals.com*, as well as: *http://magneticclay.com.* Also, *see http://www.swansonvitamins.com.* (Discussed earlier in this chapter in more detail.)

VIII. Magnesium & Ocean Water

Much of our magnesium comes right from the ocean. Seawater has all the trace minerals that our body needs. How life-sustaining is seawater? Well, in an attempt to answer this question, Dianne Jacobs Thompson says that researcher René Quinton and a group of his medical assistants actually took a dog, drained all of his blood supply and "replaced it with isotonic (diluted) seawater." They expected the dog to die rather quickly, but he didn't. Two days later, the dog was still alive and half of his natural "blood components had reappeared" (297). By the fourth day after the total transfusion, nearly "100 per cent of the missing blood components were restored...Not only did the blood completely regenerate," but the dog was soon back on his feet, jumping around with greater energy and living on for many years after the procedure (297).

Ms. Thompson says if she had to have a surgical procedure, she'd love to see "ocean plasma' in a drip bag above" her head "before the lights went out" (297). There truly is something life-sustaining about the ingredients that God placed in seawater. Nobel laureate Alexis Carroll was able to place a section of live *chicken heart* in seawater and keep it alive and beating "for over 26 years." He simply changed the water every day to "dispose of metabolic wastes," but the tissue lived (297)!

IX. Zinc Combo Stops Abdominal & Esophageal Cancers

Although we need only small amounts of zinc, a deficiency has been connected to many cancers, especially those of the esophagus and upper abdomen (255). Remarkable evidence of the link between cancer and zinc was revealed in data from a research study conducted in Linxian, China in the 1990's (255). This province holds the infamous reputation for having more throat cancer than any other region of the world (255). It was theorized that the area lacked adequate amounts of important minerals, such as selenium and zinc in their soil (255). Chinese researchers collaborated with those in the U.S. to try to determine the exact cause. Zinc, selenium, and beta carotene studies were done over a period of nine years involving thousands of Chinese participants. The human subjects, as described by Dr. Ralph Moss, author of *Antioxidants against Cancer,* were given larger doses than the RDA. He says that those participants receiving the supplements cut their gastric cancer rates by more than half (255), and those "taking beta carotene, vitamin E, and selenium [had] a 42 percent reduction in esophageal cancer" (255). I use zinc in my *Orange Wunder Formula* (see Chapters 1 and 2).

• Zinc & Vitamin A for Leukemia & Prostate Cancer

Research shows that the lifespan of *chronic myeloid leukemia* patients could be extended by minimal supplementation with vitamin A (277). It appears that Vitamin A also plays an important role in tumor prevention. Even a synthetic form of vitamin A caused dozens of APL (*acute promyelocytic leukemia*) sufferers to go into *remission*. A study from Italy involving dozens of patients revealed that deficiencies in *zinc and thymulin* could throw *acute lymphoblastic leukemia* patients into relapse (277).

Yourhealthbase.com reports that researchers in Houston, Texas, have found that *retinoic acid* and *retinal* (forms of vitamin A) could inhibit and fight cancers of the prostate, as well as *acute promyelocyte leukemias* (146).

Dr. Abram Hoffer, M.D., Ph.D., in his book, *Healing Cancer— Complementary Vitamin & Drug Treatment,* says that it is very common for cancer patients to have excessive levels of copper in their body, possibly caused by a lack of zinc (213). Excessive copper in your body will rob you of zinc.

CHAPTER 7

Selenium - Don't Fight Cancer Without It

****

I. Selenium's Role in Cancer Prevention & CURE

In her book: *Doctors ARE Dangerous Take Control Of Your Health And Escape The Sickness Industry,* Elaine Hollingsworth lauds the importance of using selenium for prevention and cure of diseases like cancer (214). She says that "cure" has become a four-letter word much like a curse-word when it comes to the health care industry:

> It has become a one-way ticket to jail, or loss of license, for health professionals who try to help patients without using the cruel burn, poison, mutilate 'cures' so loved by conventional oncologists, who earn billions in one of the most lucrative professions on earth. The brutal truth is that they do not want you to avoid cancer, and they certainly don't want you to treat it in a non-toxic way, if you have it (214).

She goes on to explain exactly what she would do if she were diagnosed with cancer:

> I would find a doctor willing to give intravenous vitamin C, with magnesium chloride. But I would lie and tell him/her it's for general health, and never mention the word 'cancer.' I would do a complete detox with lots of wheatgrass, which I can do easily, as I live at Hippocrates Health Centre...I would take large amounts of selenium --- way over the RDA...farmers...have known the importance of selenium for the health of their animals for many years. Selenium-deficient soil, and therefore feed, causes degenerative-diseases in stock,

> including cancer...Sodium selenite drench is also used to prevent and cure animals of cancer (214).

She also says that we are warned against megadosing with selenium in humans; however, she admits that:

> I know of many cases of people with 'terminal' cancer curing themselves by taking 5000 to 6000 micrograms per day of Sodium Selenite, 'for animals.' And they have taken the liquid, long term, by mouth with no untoward side effects. A man who had inoperable prostate cancer that had spread to his bones told me he was totally cured by intravenous selenium (214).

Ms. Hollingsworth also gives a website for sodium selenite where it can be purchased *for animals* at: *www.centreforce.com* or *bevan@centreforce.com* (214). I would not recommend this form of selenium for human consumption, not when there are excellent organic supplements intended for humans available (see below).

See **Chelorex™** brand selenium at *http://www.scienceformulas.com,* which contains organic selenium and many other nutrients, or if shopping at a natural health food store, purchase the **L-selenomethionine, L-methylselenocysteine,** or **selenocysteine** or get your selenium from organic brewer's yeast (287).

Also, see information in Chapters 1 and 2 in this book on why you may not even need intravenous C anymore, especially if your physician refuses to provide it and you cannot obtain it. There is now a new potent form of C on the market that could be more powerful than intravenous C, and it is known as **liposomal vitamin C.**

• Selenium Cuts Risk for All Cancers

A *JAMA* article in 1996 stated that having sufficient selenium in the diet could prevent 69% of prostate cancer cases. Leafy greens are a good source of selenium as are Brazil nuts (255), wheat germ, and eggs.

A **human** study (from the *British Journal of Urology*) involving 974 men taking selenium supplements showed a 63% reduction in prostate cancer in those who were taking 200 **micrograms** of selenium daily for 4.5 years. There were also lower cancer deaths in the men taking selenium (from all types of cancer), and lower rates of colorectal and lung cancers (123). Most health advocates recommend about 100 micrograms per day, though this is higher than the RDA. Those already fighting cancer (or wishing to prevent cancer, often use 200 micrograms per day or more as described in other places of this book).

Another **human** study described in the *Journal of the American College of Nutrition, JACN,* used the easily-absorbable organic form of selenomethionine-rich yeast for human testing, and showed that those who took "an extra 200 micrograms of selenium per day significantly lowered the risks of developing prostate, lung and colorectal cancer" (279a).

• Selenium & CoQ10 Helps Heal Breast Cancer

For optimum health, CoQ10 should be taken in conjunction with selenium (and alpha lipoic acid) because animal testing has shown that being deficient in selenium reduces liver levels of CoQ10, as well as cardiac levels (255). Selenium can be found in many food sources, such as fresh leafy greens, *garlic...egg yolks* and *Brazil nuts* (255); however, if the soil that produced the planted items is selenium-poor, there is no guarantee you will profit from eating them. Most adults find it difficult, if not impossible, to get an adequate amount of CoQ10 (ubiquinone) and selenium daily without supplementing.

Current research conducted by the Leonard M. Miller School of Medicine in Miami, under Nevain, et al, revealed that CoQ10 has the ability to kill cancer cells without damage to healthy cells. (See Chapter 10 in this book for CoQ10 levels used to cure breast cancer in human studies.) Take CoQ10 with selenium and alpha lipoid acid. The NCI (National Cancer Institute) actually **acknowledged in 2005** that CoQ10 can extend the lives of those with breast cancer and other cancers. Do YOU have cancer? Has your physician recommended CoQ10 to you? CoQ10 is used at the Issels Treatment Centers. You can reach Issels at: #888-447-7357 (135). You can find CoQ10 literally just about anywhere food is sold. Once available at only health food stores, you can now find it at most chain grocers and pharmacies, as well as internet nutritional supply stores.

Selenium Fights the BRCA-1 Gene (Genetic Mutation that Increases Breast Cancer Risk)

In a human study, described by *Cancer Epidemiology, Biomarkers & Prevention,* researchers studied subjects who were identified as having the BRCA-1 gene, which dramatically increases the risk for ovarian and breast cancer in women (as well as breast cancer and prostate cancer in men). They discovered that the chromosome damage in those who carry this gene could be normalized by giving them selenium supplements by mouth (226). Though the study was conducted over a small span of time (just 90 days), this is indeed encouraging news for those who carry this gene, as well as confirmation that nutrition can play an important role in cancer prevention, even where there is a genetic tendency. For specific details on this human study, see website: *http://cebp.aacrjournals.org/cgi/content/full/14/5/1302.* Again, we are talking humans here, not lab mice!

- ## Selenium & Vitamins A, D, E

Vitamin A and selenium have been shown to destroy bone cancer cells during in vitro testing. Vitamin E and selenium work together. Vitamin A blood levels can be maintained by juicing fresh fruits and vegetables, such as carrots, yams, celery, and leafy greens, or by taking spirulina which is high in beta carotene. Vitamin D helps to normalize the manufacture of bone cells and may help reduce the occurrence of abnormal cells; however, taking synthetic vitamin D as a supplement is not recommended. It may cause the release of calcium from bones that are already deficient from the cancer (16), or from osteoporosis. Vitamin D is manufactured in the skin when direct sunlight strikes the skin. It takes about 10-20 minutes of full-spectrum direct sunlight each day (or at the very least, 3 or 4 times per week) for sufficient vitamin D synthesis in most light-skinned individuals and usually longer if you are darker-skinned. Some researchers believe that Caucasians need (a little less) at least five to ten minutes of sunlight (without sunscreen) twice or thrice weekly in order to get sufficient vitamin D levels (275). You should consult your physician about sun exposure, especially if you have a history of, or a genetic tendency toward melanoma.

The oils in your skin help in this vitamin D "transformation" process, so avoid showering for at least one hour after the sun exposure (310).

Vitamin D not only reduces the risk for colon cancer, but now Harvard scientists and those from the Dana-Farber Cancer Institute, say that it could increase the **survival** of those already fighting the disease (62). While animal studies indicate that vitamin D is critical for slowing the progress of cancer, a **human** study (involving more than 300 people with colon cancer) found that those patients with the *highest* levels of vitamin D had dramatically lower chances of *dying from the disease* (62). It is already known that deficiencies of vitamin D can cause colon cancer, as can insufficient calcium intake.

• Selenium & Iodine Deficiencies Cause Breast Cancer

Selenium fights cancer in at least two ways: it defends the body by destroying free radicals, and it prevents the growth and spread of tumors (44). There are at least three diseases directly caused by a lack of selenium in humans: *Keshan's Disease*, where the heart enlarges, *Kashin-Beck Disease,* "which results in osteoarthropathy", and *Myxedematous Endemic Cretinism*, which causes "mental retardation" (44). Studies also show that victims of HIV die younger when they have insufficient levels of selenium in their blood (44).

Besides the work of super antioxidants (like selenium and vitamin C) in preventing and curing cancers, such as breast cancer, the problem is that many of our soils are leached of vital cancer-preventing nutrients, such as iodine and selenium. See Dr. Mark Sircus' book on *Iodine Bringing Back the Universal Medicine* at website: *http://www.winningcancer.com* and information on a gentle, superior form of oral iodine called *Magnascent©* Iodine (287). See Chapters 1 and 2, earlier in my book, for how I used this form of gentle iodine in my **Orange Wunder Formula.**

• Selenium Fights Cervical & Ovarian Cancer

Selenium is gaining much attention for its ability to fight cancer, and combined with vitamin E, it has powerful anti-inflammatory properties (133). When two different universities conducted research over several years on this mineral, they discovered that it only took ***200 mcg [micrograms] of selenium daily* to slash all incidences of lung, prostate, intestinal, and rectal cancers** (133). [Emphasis mine.] Selenium helps prevent just about every cancer imaginable and insufficient levels of this mineral increases the risk for malignancies, metastases, and death (133). Have you noticed that the RDA allowance for selenium is a meager 40-55 micrograms? The studies above used 4 times that amount!

Don't depend on the FDA to keep you healthy. They are not concerned with the health and well being of American citizens. Only when they are thrust in the public spotlight do they suddenly become staunch warriors against all those evil vitamin and herbal producers! They are concerned with keeping the pharmaceutical industry afloat and they are in bed with the ADA, the AMA, ACS, NCI, and companies like MONSANTO, who gave us all those *wonderful* additives and cheap growth hormones that are slowly killing us, used to fatten the beef and chicken that is now in the food we bring to our tables, not to mention their atrocious GMO products, which accounts for why so many people are now buying ORGANIC or planting their own gardens! If you want to see the most eye-opening video about exactly what MONSANTO has done to the food supply in India, the U.S., and many other countries, and the revolving door of politicians who have been involved in this debacle, please see this video before it is removed from the internet. It will probably be scrubbed soon. Watch it while you still can!

http://thelastoutpost.com/video-1/genetically-modified/the-world-according-to-monsanto.html

- **Selenium & Liver Cancer**

Selenium is vitally important for liver cancer prevention and overall liver health. Testing of 100,000 humans in China revealed that this mineral could reduce liver cancer deaths by more than one-third! The study lasted eight years. Remember, this is **humans** we are speaking of, not lab rats. This mineral is particularly important for anyone fighting *hepatitis-B* (84). Though too much selenium can be toxic, most people don't get enough of this mineral on a daily basis, and it takes large amounts for most people before toxicity occurs.

• Selenium Prevents Lung Cancer

During 1973 in a scientific study known as *The Willett Study*, blood was drawn from over four thousand healthy men, after which they were followed for *5 years*. Cancer was later found in more than a hundred of the participants (255). Blood comparisons were made to the men who were still healthy. It was found that those men who developed cancer had very little selenium in their body. Those having the lowest levels of selenium were twice as likely to have cancer as the men with higher amounts. Their greatest risk was for gastric and prostate cancer (255). The *Willett study* generated so much interest that the National Cancer Institute sponsored yet another study on selenium that lasted for eight years, whose primary intention was to test the mineral's effects on skin cancer. They wanted to see if selenium could help prevent melanoma. They were in for a surprise; however, because the mineral did not influence the incidence of melanoma, but the participants given selenium experienced half as many deaths from deadly *lung, colon, rectum, and prostate* cancers as those not receiving the selenium (255).

It has also been discovered, in **human** research, that sufficient levels of selenium can dramatically reduce your risk for asthma. In taking selenium supplements, it is always good to do so in combination with *vitamin E* (86), alpha lipoic acid (ALA), and CoQ10. Use organic selenium forms discussed earlier in this chapter (not the inorganic form which will be identified as sodium selenite, sodium selenide, or sodium selenate), and use the natural vitamin E, not the synthetic form.

• Selenium & Vitamin C Heal a "Fatal" Lymphoma

Selenium and vitamin C are crucial in treating severe lymphoma. Dr. Abram Hoffer, M.D., Ph.D., in writing about the importance of these two supplements, believes that selenium has been much maligned in the medical community and that higher levels are not toxic as has been claimed (212). He recounts the experience he had in treating a patient from Chile who was told that he had fatal lymphoma. The patient had surgery, but the cancer returned. **He received radiation and still the**

cancer returned. He was told that he had just a few months left (212). Dr. Hoffer started him on 600 **micrograms** of selenium a day; however, the patient, on return visit, admitted that he was not taking 600 mcg per day, but **2,000 micrograms** per day! Of course, Dr. Hoffer was alarmed about such a huge dosage of selenium, and recommended that he decrease the amount by half; however, it was too late! The higher dose had already worked and the patient went into total remission and survived many years without further trace of cancer (212).

Dr. Hoffer uses selenium, zinc, vitamin E, beta carotene, the B complex vitamins, and megadoses of vitamin C. He is convinced that the most vital ingredient for fighting cancer is vitamin C. In his experience, he says that doses of *12 grams per day (sodium ascorbate or calcium ascorbate)* can be tolerated. He starts his patients off with a *teaspoon three times per day*, then has them increase the dose until they develop diarrhea, at which point, they cut back just below the dose that caused the diarrhea. This was discussed earlier as the *bowel tolerance level* (212). You can get powdered vitamin C in health food stores. Some of the brands have 1000 mg of vitamin C in one teaspoon, while others have 5000 mg of vitamin C in one teaspoon. Remember this: the ascorbic acid crystals will be very bitter-tasting. There is a way to remove the bitterness. Take one teaspoon of the C crystals (or powder) and put them in a glass with four ounces of distilled water, then add ½ teaspoon of soda bicarb (*Arm & Hammer®* brand works great). Wait until the fizzing stops. Once the fizzing stops, stir to completely dissolve. You have just changed your ascorbic acid vitamin C into sodium ascorbate vitamin C, and the bitterness will be gone, but your vitamin C is still intact! This change does add salt to the mixture and will taste a lot like *Alka-Seltzer®*. (You can add it to orange juice for better flavor, if you like.)

II. Selenium & Chronic Illnesses

Scientific studies have shown that being deficient in this valuable mineral can be a major factor in many chronic disorders, including: schizophrenia, SIDS, cystic fibrosis, all cancers, muscular dystrophy, diabetic retinopathy, cataracts, fibrocystic breasts, asthma, arthritis, birth defects, pancreatic disease, rheumatoid arthritis, acne, seborrheic dermatitis, and thyroid dysfunction. It can help with heavy metal detox and can be important for those with Down's Syndrome (304). Most adults, especially those with cancer, need at least 200 **micro**grams a day of selenium, though (as noted earlier in this chapter); some cancer patients have used much higher dosages to cure their cancer without negative side effects.

• Selenium & Diabetes Link

Human studies have shown that insufficient levels of selenium in the diet can lead to type II diabetes, as well as gestational diabetes. If you do not wish to take selenium in supplement form, eat a good handful of Brazil nuts every day. Just find out if they were grown in soil that was selenium-rich. Always choose organic when possible.

• Selenium, ALA & Silymarin Enable Patients to Cancel Liver Transplants

When three men with hepatitis C were involved in a study where they were treated with ALA (alpha lipoic acid), silymarin (milk thistle), and selenium, they had such dramatic improvements, that they were able to go off the liver transplant-waiting-list. For details on this study, see the National Library of Medicine's website article: "A Conservative Triple Antioxidant Approach to the Treatment of Hepatitis C. Combination of Alpha Lipoic Acid (thioctic acid), Silymarin and Selenium: Three Case Histories by Berkson, B.M." See PubMed website (National Library of Medicine) at website: *http://www.ncb.nlb.gov/pubmed/10554539?dopt =abstract* (169) for the research details. Remember too, that hepatitis can progress into liver cancer. When purchasing selenium supplements, read the label. It will tell you what form of selenium you are purchasing. You want the L-selenomethionine, selenocysteine or the methylselenocysteine.

Although chemo drugs can cause peripheral neuropathy, new evidence shows that alpha lipoic acid may help reduce this risk in chemo patients, especially in those using *Cisplatin* and *Paclitaxel* (241). You can find ALA (alpha lipoic acid) supplements at health food stores, some grocery chains and pharmacies, as well as on the internet.

• Selenium, Keshan's Disease & HIV

Dr. Ralph Moss, author of *Antioxidants Against Cancer*, says that selenium is so important that Chinese scientists are using it to heal a virus known as *Keshan's disease. Vitamin E* helps as well (255). Though the RDA is 40-55 **micro**grams per day for adults and adolescents, much higher levels have been used in some cancer patients, and those wishing to avoid cancer. It is difficult to overdose on selenium through dietary measures (eating certain foods). Overdosing usually occurs from taking too much in supplement form. This mineral has also been helpful with HIV patients. See the documented case earlier in this chapter of a patient using **2000 micro**grams of selenium daily to cure his cancer. Many times, alert physicians will be able to tell how pervasive a person's cancer is, simply by looking at their selenium levels. Cancer patients are usually deficient in selenium.

As I discussed in my last book, when taking selenium, always take it with natural vitamin E, CoQ10, and alpha lipoic acid. Not only do these ingredients boost the immune system, but they also raise the body's levels of the critical antioxidant, glutathione. This alone should tell us that not only will these nutrients treat those with cancer, they are also important in the prevention of all cancers and chronic illnesses.

• Virus Mutations – How Selenium Kills Viruses

In a study reported by *Science News* on the importance of selenium for killing viruses in the body, it was revealed that if mice were kept on a very low selenium diet, then exposed to what is usually a harmless *coxsackievirus B3*, they developed inflammatory changes and "heart disease," while the mice fed normal levels of the mineral stayed completely healthy (159). They determined that because of selenium's ability at protecting the immune system, lack of the mineral induced the heart disease in the deprived rodents. They also stated that this could explain why selenium-deficient regions of the world (such as China), keep having outbreaks of so many "new strains of influenza virus," and why some viruses (like HIV) mutate and cross-over from animals to humans (159).

According to Edith Gaylord, editor and writer, *Health Sciences Institute Newsletter*, it's not just *flu viru*s that selenium may protect against. Some researchers believe that mad cow disease, Ebola, HIV, and others are able to spread through populations because the people are deficient in this valuable mineral (122). Even diseases like arthritis, hepatitis, CAD, and most cancers have been found in individuals who do not get enough selenium in their diets. One double-blind study in particular that involved more than 1300 humans who received 200 mcg of "yeast based selenium per day for 4.5 years... [resulted in a] 50% drop in cancer death rate," in comparison to those who were not given the mineral (122).

• Best Choices for Selenium Supplements

When using selenium supplements, be sure to use L-selenomethionine, selenocysteine, methylselenocysteine, or get your selenium from organic brewer's yeast (287). You could also choose the brand known as **Innate Response™** which has as much as "100 times the bioavailability of selenomethionine" (70). You can find this formula at *http://www.healthtruthrevealed.com/articles/11535928110/article*. Be sure to check the label of contents on the selenium you are about to purchase. It should clearly tell you what form of selenium you are getting.

Dr. Mark Sircus Ac, OMD, recommends a "natural chelation formula from *Science Formulas* called **Chelorex™**," which you can find at website: *http://www.scienceformulas.com*. It contains not only organic selenium, but many other nutrients (287). You can also find Chelorex™ at *http://www.rangeguide.net/chelorex.htm*, as well as some detailed information on their product (117).

Do not use inorganic forms of selenium, which have been shown to cause *cataracts* in test animals (287). It is best to take selenium with vitamin E, ALA, CoQ10, and vitamin C (if you are using the organic selenium) to increase effectiveness. Dr. Emanuel Revici cured many of his cancer patients using a formula that incorporated selenium, until he was driven out of practice by his local state medical board, mostly because they undoubtedly had too much of their money invested in the pharmaceutical drug industry with their $20,000 chemo drugs, and were unwilling to compete with Revici's cure rate using a common mineral available to the general public (with little expense), that they could not patent for their own exclusive use!

- **Estrogen/Testosterone, Selenium & Thyroid Health**

Since selenium is needed to manufacture an enzyme which "breaks down estrogen," insufficient levels of this mineral in your body will cause excess estrogen and "depress thyroid function" (140). Excess estrogen has also been implicated as a major cause of several types of cancer, cystic breasts, menstrual disorders, uterine fibroids, obesity, acne, osteoporosis, and many other health conditions.

Selenium is needed in order for the body to produce the hormone, testosterone, low levels of which can lead to osteoarthritis (140). Low levels of selenium can also lead to hair loss and the "degeneration of the knee joint (seen in Kashin-Beck disease)" (140).

As noted by *www.greenwillowtree.com*, other problems associated with low levels of selenium include:

> …anemia…fatigue…myalgia…muscular dystrophy…cardio-myopathy (sudden death in athletes), heart palpitations, irregular heartbeat, liver cirrhosis, pancreatitis, Lou Gehrig's and Parkinson's diseases (mercury toxicity), Alzheimer's Disease (high intake of vegetable oil), sudden infant death syndrome [SIDS] (and possibly 'breathlessness' in adults), cancer, multiple sclerosis, and sickle cell anemia (140).

It is possible that the palpitations caused by low levels of selenium could be from the fact that low selenium will "increase T3 in the heart," as discovered in animal testing (140).

For those people with hypothyroid disorders, studies show that you may be deficient in iodine and selenium. Selenium helps the body absorb iodine. If you are taking iodine, but you do not have enough selenium in your cells, your body may not be able to use the iodine (140). If you are low in selenium, your deficiency of iodine will keep getting worse and worse (140). It is also possible for low selenium levels to cause hyperthyroidism, though taking high levels of selenium will **not** cause this disorder (140).

III. Vitamin E & Selenium – Latest Controversy

Though prior human studies showing that having adequate selenium & vitamin E could cut the incidence of prostate cancer by at least *30 percent* (270), newer studies are saying that this may not be the case, but those studies do not say whether a natural or SYNTHETIC form of vitamin E was used.

Apparently, keeping high levels of vitamin E in the body can protect against bladder cancer (266). In one particular study, vitamin E from alpha-tocopherol and gamma-tocopherol sources was used (266). Some researchers believe that the gamma form of vitamin E is superior to the alpha-tocopherol form in cancer prevention. If using the alpha, do not get vitamin E in the synthetic form which is called dl-alpha. Use the **d**-alpha. Others believe that for best results, you need both: the vitamin E that is d-alpha with gamma-tocopherol and mixed tocotrienols. Just do not ever use any form of vitamin E that has the **dl** in the label of contents. Use the form with the **d** only.

Some good **natural sources** of vitamin E are: wheat germ oil, olive oil, sunflower oil (and seeds), dandelion greens, spinach, broccoli, turnip greens, almonds and other nuts, eggs (205) (252) (266), kiwi, and mangoes, fortified cereals and fresh sprouts, especially wheat berry sprouts.

IV. The Mercury Poisoning Mystery & Help From Selenium

One of the major ways that people are getting mercury contamination is in the form that the government is strangely quiet about. It is the mercury vapors released from dental amalgam mercury fillings that have been placed in the mouths of millions of people and still continue to be done. It is a strange mystery that a dentist can put a metal in your mouth as a dental filling and tell you it's completely safe and harmless, and in the same breath, tell the dental hygienist to be sure and put the filling they just removed from your mouth in the hazardous waste disposal in order to be compliant with government regulations for disposing of toxic and hazardous waste substances!

According to Dr. Mark Sircus, Ac., OMD, in his e-books on Magnesium, the best antidote for mercury poisoning is the mineral, selenium (287). Selenium is also vital for the functioning of the thyroid gland. If you want to prevent cancer or kill the cancer you already have, you need at least 200 **micrograms** of selenium a day. Be sure that you are taking a form of selenium that is easily absorbed by the body: the

L-selenomethionine, selenocysteine, or methylselenocysteine organic forms of selenium. You may see it combined with zinc as zinc-L-selenomethione, which simply means you are getting extra zinc.

• Cilantro for Removing Heavy Metals

Cilantro is a mild herb that gets little attention, but it is powerful. The herb acts like a chelating agent to remove toxic substances (e.g., *heavy metals*) from human cells (34). (I.V. chelation therapy is common in alternative medicine as a way to get toxic metals, such as aluminum, cadmium, mercury, and other free radicals out of the body.) One physician in particular, Dr. Yoshiaki Omura, discovered that using *fresh cilantro* can cause the body to excrete these toxic metals within 14 days, and this is one chelating agent that you can take orally, rather than intravenously, without toxic side effects. He used this herb when he found out that he himself had been accidentally over-exposed to mercury (35). He heads up a research team at the *Heart Disease Foundation* (and is also President of the *International College of Acupuncture,* New York). He says that a "lightly cooked form of cilantro causes a massive excretion of mercury via the urine" (35).

Dr. Dietrich Klinghardt, MD, says that according to his research findings, "one of the best" ways of ridding toxic mercury from your brain is by ingesting "5 grams (teaspoonful[s]) a day" as "the minimum dose" (35) of cilantro. Do not cook it in metal pans or use metal utensils. "Use only Pyrex or Corningware!" (35). Chop up "eight or more heaping teaspoons" and steep in about "one quart" of water that has just been boiled. It should be "covered for twenty minutes" (35). One study in particular revealed that cilantro (often called *Chinese parsley*), not only rids mercury from cells, but it "protects the body from pre-cancerous lesions" (101). Be sure you are using organically-grown cilantro. Other items that help the body detox from mercury (besides cilantro and selenium) are: chlorella, vitamin E, glutathione, garlic, vitamin C, all the leafy green vegetables, and hyaluronic acid.

• Mercury Kills the Heart

For some reason, the heart is particularly sensitive to mercury, more so than the rest of the body. When patients with *idiopathic cardiomyopathy* were studied, it was discovered that they had 22,000 times more mercury in their *heart muscle* than the group of *the same age* without this fatal disorder (102)! This disease eventually leads to *heart failure,* and patients will usually die unless they have a heart transplant (102). For those who already have heart problems, especially prevalent in the elderly population, this is why vaccines with mercury can be so dangerous for them, especially *the flu vaccines*, which still *contain mercury* (102). As described at www.yourhealthbase.com/amalgams.html, scientists from the University of Kuopio, Finland, just finished "a major study which clearly implicates mercury as a major cause of heart attacks and other coronary and cardiovascular diseases" (261). They believe that it creates free radicals, wipes out glutathione levels [which we desperately need for good health], and *binds with selenium,* making the mercury useless (261). *Selenium and vitamin E* guard against mercury toxicity (261).

See later in this book for more information on mercury and why it is harming every living person on the planet and causing untold misery through diseases like cancer, autoimmune disorders, and death.

V. More Deadly Chemicals that the FDA Has Allowed in the U.S. Food Supply - ALLOXAN – Food Additive for Making Bread White

For years, you probably have heard nutritionists warn that eating white bread is just like ingesting sugar, but there are other reasons you need to be wary of white flour! Yes, difficult to believe, but TRUE. There is a chemical substance that is added to flour to bleach it white, called *alloxan,* but many people don't know that they are better off eating natural, unbleached flour products free of this useless, toxic chemical! Alloxan is just one of the many thousands of chemical poisons that the FDA believes is SAFE for us, because we only use small amounts of it. Of Course! Again – a LITTLE poison won't hurt, right? As long as it is in small doses! So, every time you eat a slice of white bread, you or your child could be getting a dose of alloxan, a chemical that has already been linked to causing insulin-dependent diabetes and gum disease! And it isn't just in bread, it is also found in cakes, pies, donuts, and hamburger buns—anything made with bleached white flour. You are better off eating organic, unbleached whole grain, flour, cereals, and bread products. Use gluten-free if available.

In a research article from Sao Paulo University in Brazil, it was proven that rats would develop diabetes simply by feeding them alloxan "42 mg/kg" (187). The alloxan caused an inflammatory reaction, diabetes, and periodontal disease in the animals (187). Is this why so many diabetics have a problem with gum disease? Alloxan is so toxic to the B cells in the pancreas, **when research scientists want to induce diabetes in test animals; they simply feed them alloxan** (258)! [Emphasis mine.] When research was done to check alloxan levels in children, it was shocking to discover that diabetic children had much higher levels of the chemical in their blood than non-diabetic children, indicating that indeed, alloxan is a culprit in causing insulin-dependent diabetes in children (258). When alloxan is digested in the body, it produces destructive free radicals which promote "diseases from autoimmunity" (258). Alloxan also causes Type II diabetes (302). Remember that diabetics have high levels of glucose in their cells and this raises the body's acidity. High acidic levels over long periods of time promote all chronic diseases.

You may want to re-think that fourth cup of caffeinated coffee in the morning. Studies show that when you ingest caffeine, the caffeine has the capacity to create alloxan in the body, which means that eating foods rich in caffeine can increase your risk for diabetes (137).

• Drowning In a Chemical Sewer

When was the last time that YOU as a consumer got to vote on which chemicals and small levels of POISON could be added to your flour supply? Your water supply? Why are such decisions made without the majority of citizens knowing anything about them? Alloxan is a chemical that is added to flour to whiten it so that it appears cleaner, brighter, and more attractive! The same thing is done with fruits. They are often sprayed with chemical waxes to make them shiny and more appealing to the eyes, but who wants to eat wax on their fruit? Did anyone ask YOU if you minded having wax sprayed on your fruit?

We are constantly being bombarded with chemicals just like alloxan, many worse than alloxan, on a daily basis in our environment. It is in the air we breathe, in the food we eat, in the crops we harvest, in the water we drink, in our dental fillings, and in pharmaceutical drugs, and more and more of these chemical poisons are being added to our lives everyday under the guise of social improvement—for the good of all—of course! Are you tired of all the poisons? Are you SICK of all the poisons? Where does it end? When does it stop? When do we say: enough is enough?! When does the FDA become accountable to the citizenry of this nation for all their devilment? When are they going to be scrubbed and replaced with people who truly CARE about the health of our citizens?

VI. Safe Daily Intake of Selenium

In an article by Dr. Richard A. Passwater, Ph.D., he says that "many natural diets contain more than 600 micrograms of selenium daily," and that in "Northern Greenland, many residents consume about 1,300 micrograms of selenium daily" (264). When people in China realized selenium could prevent them from a multitude of diseases, many began taking "1,000 micrograms of selenium daily..." The only side effects they had were thickened fingernails and a garlic-like breath," and one woman who took an incredible "2,400,000 micrograms of selenium daily for seventy-five days" had "only mild and reversible side effects." The writer pointed out that this was "12,000 times the recommended upper limit for supplementation for healthy people" (264). Now THAT is a LOT of selenium and it killed no one!

CHAPTER 8

Iodine, Lost Treasure, Medical Marvel

****

I. Skimping On Iodine Can Kill You

Iodine is as essential to the body as vitamin C, magnesium, and every other vitamin and mineral discussed in this book and my first two books. New studies have come out showing that iodine, the type found in dietary seaweed, could be a major help in reversing metabolic syndrome. Results of human studies showed that consuming just "4 to 6" grams per day of "seaweed, typical for most people in Japan, may be associated with low metabolic syndrome prevalence" (294).

Iodine isn't just for the thyroid gland. According to Dr. Michael Donaldson, "Iodine stabilizes the heart rhythm, lowers serum cholesterol, lowers blood pressure, and is known to make the blood thinner…and improves glucose metabolism…" (73). The country of Finland has been given as an example of what happens when half a nation becomes iodine deficient. In studies during the 1950's, those living further from the sea in eastern Finland were plagued with goiter problems [lack of iodine] (73), and those suffering from goiter had a "3.5 times higher…risk of death from coronary heart disease…" than those in western Finland with normal dietary intake of iodine (73).

Most people in the U.S. have no idea how deficient this nation is in iodine. How did this happen? Well, according to physician, James Howenstine, M.D., a Board Certified Internal Medicine Specialist, one problem began four decades ago when "the food industry decided to remove iodine from baked goods and replace it with bromine" (218). These two ingredients look alike to the thyroid, so the thyroid sucks up the bromine without hesitation; however, there is one really BIG problem! Bromine has absolutely no value at all and it has some very bad affects on the human body, unlike iodine, which every cell in the body desperately needs. As noted by Dr. Howenstine:

> Bromine inhibits the activity of iodine in the thyroid gland. Bromine also can cause impaired thinking and memory, drowsiness, dizziness and irritability. This substitution of bromine for iodine has resulted in nearly universal deficiency of iodine in the American populace. Iodine therapy helps the body eliminate fluoride, bromine, lead, cadmium, arsenic, aluminum and mercury. **Could this substitution of bromine for iodine have been carried out to increase diseases and thus *create more need for pharmaceutical drugs*** (218)? [Emphasis mine. Consider that last sentence carefully!]

Some good natural sources of iodine include "sardines... brown and red seaweeds" (such as *kombu* (218), dulse, nori and laminaria), as well as "most seafoods...shellfish, especially oysters...unrefined sea salt, kelp...fish broth, butter, pineapple, artichokes, asparagus, dark green vegetables and eggs" (286).

Dr. D. Brownstein said that as he began using "12.5-50mg/day" in his patients: "I began to see positive results...goiters and nodules of the thyroid shrank. Cysts on the ovaries became smaller and began to disappear... [people reported] better sleep...I realized what I was taught in medical school was incorrect. The iodization of salt was adequate to lessen the prevalence of goiter, but it did not address the rest of the body's need for iodine" (180). Is it any wonder that he observed that "as iodine levels have fallen over 50% in the last 30 years in the United States, autoimmune disorders and hyperthyroid symptoms have been increasing at near epidemic proportions" (180)?!

II. Iodine for Cancer Patients

Lugol's iodine was made in 1829 by J.G.A. Lugol, a physician in France, and it contains "5% iodine, 10% potassium iodide and distilled water" (267). It is sometimes used during natural disasters for drinking water purification at the rate of "three drops of Lugol's iodine per liter of water" (267). Never take this form of iodine if you are allergic to iodine, nor should iodine be taken by those with "pulmonary edema, bronchitis or known tuberculosis unless" ordered by their doctor (267).

You can only get the 7% Lugol's now by prescription; however, it is available on the internet in weaker solutions, such as 2%, at some online health stores. The best iodine for topical use on the breasts (for women with breast cancer), is Lugol's 7%. Topical magnesium oil should also be used for anyone with cancer. If you are looking for a 2% Lugol's solution, you can find it at Swanson Health Products: *swansonvitamins.com*.

(For a website with a link that will give you directions on making your own Lugol's Solution, see: *http://www.veggieterryann.com/?q=node/39)* (74).

The most gentle and effective iodine that I have found, and use myself for oral consumption is *Magnascent© Iodine*, available at *www.magnascent.com*. You can write them at: Shield Bearer, Inc., 11320 Mountain View Drive, Azle, Texas 76020, or call them with your questions at: (817) 444-4204. Their iodine is available in 1% and 2% solutions.

• Iodine & Yeast

During the early fifties, Dr. Orion Truss saved a man's life by giving him "six to eight drops of Lugol's solution four times a day," when "Candida infestation of the blood" from taking antibiotics for a finger cut had nearly killed him (74). Website *nourishedmagazine.com*, lists other good sources for killing Candida: *clover oil, coconut oil, garlic, oil of oregano, Pau D'arco*, the last two to be avoided by women who are pregnant (310). They also suggest "all the cabbage and onion families..." as good Candida killers (310). You can significantly reduce fungal growths in your body with a diet of fish and fish oils, fresh herbs, spices, yogurt, garlic, onions, leafy greens, chlorella, spirulina, wheat grass juice, barley grass juice and fresh sprouts (use organic whenever possible), and keeping the body in an alkaline state.

Well, if as Dr. Simoncini believes (see Chapters 10 and 11 in this book), that cancer is a FUNGUS, does it not make sense to use this valuable mineral against cancer, when you realize that iodine will kill fungi and parasites on contact? Dr. Simoncini has used 7% iodine several times a day, painted on his skin cancer patients (the lesion is painted), until the growth shrivels up and falls off. See his website at: *http://www.cancer fungus.com*.

There are also specific fungicidal drugs used to kill fungal infections. Fungi are hard to kill because they are not like bacteria. *Fungi* are a closer kin to *animals*...than are bacteria, one reason they are so difficult to treat (56). They can quickly exchange genetic material, morphing into new strains and building up resistance to fungicides, much like bacteria build up resistance to antibiotics (56). Of Lugol's solution, Dr. Daniel H. Duffy asks: "Why did doctors quit using Lugol's solution, the sure cure for thyroid disease? Why did the medical quacks bring in anti-thyroid drugs and goitrogens to kill the thyroid gland when iodine was being used so successfully for so long" (286)?

When sixty people with different forms of cancer were checked, it was discovered that every single one of them had very "serious iodine" deficiencies (217). Dr. James Howenstine works mostly with thyroid patients. He says that you can't make up for deficiencies in iodine by taking iodized salt, because you would have to take "20 teaspoons" per day for sufficient amounts! He describes a type of iodine to correct this deficiency that was developed by Dr. G.E. Abrahams called "Iodoral." It is a tablet made of "dried Lugol's solution containing 12.5 mg of iodine per tablet" (217). He says that if you have sufficient iodine in your body and you ingest "4 of these tablets (50 mg.)," you will "excrete 90% of the iodine in" the urine (217).

Dr. Abrahams believes that in order to keep "sufficient amounts of iodine in the body," we need to take in "13 **mg** daily," and "this is 100 times more than the government recognized RDA for iodine" (217). He says that the thyroid needs *six mg*, females need *5 mg* for their breasts, and the other *2 mg* is for the rest of the body, with men using a little less iodine than women (217). (Women with larger breasts need more iodine.) Dr. Howenstine also mentions another form of iodine known as *Triodide*, which is produced by Scientific Botanicals, Seattle, Washington, and says that it "has the same dosage of iodine and iodide combined with a sea vegetable called bladderwrack," as is found in Iodoral (217).

In order to get started, Abrahams "recommends taking 50 mg of Iodoral (four 12.5 mg tablets) [or] Lugol's solution [7%] (8 drops) or Triodide (8 drops) daily for 3 months as a loading dose," then to gradually lower the dosage "to the 12.5 mg maintenance dosage under the supervision of a knowledgeable health care professional" (217). He believes "that 14 to 15 mg. of iodine/iodide daily is the upper maximum of safety" (217). However, the article also notes that scientists in Japan found hypothyroid patients "who were taking 20 mg. of iodine or more daily" (217) without problems.

• Iodine Resources

See website *www.magnascent.com* for information on Magnascent© iodine. This is a very gentle form of iodine, less harsh than Lugol's iodine. Just remember that iodine can kill viruses (as well as bacteria and fungi), but antibiotics will not kill viruses. You can get Lugol's 7% iodine only by prescription. At one time, you could walk into a pharmacy and purchase 7% Lugol's without a prescription. You can, however, get the 2% Lugol's from *Swansonvitamins.com*.

• High Iodine Consumption = Low Statistics for Breast Cancer

Dr. G.E. Abrahams described two breast cancer remissions that occurred in women who took "75 mg of Iodoral daily," and he believes that "iodine deficiency" is largely responsible for the formation of "breast cancer and prostate cancer" (215) (217). Also, being deficient in iodine greatly increases the risk for not only breast and prostate cancers, but ovarian and endometrial cancers as well (215) (217). And for women who take "thyroid hormone therapy," their risk for breast cancer increases with each year that they are on the hormone therapy (215) (217). These studies could very well mean that instead of thyroid hormone replacement, women might be better off correcting an "iodine deficiency," which could "eliminate the need for thyroid hormone," thus reducing their risks for breast cancer (215) (217). A good verification of this approach could be made by comparing breast cancer rates of Japanese women to those of women elsewhere in the world. Japanese women ingest high amounts of seaweed and "have the highest iodine intake (13.8 mg. daily) of women anywhere in the world," with fewer cases of breast cancer of any other country (215) (217). It is amazing that the Japanese actually ingest "100 times more iodine than Americans," per day, and most of their iodine is from seaweed (251).

Dr. Donald W. Miller teaches cardiac surgery at the University Of Washington School Of Medicine and the Seattle VA Medical Center.

You can reach his website at: *http://www.donaldmiller.com*. He says that the people of Japan are "clear evidence that large amounts of iodine cannot be very bad for a population (251). To get the amount of iodine the Japanese consume in one day, if you were eating fish as your iodine source, "you would have to eat 10-20 pounds of fish per day" (251). U.S. consumers ingest about "240 micrograms...of iodine a day...people in Japan consume more than 12 milligrams (mg) of iodine a day." This is 12,000 micrograms eaten by the Japanese in their daily diets in comparison to the 240 micrograms ingested by Americans (249). Is it any wonder that the breast cancer rate in the U.S. was "1 in 20 women" three decades ago when they ingested twice the iodine they do today? Compare that to statistics today that show women in the U.S. developing breast cancer at the rate of "1 in 7" (249) and higher in some areas. Dr. Miller says that the human body needs iodine "in microgram amounts for the thyroid, mg amounts for breast and other tissues, and can be used therapeutically in gram amounts" (251).

Dr. Miller further explains that the reason for most of the resistance to using milligram amounts of iodine from physicians who treat thyroid disorders is because of the "Wolfe-Chaikoff Effect," which is a "temporary depression of thyroid hormone synthesis when you take large doses of iodine. But, this effect is not of clinical significance," and because "TSH can go up," this only happens in very "few people..." and he adds "there are no clinical symptoms of hypothyroidism" (251).

- ## Iodine/Selenium Deficiencies & Breast Cancer

Besides the work of super antioxidants in preventing and curing cancers, such as breast cancer, the fact that our soils have been leached of minerals is the focus of much concern in cancer prevention. Maureen Kennedy Salaman, popular nutrition author and health advocate, warns in her excellent book, *Nutrition: The Cancer Answer II,* of the disastrous consequences we face as a nation due to the lack of essential minerals in our soils (278). Many of our soils are leached of vital cancer-preventing nutrients, such as iodine and selenium, both important breast cancer preventatives (278). Ms. Salaman has an excellent line of health products, including an easily-absorbable, good-tasting, mineral drink called *Mineral Rich®* that you can find along with many other nutritional products at her website: *www.mksalaman.com*. Her health products are also available at many health food stores.

Human studies have shown that insufficient levels of selenium in the diet can lead to type II diabetes, as well as gestational diabetes. A recent study involving men, who took selenium for cancer prevention, stated that those men who took selenium only (as opposed to those who took it with vitamin E) had a higher incidence of diabetes. It is apparent from looking at both studies, that we need **all** the nutrients and vitamins as given by our Creator, not just isolated supplements working alone.

We also need to be asking what kind of vitamin E was used in these human studies? Synthetic E or natural vitamin E as given by God, and what kind of selenium was used? Was it organic as found in L-selenomethionine, selenocysteine, methylselenocysteine, or inorganic selenate, selenide or selenite? Trying to compare the naturally organic easily-absorbable supplements with inorganic, poorly-absorbed supplements is like trying to compare apples with oranges.

Studies have shown that if you have sufficient levels of selenium in your diet, this will give you some protection against iodine deficiency (163), but not indefinitely. Iodine is much underrated. We are told that only very tiny amounts of iodine are needed by the human body on a daily basis, when in fact, this mineral is needed in every single function in the body.

In an article by Dr. Bruce West at *www.oasisadvancedwellness.com/learning/iodine-fulfillment-therapy.html*, it is revealed that:

> In addition to thyroid therapy, all thyroid patients should be on iodine therapy with the goal to reach a whole body iodine sufficiency [and] Synthroid or thyroid-destructive therapies should never be taken without iodine therapy – something you will never hear from your endocrinologist. If all Thyroidologists and endocrinologists were forced to fluorescence scan their patients' thyroid glands, they would then have to fact up to the damages they are causing to these glands and their patients (305).

Dr. West admits that in the first 60 years of the 1900s, nearly "every single U.S. physician used Lugol's (iodine) supplements in his or her practice for both hypo- and hyperthyroid, as well as many, many other conditions – all with excellent results" (305). He says that doctors could get as much as a "90% cure rate" with both hyperthyroid and hypothyroid in using [iodine] "doses of six to 37 mgs daily," doses that were "once considered normal" (305). "Expert Thyroidologists like Dr. Abraham are convinced that the medical iodine phobia has a great deal to do [with the] "epidemic of cardiac arrhythmias and atrial fibrillation in this country" (305). He also adds that:

> Whole body iodine sufficiency is also a critical means to counter the side effects of thyroid hormone medications (Synthroid, etc). Long-term use of these drugs is associated with depletion of thyroid and tissue iodine levels as well as **increased rates of cancer**. Fluorescent scanning of the thyroid clearly shows how drug and other medical thyroid therapies deplete the gland and body of critical iodine (305).
> [Emphasis mine.]

Iodine also rids the body of dangerous mercury and other heavy metals. You can apply iodine topically for absorption using Lugol's iodine that can be found at some health food stores, but only at 2% strength. It takes a prescription to get Lugol's at 7% strength; however, I believe the best form of taking iodine is a gentle food grade form known as *Magnascent© Iodine*. See Appendix II in the back of this book for suppliers of this iodine source. It is the original *Nascent Iodine*. Much of the body's iodine in women is concentrated in the breasts, thyroid, and ovaries. Is it any wonder then that iodine deficiencies also show up in cancers that affect these organs? Hello? Why is 99% of the medical profession failing to connect-the-dots here?

• Iodine, Magnesium, Soda Bicarb & Cure for Invasive Prostate Cancer

For an amazing study on the importance of alkalizing the body with a rapid, powerful ingredient as simple as sodium bicarbonate, see Chapters 10, 11 and 15 of this book. You can get *Arm & Hammer®* soda bicarb at your local grocers rather inexpensively. They do not advertise the product for cancer use, but it is used for alkalizing a "sour stomach". There has been some controversy about aluminum in baking soda, but *Arm & Hammer®* says that their product contains no aluminum. For a company that sells a soda bicarb that they guarantee to be aluminum-free, see Bob's Red Mill products at: *http://www.bobs*

redmill.com (288). (I have used both.) Simply use pH testing strips that you can get at your local health food store to quickly and easily check your urine or saliva pH.

You can also alkalize rapidly with little packets of *Alka-Seltzer® Gold*, which contain not only soda bicarb, but potassium bicarb as well. Don't take alkalizers like soda bicarb or *Alka-Seltzer® Gold* if you have a stomach full of food because they neutralize stomach acid and your food will just sit there and not digest! Do NOT use regular *Alka-Seltzer®*, as it contains aspirin.

• Zapping Cancer with Iodine & Magnesium

Dr. Mark Sircus has much to say about the pervasive lack of magnesium and iodine in the average diet, and why these deficiencies are causing heart disease, cancer, and many other diseases. See his books: *Magnesium The Ultimate Heart Medicine* and *Magnesium Medicine The Lamp of Life,* available at: *http://www.magnesiumfor life.com,* and *Iodine Bringing Back the Universal Medicine,* available at website: *http://imva.info* (287). These books are great! I have read them and I highly recommend all of them.

III. Iodine for Other Diseases

Nascent iodine has been used in successfully treating malaria, dengue fever, influenza, GI problems, urinary infections, high blood pressure, venereal diseases, throat infections, sinus, ear, and eye infections, tonsillitis, asthma, bronchitis, pharyngitis, poison ivy, arthritis, and other diseases (74). For "severe eye inflammation," the dosage of Nascent used is "Five to ten drops of nascent iodine into one ounce of water" as an "eye lotion" (74). For the original Nascent iodine supplement, see website: *www.maganascent.com.*

As described at website *www.vitamincfoundation.org,* apparently once again, the public has been misled by conventional medical beaurocrats severely understating the levels of a nutrient that is vital for our survival (75):

> According to Dr. G. E. Abrahams, 'Of all the elements known so far to be essential for health, iodine is the most

misunderstood and the most feared. Yet, it is by far the safest of all the trace elements known to be essential for human health. It is the only trace element that can be ingested safely in amounts up to 100,000 times the RDA. For example, potassium iodide has been prescribed safely to pulmonary patients in daily amounts of up to 6.0 gm/day, in large groups of such patients for several years. It is important however to emphasize that this safety record only applies to inorganic nonradioactive iodine/iodide, not to organic iodine-containing drugs and to radioiodides' (75).

• Iodine for Fibrocystic Breast Disease

Dr. Donald Miller also discusses a study in Russia from the 1970's revealing that "iodine cured FBD [fibrocystic breast disease] in 70% of women (251). He also notes that women diagnosed with an "iodine-deficient goiter have three times the rate of breast cancer," and agrees with other physicians who believe that "Fibrocystic Breast Disease and Breast Cancer are iodine-deficiency disorders, just like goiter and cretinism" (251). If you start taking iodine supplements or drops, you may initially develop acne and a "brassy taste" in the mouth. This is because taking in iodine kicks the bromide (also referred to as bromine) out of your body and bromide is toxic and useless. Iodine also helps rid the body of fluoride (251). Dr. Miller believes that the view that "iodine should not exceed 300 mcg per day…is without good evidence. Studies that show that iodine in mg amounts can cure FBD [fibrocystic breast disease] are ignored" (251). Iodine in milligram amounts is needed for health (251), not microgram amounts.

    Dr. David Derry considers "fibrocystic disease of the breast" as the "first phase of [breast] cancer, and says that it only takes "One drop (6.5 mg per drop) of Lugol's [7%] daily in water, orange juice or milk" to "gradually eliminate the first phase" of this "cancer development" (286). He insists that this dosage also works for cancer of the prostate, as it "is similar to breast cancer in many respects," and "will help with most cancers" (286). He adds that "higher doses of iodine are required for inflammatory breast cancer," and says that taking high dose iodine by I.V. is perfectly safe (286). Dr. Derry says that "Iodine is by far the best antibiotic, antiviral and antiseptic of all time," and calls it the "Universal Pathogen Killer," that "has been completely ignored by modern medicine" (193). He further explains that "only iodine is capable of killing all classes of pathogens: gram-positive and gram-negative bacteria, mycobacteria, fungi, yeasts, viruses and protozoa," and it kills "Most bacteria" in just "15 to 30 seconds of contact" (193). A *missionary in Zambia* used iodine to kill **malaria** by placing "20 drops of Nascent Iodine in a half glass of water given 4 or 5 times during the first day and then decreased the dose to 10 drops of Nascent Iodine 4 times a day for 3 more days" (193). This same article by Dr. Derry also states that this "protocol can be used for the swine flu or any other type of influenza," and often much higher doses have been given (e.g. using "Lugol's and Iodoral for cancer treatment") (193).

As noted earlier, be aware that when you begin taking iodine, you may experience a side effect known as *bromism,* where the iodine is flushing toxic bromine from your body (17). Symptoms can include: "lethargy, depression, 'dark' thoughts, 'brain fog,' constipation, leg and hip pain, acne, rashes and other symptoms," which can be reversed in a day or two by stopping the iodine dose and using a "washout" of "Celtic salt in water" (17). See the details on how to do this under **The Iodine Protocol** of ***BreastCancerChoices.org*** later in this chapter.

In an article from the *Journal of American Physicians and Surgeons,* Vol 11, Number 4, Winter 2006, Dr. Miller stated that "The recommended dietary intake [RDA] of 100-150 mcg [of iodine] is perhaps 100 times too low" (251). He says that the "ductal cells in the breast, the ones most likely to become cancerous, are equipped with an iodine pump…the same one that the thyroid gland has" for soaking up iodine (141).

Some physicians are now questioning the wisdom of chemo for breast cancer patients. Drugs known as "anthracyclines are a breast chemo staple despite" the fact that "they **weaken women's hearts** (141). As noted by Duke University cardiologist, Dr. Pamela Douglas, "In the process of curing their breast cancer, we've exposed them to some pretty nasty things. And it's not just one nasty thing, it's a sequence of nasty things" (141). Even Avastin (with all its potential deadly side effects, is being discontinued as a chemo drug for breast cancer).

• Iodine & Cancer Rates

Thailand and Mexico have deficient iodine and "high rates of breast cancer and goiter" (215) (217). People in Iceland have a "high iodine intake" and "low rates of goiter and breast cancer" (215) (217).

Dr. Robert Rowen, M.D., studied 60 cancer patients, all having *various types* of cancer. Every single one of them had excessive levels of bromine in their body and critically low amounts of iodine (274)! Since 100% of his cancer patients were iodine deficient, what should that tell us about the rest of the cancer sufferers in the world (274)? Does it not seem likely that the medical profession in the U.S. and other high breast cancer rate countries would connect-the-dots with these statistics and reach the obvious conclusion that IODINE prevents breast cancer and other cancers and has even cured the disease?! Yet, how many physicians are telling their cancer patients (and women at risk for breast cancer) to take iodine in **milligram** dosages, rather than **micro**gram amounts? Ask YOUR doctor about this. Take this book with you and point out this chapter to your physician. If your concerns are merely dismissed as insignificant, find a physician who will listen, or a good Naturopathic doctor. (See Appendix II in the back of this book for resources.)

Dr. W. W. Greene, D.C. says of iodine:

> Of all the elements known so far to be essential for health, IODINE is the most misunderstood. Yet, it is by far the safest of all the trace elements known to be essential for human health. It is the only trace element that can be ingested safely in amounts up to 100,000 times the RDI. It is estimated by myself and other clinicians that probably 90% or more of the population of the United States is grossly deficient in Iodine. In fact, it must be noted that Iodine is the single most deficient nutrient in the world --- **with approximately 70% of the world's population deficient** (76). [Emphasis mine.]

In his e-book, *Iodine: Bring Back the Universal Nutrient Medicine*, Dr. Mark Sircus AC., OMD quotes Dr. H. Duff who says that "I was shrinking tumors in the early 70's by using thousands of times the RDA on iodine. Iodine along with the proper essential fat will fix just about any thyroid problem" (285), and according to him: "There is one form of iodine...called Magnascent©, which is safe to give even to babies, even at much higher doses than are on the label for adults" (285), and for people who say they are allergic to iodine, perhaps they are using harsh forms. Magnascent© is a very gentle form of iodine. Dr. Sircus adds:

> J. Edgar Hoover said: 'The individual is handicapped by coming face-to-face with a conspiracy so monstrous he cannot believe it exists.' When it comes to iodine suspect the worst from top government health officials who only seem to want to poison the public. What can one say about an FDA that, for example continues to assert the safety of aspartame when scientists around the world are finding it to be the worst food additive ever used? Now that there is an iodine revival going on expect the FDA to clamp down on its availability (286).

I always advise my readers to consult with their physician or pediatrician about iodine intake for themselves or their children, but be prepared for an argument and a total dismissal of your concerns, because most conventional doctors would never go above or beyond the RDA for iodine. Mention any of the amounts recommended by the physicians in the research articles in this book (for specific conditions and prevention measures) and you may get a blank stare and dismissive shrug from your physician or this comment: ***"As long as you are eating a balanced diet and feeding your children a balanced diet, and using iodized table salt, and eating seafood once in a while, you will get plenty of iodine. You don't need to supplement."*** That is the "PAT" answer that most physicians give to their patients, because they do not want to deal with iodine supplementation, so be prepared for it! Most people do not realize that a great deal of the iodine in their iodized table salt has already evaporated from the salt in their container, and many others have cut back so drastically on their salt intake, it wouldn't matter if it DID have iodine in it – they don't get it anyway! (And how many Americans and their children actually get a healthy "balanced diet" in this fast-paced world we live in?) Opting for a Naturopathic physician, who can advise you on iodine, may be your best choice.

• The Diabetes, Iodine Link

Some very interesting studies have been done showing that keeping sufficient levels of iodine in the body may help prevent the development of diabetes, because iodine (in a way that is not fully understood) increases the body's sensitivity to insulin (78). In one human study in particular, Dr. Jorge Flechas, who sometimes uses Iodoral "to treat fibrocystic breast disease," discovered that he was able to wean 6 out of 12 of his diabetic patients off all of their diabetic medications by simply giving them "50 mg to 100 mg per day of iodine" (78). These are **milligrams** we are speaking of, not **micrograms!** One of his "insulin dependent diabetics was able to reduce" their "Lantus insulin from 98 units to 44 units per day within a period of a few weeks" (78). He also said that he was able to help some of his Type 1 diabetics to "get off their insulin," or assist them in decreasing "the total amount of insulin needed to control their glucose," if their "C-peptide is measurable" meaning that they were "making their own insulin" (78). See Dr Flechas' website at: *http://cypress.h e.net/~bigmacnc/drflechas/index.htm/IOD50.htm* (78). Note that Iodoral is "the Lugol's formula in tablet form," which is gentler and less irritating to the stomach (77). See website *www.magnascent.com* for an even milder, easily absorbed form of iodine, *Magnascent©*.

Dr. John Young, a Florida physician and diabetic researcher, puts his diabetic patients on "alkaline protein and minerals with a form of iodine that he says reverses the process in [Type II] diabetes patients in eight to 12 weeks." He says that he "resets the pancreas and permanently returns patients to normal" (238).

IV. The Iodine Protocol

Guy Abraham, MD, David Brownstein, MD, and Jorge Flechas, MD., have cared for more than "4,000 patients with iodine supplementation," and they recommend the below protocol from *breastcancerchoices.org*, not merely for those with breast cancer (77):

BreastCancerChoices.Org Iodine Protocol
Developed & Published From Their October 2007 Iodine Conference
(Reprinted with their permission)

- 50 mg Iodoral minimum for breast cancer (may start with 12.5 mg). Some practitioners may recommend another form of Iodine such as Lugol's...
- Vitamin C – 3,000 mg per day (more may be necessary to detox bromide)
- 300-600 mg magnesium oxide or comparable magnesium supplement.
- 200 micrograms selenium
- 500 milligram niacin (B3) twice a day. (NOT niacinamide) Start lower to avoid flush...[you can also use an alternative known as ATP Cofactor and it is available at *www.breastcancerchoices.org*].
- 100 mg Vitamin B2 three times a day [See above about using the ATP Cofactor instead].
- A comprehensive vitamin and nutrition program. [Note that you can purchase Iodoral and ATP CoFactor, as well as Lypo-Spheric™ Vitamin C at *breastcancerchoices.org/order.html.*]
- (Feb 2008) Dr. Guy Abraham cautions that 'excess calcium supplementation (2,000-3,000 mg/day) has been the most common cause of poor response to iodine supplementation' (see *Vitamin Research News* Vol 22, Number 2.) (77).

BreastCancerChoices.Org recommends that you should have the "**24 hour Iodine Loading Test** before beginning iodine supplementation to see if you might have a possible iodine absorption defect" (77).

I had not seen this protocol before I developed the *Orange Wunder Formula* that I used in Chapter 2. I was surprised to see two of the ingredients that I had already been using in my formula.

• Fighting the Bromide Problem

In order to help prevent the side effects of the iodine as it pushes toxic bromide out of your body when you begin an iodine protocol, such as the one above, "Many iodine takers found the *Salt Loading Protocol* devised by Dr. William Shevin (and presented at the February '07

Iodine Conference) to be effective in eliminating the side effects such as bromide sedation, acne, brain fog, brassy taste, mouth sores, frontal headache or other symptoms which occur in a small percentage of patients" (77). If interested, you can find the formula for the Salt Loading Protocol at *BreastCancerChoices.Org* website. How many people are aware that iodine has been shown to kill more breast cancer cells than *Fluorouracil,* a common chemo drug, but without the side effects (77)? Fluorouracil is sold under several different brand names.

V. Iodine & The Brain

In a presentation at the 24th Annual Meeting of *Doctors of Disaster Preparedness* at Portland State University in August of 2006, Dr. Donald W. Miller, Jr., M.D., reported that it is estimated that as many as 50 million children "including 10 million in China," suffer from mental retardation due to severe iodine deficiencies (250). A study in Sicilian children revealed that "two-thirds" of those "born in an iodine deficient area had attention deficit and hyperactivity disorders (ADHD)," yet none of the kids born in an area with sufficient iodine were afflicted with ADHD (250). What do physicians in the U.S. resort to for ADHD? Certainly not iodine. No, they give prescription drugs instead!

The most severe lack of iodine in the diet causes one of the worst types of mental retardation known that also includes severe "physical deformities," and it is known as *Cretinism* (250).

From website: *www.thyroidnascentiodine.com/cancer.htm* for help killing a sore throat:

> Painting iodine on my wrist gets rid of my sore throat every time! Iodine definitely works for me, however, I find it best to use the clear 'decolorized' iodine, available at most drugstores. I paint it on the inside of the wrists (where the veins are closest to the skin) and on the sides of the throat (141). [Note that this is NOT a type of iodine that can be diluted with water and taken by mouth.]

Dr. John Myers recommends "iodine sprayed on the mucous lining of a woman's vagina" [for women with cystic or lumpy breasts], which he says will "be absorbed and will soften [the] breasts in a matter of 5 minutes" (141).

Even if you supplement with iodine, there are many environmental poisons that will strip iodine from your body on a daily basis. These include: fluoride, chlorine, bromide, mercury, "aspirin...steroids, and unfermented soy products" (215) (217). Be aware that people with kidney problems cannot use iodine therapy unless closely supervised by their physicians.

VI. Check Your Thyroid Function

Dr. Mark Sircus points out that a good way to check your thyroid function is by measuring your "oral temperature before getting out of bed in the morning" (286) [your basal body temperature], and if it is below 97.6 degrees Fahrenheit, you should be concerned. Your "mid-afternoon... temperature should be 98.6" (286). The report also says that the body's blood supply passes through the thyroid "Every 17 minutes... and if our thyroid has an adequate supply of iodine, blood-borne bacteria and viruses are killed off as the blood passes through the thyroid" (286). Can you see how the thyroid acts like a filter in your body, filtering out and killing germs, but only when it is well-supplied with iodine?

CHAPTER 9

Glutathione (GSH) Cellular Warrior

****

I. Keeping Levels of GSH High

Glutathione is one of the most important cell defenders in the body, a nutritional substance that is found in every cell, without which we would soon die. It is the most important nutrient within the cells, and vitamin C is the most important nutrient outside of the cells (231). How much of this nutrient is found in your cells is a good indicator of your potential longevity. If levels drop too low, you will die. GSH is made up of "three...amino acids...cysteine, glycine, & glutamic acid" (57).

Though vitamin C is the king nutrient outside the cell walls, and GSH inside the walls, you must have sufficient amounts of one to effectively regulate and allow the other to do its job. In his book, *GSH MASTER DEFENDER Against Disease, Toxins, and Aging,* Dr. Thomas E. Levy goes into great detail describing the importance of this vital nutrient in all cellular processes. It helps neutralize heavy metals (like mercury and lead to name a few), toxins, viruses, bacteria, fungi, parasites, boosts the body's natural immunity, protects other antioxidants from destruction, such as vitamin C and vitamin E, and helps protect the heart against damage, abnormal rhythms, and high blood pressure (231).

This miraculous nutrient also lessens the likelihood or the severity of asthma, and insufficient levels will increase your risk for COPD, cystic fibrosis, ARDS, arthritis, cancer, cirrhosis, hepatitis, rapid aging, and many other chronic diseases (231). In combination with vitamin C, glutathione can also prevent and treat cataract formation and glaucoma (231). Dr. Levy also discusses a new state-of-the-art delivery system for getting maximum absorption out of the glutathione (GSH) that you take. It is **liposomal GSH** and can be found from the same laboratories that produce the famous liposomal vitamin C known as ***Lypo-Spheric™ C***. Their product is available at website: *http://www.livonlabs.com*. I went into more detail in other areas of this book on the high absorption capacity that the human body has for liposomes, as opposed to taking pills.

One thing to remember is that glutathione breaks down in stomach acid and much of it is lost that way. Taking it in the form of liposomes protects it and allows it to reach the fat-loving cells, unhindered by gastric acid (231).

Note that there are many ways that you can boost your glutathione levels in the body naturally, besides taking the liposomal GSH. This can be done by including glutathione-rich foods (such as asparagus and avocados) in your diet, as well as the following (231):

- B6
- B12
- CoQ10 supplements taken with L-Carnitine & ALA (Alpha Lipoic Acid)
- Folic acid
- Garlic
- Glutamine
- Immunocal (a form of undenatured whey protein)
- Magnesium
- NAC (N-acetylcysteine)
- SAM (S-adenosyl-L-methionine)
- Selenium
- Sesame oil
- Taheebo tea
- Vanadium
- Vitamin C
- Vitamin E
- Zinc (231).

Always take GSH with selenium and B2 to enhance its absorption (255). According to Steven Petrosino, Ph.D., at website *www.nutritionadvisor.com*, you can increase your body's glutathione levels *with undenatured whey protein isolate*, as well as with "the herb milk thistle...[and] curcumin...riboflavin... selenium... asparagus, avocados, squash, okra, cauliflower, broccoli, potatoes, spinach, walnuts, garlic, and raw tomatoes...." (36) Other nutrients that increase the body's production of glutathione (besides vitamin C), are natural nutrients that can be found in the sulfur and cruciferous veggies (165) (166).

You can find undenatured whey protein isolate at *www.nutritionadvisor.com* in a brand known as *Immunocal,* as well as more information on the scientific studies performed on this supplement. It is the only whey protein isolate listed in the *Physician's Desk Reference* (PDR), but you do not need a prescription to obtain it. Most health food stores carry this nutrient. You can also find an excellent non-GMO whey protein formula at Dr. Mercola's website: *http://proteinpowder.mercola.com/Whey-Protein-With-Aminogen.html.* This whey formula also contains an amino acid known as *Aminogen,* which helps the body digest the protein.

See other sources of glutathione below and other ways to raise your levels. Whey protein is important because it is so high in glutathione. I use this protein mix in one of my recipes in Chapter 2 of this book.

Animal studies show that several spices and plants can raise glutathione levels in the body. Scientists concluded from their studies that these phyto-compounds can help play a role in the prevention and suppression of cancer (e.g., the next time you bake bread, you may want to add some poppy seed or flax seed). Flax seed can be used for cooking, if you soak them "in water for at least an hour before using them..." (207).

• GSH & Liver Protection

GSH is very protective of the liver, but it is the liver that produces large amounts of this essential nutrient, as long as the liver is healthy and functioning normally. As we age the liver ages too and GSH production is drastically decreased. This is why the older we are, and the more compromised our immune systems become, the more GSH we need (231). Glutathione slows down the entire aging process, reducing the onslaught of "premature aging" and the chronic conditions that accompany it. In a nut shell, high amounts of GSH in your body are a good indicator that you will have a *longer* and *healthier* life. Studies have shown that people who live 100 or older have high GSH levels (231).

NAC is a "precursor" to GSH, so taking *NAC (N-acetylcysteine)*, will also elevate glutathione levels, which is important, because adequate amounts of GSH and vitamin C can make a life or death difference in patients battling liver disease (231). GSH re-vitalizes or "recycles" vitamin C, making the vitamin C that we have last longer and fight free radicals more efficiently (231). It has recently been discovered that insufficient amounts of glutathione contribute to the onset of Parkinson's disease, bi-polar disorders and schizophrenia, and that supplementing with GSH can improve these conditions (231). Studies have also shown a link between magnesium deficiency, depression, and schizophrenia (38). It is noteworthy how all of these nutrients are inter-dependent upon each other. If you are lacking just one of them, it can make a major health difference for you.

II. Glutathione Prevents Lung & Other Cancers

Glutathione is another amino acid important in cancer prevention that the body is able to produce if we are not nutritionally-deprived (165). This nutrient helps fight obesity, food addictions, cataracts and several forms of cancer, including those of the urinary system and the lungs (165).

It may not be wise to take glutathione in supplement form (orally) (because of poor absorption) unless you use the liposomal GSH. Taking Vitamin C keeps GSH levels elevated, but does not produce more (165). Glutathione helps the body maintain constant supplies of vitamins C and E by *recycling* these vitamins once the body has *oxidized* them (165). Cooking destroys much of the glutathione in foods. Some excellent sources of this nutrient include: avocados, asparagus, uncooked spinach, apples, carrots, and tomatoes.

• **Glutathione & Vitamin E Prevent Cervical Cancer**

The risk for invasive cancers can be greatly decreased by simply supplementing with 200-400 IU per day of mixed tocopherols (vitamin E) (27). Some researchers believe that the gamma form of vitamin E is superior to the alpha-tocopherol form; however, it is best to have mixed tocopherols and tocotrienols. Do not purchase vitamin E unless you see **tocotrienols** on the list of ingredients! If you decide on the alpha-tocopherol vitamin E, use the **d**-alpha (which is natural), not the **dl**-alpha (which is synthetic), and be sure it is mixed with tocotrienols.

Some good **natural food sources** of vitamin E are: wheat germ oil, olive oil, sunflower oil (and seeds), dandelion greens, spinach, broccoli, turnip greens, almonds and other nuts, eggs (205) (252) (266), kiwi, mangoes, fortified cereals, and fresh sprouts (especially wheat berry sprouts).

Insufficient levels of *glutathione* can mean an increased incidence for cervical cancer (27). Having a pap test with abnormal cells, however, does not necessarily mean a cancerous condition. Lesions that are suspicious in the cervix will lighten in color or whiten if coming into contact with *vinegar* (a way that they can be tested) (27).

III. Glutathione, Endometriosis, Milk Thistle & Skin Disorders

As noted earlier, glutathione is a major antioxidant found throughout the human body, and there are a few substances you can take that will increase its production. Milk thistle is one of them. Milk thistle also helps raise the body's amount of *superoxide dismutase, (SOD),* another potent antioxidant (290). Because the liver can be helped by milk thistle, it may be especially important for people with various types of liver disease (290). It also prompts the regeneration of kidney cells, improves biliary function and digestion of fats (290). Of course, you will need to check with your doctor before using this herb if you have any type of biliary problems, stone formation (290), ulcers, colitis, GERD, Crohn's or IBS.

Though vitamin C aids the body in making more glutathione, milk thistle keeps glutathione reserves from being exhausted in the liver, and it appears to be stronger than either vitamin C or E for this purpose (165). Milk thistle also acts as an anti-inflammatory for skin disorders, such as *psoriasis*. It may help relieve the painful symptoms of *endometriosis,* since it assists liver cells with estrogen use (133). Scientists have discovered that, in animal testing, if the skin suffers dangerous sun exposure, then they apply silymarin topically, melanoma formation was decreased (133). Silymarin comes from milk thistle.

No major side effects have been reported from the use of milk thistle. Though it has a reputation for being exceptionally safe, some users of the herb experience diarrhea on initial use for the first 24 to 48 hours (133). It is recommended that the herb be ingested on an empty stomach. There have been no reports of adverse effects when milk thistle was taken with other routine medications (133). (Of course, as with any herb, there is always the possibility of allergic reactions.)

Do not use this herb if you have allergies to ragweed or daisy-type flowers, dyes, or other allergies (66). Check with your doctor to be certain that milk thistle is appropriate for you. Do not use with alcohol, nor during pregnancy or breast feeding (66).

IV. Glutathione (GSH) & Glutamine

Glutathione helps protect the brain and gastric wall (against toxins) and enhances the body's immunity (255). If you do use glutathione supplements, it is best to combine them with *selenium and vitamin B2* to enhance its function (255). Use natural sources of glutathione, such as raw veggies of every color (e.g., carrots, tomatoes, avocados, asparagus, and spinach). Just remember that cooking and freezing food kills glutathione. This is also true of canned foods (63). This is another reason to consume your veggies and fruit raw, their most nutritious state. Eat tomatoes, both cooked and raw. Cooking appears to increase their lycopene availability, but eating them raw means more glutathione. Eat fresh WHOLE fruits on an empty stomach. Don't mix them with other foods like vegetables and cooked foods, or they will simply ferment in the stomach.

Avocados are not only very rich in glutathione, but they are also high in beta carotene, a better source of *potassium than bananas*, and they may be important in protecting the liver, as well as fighting *viral hepatitis* (24). Avocados are also high in lutein. Another excellent source of beta carotene, which is also high in lutein and other carotenoids, is chlorella. Just be sure to get the broken cell-wall chlorella. Chlorella has the highest amount of chlorophyll of any green food. Try to use LIVE FOODS or whole food sources for your best vitamin/mineral source. Chlorella is one of them. Other whole food sources include: spirulina, brewer's yeast, sesame seeds, wheat germ, whole vitamin C (which contains bioflavanoids), sunflower seeds, pumpkin seeds, sprouts, bee pollen, ginger, wheat grass, barley grass, and organic fruits and vegetables.

An amino acid, known as *glutamine,* is essential for the human body. Tumors feed on glutamine to grow (255). They seem to need excessive amounts of this amino acid, and they absorb it to the extent that the patient's own body is depleted of the nutrient, causing the patient to waste away, a disorder commonly found in cancer patients, called *cachexia* (255). Glutamine appears to boost immunity. Rats with tumors had a remarkable decrease in cancerous growths after just *seven weeks* of "glutamine supplements" (255). Beans, fish, and whey protein contain glutamine. This amino acid is also available in supplement form at health food stores, and is one of the ingredients in my **Orange Wunder Formula** in Chapter 2 of this book.

V. Cancer & THC

A study noted in *ScienceDaily.com* revealed that a substance in marijuana (THC) can shrink lung tumors down to half their size and help prevent them from spreading (4). Medical marijuana has successfully treated "glaucoma, asthma, inflammatory bowel disease, migraines, multiple sclerosis, arthritis, epilepsy, depression, hypertension and Parkinson's disease" (234). It has also been helpful in stimulating the appetite in cancer patients (234). Hemp seed oil is very high in GLA, a natural cancer fighter. Just remember that before you ask your physician about using this substance medically, you must be aware of its potential addictive nature.

CHAPTER 10

CoQ10 – Longevity Yardstick, Cancer Killer

****

I. Coenzyme Q10 – Working Miracles

Cardiologist, Dr. Stephen Sinatra, M.D., F.A.C.C., in his book, *Coenzyme Q10 and the Heart,* considers this super antioxidant miraculous, and says that he would not even think of practicing cardiology without it (282). Though he says that this nutrient is a great remedy for heart disease, he states that most physicians have no idea it exists (282). I can understand where he is coming from. When I had a relative hospitalized for heart disease and took CoQ10 to her physician, and asked him to put her on it, he asked me what it was! He really had no idea. He was a cardiologist, and this was more than five years ago. He refused to allow it. It was not on the hospital formulary!

CoQ10 is useful for many degenerative disorders, hypertension, cancer, gum disease, diabetes, and many others (282). Even more amazing is the fact that the discovery of CoQ10 was accidental.

Apparently, cancer cells absorb substances in a different way than normal healthy cells. According to Dr. Ray D. Strand, author of *What Your Doctor Doesn't Know About Nutritional Medicine May Be Killing You,* normal cells only consume the nutrients that they need, whereas cancer cells don't know when enough is enough. They keep on absorbing nutrients even when they are not needed, as though they haven't the sense to stop (292). In a nutshell—the right nutrients can kill them! Perhaps this accounts for why antioxidants like CoQ10, lycopene, alpha lipoic acid, resveratrol, beta carotene, quercetin, iodine, vitamin C, D, E, magnesium, selenium, and ellagic acid are so powerful. It may also explain why Johanna Brandt's grape cure was so effective. (See Chapter 13 later in this book.) Cancer cells thrive on sugar. The grape diet requires a few days of fasting before starting.

Then when you start drinking the grape juice, the cells suck it up very rapidly in their hungry state. In the case of the grape diet, you are using a type of nutrient (high in resveratrol) that will kill the cancer cells, because they absorb more nutrients than they need, and in so doing, they also absorb excess antioxidants, sealing their own doom. Realize too, that there are other substances (besides grape juice) that contain sugar and still kill cancer cells. It really depends on what you are mixing with the sugar and what type sugar it is! (The Budwig Formula contains natural sugar.)

Antioxidants destroy free radicals, sometimes by giving up one of their own electrons in the process. Another way of looking at how antioxidants work is to remember that a molecule of oxygen is made up of 8 *electrons* (221). Because of everyday stress (e.g., toxins in the environment, lack of sleep, vitamin/mineral deficiencies) and the normal aging process, the oxygen molecule loses an electron and the result is a *free radical* (221). This new renegade goes about trying to steal an electron to substitute for the one that was taken. Once it succeeds in stealing an electron from another molecule, another *free radical* forms and a vicious cycle begins (221). This stealing of electrons starts to weaken the cell membrane and eventually the cell begins to deteriorate. After this happens, as explained by Lynn Keegan, Ph.D., R.N., in *Healing Nutrition*, the cell is then left vulnerable to attack (221).

Antioxidants can enter cellular tissues and willingly donate an electron, but they do so without attacking healthy cells. This puts a stop to the vicious cycle of electron theft, says Ms. Keegan, and the chain reaction comes to a halt. The cell wall is saved from destruction (221). (Note that not all free radicals are bad. Some are essential to normal bodily processes.) Ms. Keegan further points out that no cell in your body is over "7 years" old, and that you have "no blood cell…that is more than 14 days old." Your own body is able to "rebuild a new heart every 30 days" (221). This means that at least once a month, you get a new chance to turn any bad habits around and provide your body with the nutrition to re-energize and regain your health (221). I believe that super antioxidants, such as CoQ10 and others discussed in this book, can help you do just that. Simply think of it this way: the quality of many of the cells that you have a month from now will be the result of **what you are eating today!**

• CoQ10 & Statins – the Controversy

Research has found an alarming rise in breast cancer cases in women taking drugs for cholesterol-lowering effects. Apparently, they lowered cholesterol, but increased their risk for breast cancer (283). Recent news reports say that statins (cholesterol-lowering drugs) do not prevent plaque build-up in arterial walls. Much research has been done showing that cholesterol-lowering drugs strip CoQ10 out of the body. (Are you taking cholesterol-lowering drugs? Does your physician have you on CoQ10?) Did you know that a major side effect of statins is damage to muscles? Well, the heart is a major muscle in your body. Many people on statins complain of increased muscle weakness, yet most doctors dismiss such complaints as unrelated to the drugs that they are giving their patients, not recognizing the fact that it is because they are losing all the CoQ10 from their cells. Ask your physician or Naturopath about placing you on CoQ10 with your cholesterol-lowering medication, or better yet, guide you to using natural LDL cholesterol lowering nutrients.

There are many natural ways of lowering blood cholesterol (discussed in this book and my last two books) that are just as effective as drugs, but without any side effects. Here are some examples: policosanol, niacin, *Ecklonia Cava,* Calcium D-Glucarate, krill oil, ginseng, barley, garlic, celery, shiitake, red grapes, resveratrol, cernitin, vitamin C, and Chinese red yeast rice with guggal. Some reports are saying that certain statin drugs (e.g., Vytorin) could increase your risk for cancer by 50%, and that the statin drug, Zetia, can cause liver damage. Reports are already filing in that Vytorin can cause strokes, liver damage, and heart attacks. Let your physician know of your concerns if you are taking statin drugs. Do not take red yeast rice or red yeast rice products if you have liver disease, or if you are already taking cholesterol-lowering drugs.

Statins have also been responsible for the development of peripheral neuropathy or polyneuropathy. (This is an illness that attacks several nerves at the same time.) This was confirmed by a human study in Denmark on half a million people. Those who took statins the longest had the highest incidence for the development of neuropathy, the effects of which are often permanent and *irreversible.* Even patients taking the drugs for only one year had a 15% increased risk for nerve damage (198) (neuropathy).

And for those who think it is okay to take an aspirin a day to prevent heart attack and strokes, this may not be such a good idea for those who are healthy, without angina, and no prior history of heart attack. A study says that if you are healthy, you may not need that aspirin, because you can double your "risk of dangerous internal bleeding," yet without reducing your chances of having a stroke or MI (237).

The *Journal of the American College of Nutrition* published a report in their October 2004 issue which said that "the beneficial effects of magnesium could outweigh those of statin drugs," and while physicians in the study noted that statins "help to prevent blood clots, lower inflammation and protect against atherosclerosis, they can elevate liver enzymes and cause myopathy [muscle damage, muscle wasting, muscle weakness] as well as other side effects" (91). Statins are likely to cost you around *$100.00 per month,* while most magnesium supplements will run you *no more than $20.00 for a month's supply* (91). Another thing about magnesium, if you do get some diarrhea, simply lower the amount you are taking, take it in divided doses, rather than all at once, or switch to a different form of magnesium. You may even wish to try the new magnesium oil spray that is absorbed right into the skin, bypassing the G.I. system with no diarrhea side effects. See Appendix II for sources and Chapter 6 in this book.

II. CoQ10 & Cancer

You may want to consider adding CoQ10 supplements to your daily diet if you are fighting cancer. This amazing nutrient has even helped those with cancer of the breast to experience total regression (283). CoQ10 is also known as *ubiquinone*. The late Dr Karl Folkers, U.S. physician and one of the researchers who first isolated CoQ10 (along with Dr. Frederick L. Crane from the University of Wisconsin), named it *COENZYME Q10*. Dr. Folkers believed that insufficient amounts of CoQ10 and B6 could induce cancer in humans. He tested 83 people who had many different types of cancer. Every single one of them was deficient in CoQ10 (283). They were also deficient in vitamin B6. It appeared that those having breast cancer, pancreatic cancer and leukemia had the lowest levels of CoQ10 (283). Dr. Folkers was also one of the scientists credited with isolating and naming vitamin B12 (cobalamin), along with Dr. Alexander Todd, an English researcher. B12 is the vitamin that prevents pernicious anemia.

For optimum health, CoQ10 should be taken in conjunction with selenium, because (in animal testing) being deficient in selenium reduces liver levels of CoQ10, as well as cardiac levels (255). Selenium can be found in many food sources, including leafy greens, garlic, and Brazil nuts (255), if they are grown in soil rich in selenium. Most adults will find it difficult, if not impossible, to get an adequate amount of CoQ10, vitamin C, selenium, and alpha lipoic acid daily without supplementing.

Current research conducted by the Leonard M. Miller School of Medicine in Miami, under Niven R. Nerain, revealed that CoQ10 has the ability to kill cancer cells without damage to healthy cells. Not only that, but the National Cancer Institute acknowledged in 2005 that CoQ10 can extend the lives of those with breast cancer and other cancers. Issels Treatment Centers use CoQ10. Their phone #888-447-7357 (135).

For one of America's largest alternative health care centers, the Whitaker Wellness Center, which is in Newport Beach (4321 Birch Street), California, see this link: *http://whitakerwellness.com/about_us/medical_team.* Dr. Julian Whitaker, who runs this health care center, has written many books on alternative healing. He has an excellent website with a great deal of helpful information. They use many of the alternative health treatments that I have mentioned in my books, including chelation, hyperbaric oxygen, and various intravenous therapies.

• The *390 mg.* Daily Dose of CoQ10 That Cured Liver, Lung, & Breast Cancer in Humans

Research has shown that high dose Coenzyme Q10 given to cancer patients may help them win the fight against several types of cancer. In a 1994 study, two women having breast cancer experienced complete remission during a clinical trial where they were given either *300 mg or 390 mg* of CoQ10 daily (235). In the patient receiving 390 milligrams, the tumor completely vanished within a 60-day period (235). A year later, another human study was conducted, and a middle-aged patient experienced total remission of a liver cancer previously marked by multiple tumors. Every single tumor vanished. Another patient on CoQ10 enjoyed complete remission of lung cancer after a period of several months. An elderly patient with breast cancer experienced no further cancer after she had lump removal and was on the CoQ10 treatment (236). CoQ10 supplements are available in health food stores, pharmacies, popular grocery chains, and many internet sites.

Most nutritionists will recommend that you start off with a low dose of CoQ10, such as 50 mg per day, and then progress to higher doses as your body adjusts. For example, start with 50 mg/day; after two weeks, take the 50 mg twice a day; two weeks later, take it three times a day. Depending on your situation, you may want 100 mg/day, 200 mg/day or more. If you are fighting cancer, you will probably want to work up to 300—500 mg daily. Always check with your physician or Naturopath. If you have a conventional doctor, I would advise getting an opinion from an alternative medicine physician because many conventional physicians are still totally in the dark about CoQ10 (see below).

CoQ10, though not a vitamin, has often been referred to as a vitamin because it is so essential to every cell in our body. All cells have some amounts of CoQ10, but unfortunately, as we grow older, our bodies manufacture less and less of this nutrient. How healthy you are can often be determined by how much CoQ10 is in your body (283). CoQ10 is such an important nutrient, it has even been used to cure breast cancers that have metastasized.

Stephen T. Sinatra, M.D., tells in his informative book, *The Coenzyme Q10 Phenomenon,* how antioxidant CoQ10 affects breast cancer so dramatically, that *390 mg per day* produced total *remission* in several women having late stage disease (283). For prevention purposes, a starting dose is usually recommended at 30—50 mg per day, and then gradually working up to higher doses over a period of time, depending on what your health care practitioner has determined. I do recommend that you see a naturopath or alternative health physician about going on CoQ10, if your conventional doctor has no idea what this nutrient is, or is not familiar with research proving that it fights cancer.

One major factor present in nearly all cancer patients (discovered by the late Dr. Karl Folkers) has been a profound deficiency in CoQ10 (as well as B6). He discovered that the lowest levels of CoQ10 were found in those having cancer of the breast, pancreatic cancer, and children with leukemia (278) (283).

Dr. Folkers suggested *500 mg of CoQ10 daily* for any cancer patient fighting a malignancy (219). He treated two breast cancer patients with CoQ10, both of whom were also suffering from congestive heart failure brought on by their cancer, as well as four others who had lung cancer. All six of them went into remission (219)!

III. CoQ10 & Congestive Heart Failure

One of the largest research studies involving the effectiveness of CoQ10 to treat heart disorders (e.g., heart failure), was an Italian study using more than 2500 people with the disease (282). It is described by Dr. Stephen T. Sinatra, M.D., author of *Coenzyme Q10 and the Heart*. All participants in the study were suffering with congestive heart failure and were given daily doses of CoQ10, most of them *receiving 100 mg daily*. After three months of taking CoQ10, patients experienced very dramatic relief in **all** their congestive heart failure symptoms (282).

One of Dr. Sinatra's patients was an elderly woman, so severely afflicted with CHF, that she was struggling to breathe and her weight had plummeted. She had a dysfunctional valve, and her heart's pumping capacity was barely enough to get her out of bed for short periods of time (282). (EF or *ejection fraction* is a measurement of the heart's pumping ability. Normal is 70-80%, and the patient's was **15%.**) Dr. Sinatra started her on "30 mg of CoQ10 three times a day (90 mg/day)," however, she continued to deteriorate until something amazing occurred (282). Her son accidentally bought his mom "100 mg capsules instead of the usual 30 mg..." She was taking 100 mg three times a day without realizing it (a total of 300 mg). Within a month, she had improved so dramatically that she was kept on the higher dose of CoQ10, and several months after starting on the increased dosage of CoQ10, she was out and about with friends. Errors like the one made by her son are a blessing in disguise!

As a result of this case, Dr. Sinatra feels that if patients do not respond to CoQ10 at low dosing, physicians should give larger doses, especially in those who are most severely ill, until they do respond (282). Is it such a profoundly simple solution that mainstream medicine cannot grasp it? Apparently so. It is also a fact that CoQ10 cannot be patented, thus big pharma has no interest in promoting this nutrient (282). There are very few problems associated with the long term use of CoQ10. In a study of 5000 patients using the supplement, very minimal effects of gastrointestinal upset, diminished "appetite...Nausea... Diarrhea...Elevated LDH (rare)...[and] Elevated SGOT (rare)," were reported (282).

Dr. James F. Balch, M.D., in his book, *The Super Antioxidants*, discusses the story of Gina F, whose experience with CoQ10 was aired on a national news broadcast in a nutrition series. Gina was only 24 and dying from heart failure (165). She was so ill that doctors had given her only a few days to live. Her physicians were ready to give up, having already tried various powerful pharmaceutical drugs that were not helping. Finally, they suggested she try CoQ10 supplements (165). A month later, Gina was still alive. Her heart had improved so dramatically that she called the nutrient her *lifeline* (165). The mystery is why more physicians don't recommend CoQ10 to their patients.

Dr. Ray D. Strand, M.D., also questioned this in his book, *What Your Doctor Doesn't Know About Nutritional Medicine May Be Killing You*. A transplant is costly, involving hundreds of thousands of dollars. This, in comparison to a CoQ10 supplement, that will cost about seven to ten dollars a week (292), and could even save you from needing a heart transplant!

Although CoQ10 can be found in foods like *eggs, rice bran*, and *wheat germ*, Dr. Ralph Moss says that you cannot get enough of it without supplementing (255). A few other natural sources of CoQ10 are "...mackerel, peanuts, salmon, sardines, and spinach" (205).

• CoQ10 & Leukemia

This is one nutrient you will want to add to your arsenal if you are fighting leukemia or any other type of cancer.

A few years ago, I saw a report of a little boy who was given Adriamycin for leukemia. He went into remission, but a dangerous side effect of Adriamycin is cardiac muscle damage. This child had such serious damage to his heart from the Adriamycin that he went into heart failure and was forced to go on the heart transplant-waiting-list. The oncologist giving him chemo could have prevented the damage to his heart from the Adriamycin by giving him CoQ10. Indeed, it is true that what your physician does not know about natural treatments can be fatal to you or a loved one!

Current research revealed that CoQ10 can help kill cancer cells without damage to healthy cells (135). Not only that, but the National Cancer Institute acknowledged in 2005 that CoQ10 can extend the lives of those with colorectal cancers and other cancers. Issels Treatment Centers use CoQ10. Their phone #888-447-7357 (135).

• CoQ10 - Low Levels Could Indicate Increased Risk for Melanoma

A human study found very low CoQ10 levels in those with melanoma, and even lower levels in those who had melanomas that had spread to other areas of the body. This indicates that insufficient levels of this nutrient may increase a person's risk for melanoma and its spread (100).

• CoQ10 Deficiencies & Multiple Myelomas

Studies by Dr. Folkers and his colleagues revealed that patients with *multiple myeloma* and tumors of the breast often had CoQ10 deficiencies, as compared to their healthier counterparts (255). As a matter-of-fact, evidence over more than three decades revealed that taking CoQ10 increased the lifespan of many cancer patients by years (255).

• CoQ10 & Multiple Sclerosis

There are other reasons that you may want to supplement with CoQ10 besides its cancer-fighting properties. Dr. Ray D. Strand, M.D., gives an amazing account of his experience treating a patient who came to him with M.S. (multiple sclerosis) in his book, *What Your Doctor Doesn't Know About Nutritional Medicine May Be Killing You* (292). When the young man suddenly developed unexplainable weakness and numbness in his extremities, and was subsequently diagnosed with multiple sclerosis, he was fortunate enough to hear a lecture by Dr. Strand, and receive treatment that eventually resulted in complete remission (292). Dr. Strand's nutritional program included more than just using CoQ10. He also used minerals, many antioxidants, essential fatty acids, and grape seed extract, which he discusses in detail in his book (292). New evidence points to deficient vitamin D levels as a cause of MS, especially in children (152) (272).

Vegetarian diets and low fat diets significantly reduce the risk for multiple sclerosis. Research shows that curcumin may be beneficial in fighting M.S. It appears to have a protective effect on nerve cells. Do not use curcumin if you have liver disease, ulcers, GERD, or other GI problems without checking with your physician first.

• CoQ10—Low Levels Linked to Pancreatic Cancer

This nutrient, also called *ubiquinone*, has been the subject of many scientific double-blind **human studies**, and is so important in fighting cancer; it is mentioned in several cancer-specific chapters in my first two books. Some natural food sources of this nutrient are: nuts, leafy greens, and salmon (283). Dr. Karl Folkers found that patients with breast and pancreatic cancers had the lowest levels of CoQ10 than with any other cancers studied. He believed that insufficient amounts of this nutrient accounts for the high death rate in cancer of the pancreas (278). The same low blood levels of CoQ10 were discovered in children with *leukemia* (278).

• CoQ10 & Prostate Cancer

Dr. Folkers funded the work of Dr. William Judy (Brandenton, Florida) to use CoQ10 on his hormone-independent prostate cancer patients (219). Note that prostate cancers can start as hormone-dependent, then after hormone treatment, they can become hormone-resistant or hormone-independent) (219). Dr. Judy tested 30 such cancer patients giving them Dr. Folker's recommended dose of CoQ10 at 500 mg a day. Half of them had cancer that had spread to their lungs and bone and half did not. 14 of the 15 without spreading cancer enjoyed a PSA *return to normal,* while eight of the 15 patients with metastases had a PSA that also went back to *normal* (219). Dr. Judy also treated six other prostate cancer patients with the same dosage as above for four months, and all six had normal PSAs at the end of the treatment (219).

• CoQ10 Used to Cure Peritoneal Cancer in 89-Year-Old

For an amazing case study from Guisseppi A. Forgionne, Ph.D., about an 89-year-old woman who experienced total remission from advanced peritoneal cancer using an alternative nutritional approach, see website *http://www.cancerlynx.com/peritonealcase.html* (199). After having surgery, she refused chemo. According to the article, her nutritional regimen included *2 grams of wheat grass* per day (a week after her surgery), then **100 mg of CoQ10** daily a week after that, and within 2 more weeks, the addition of *9 grams of bovine cartilage*/day. *Nine months* later, her CoQ10 was changed to *150 mg per day* (199).

Remember this; age is no limit when it comes to curing disease! I have heard people remark that because their grandmother or their dad was in his seventies or eighties and had "lived a full life," their physician felt that nothing further should be done to help cure them from this terrible disease! Just let Hospice take over and let them die! I have many documented cases of people in their late seventies and eighties who were CURED of cancer using natural, non-toxic therapies! Do not let someone tell YOU that because you have already lived 70, 80, or 90+ years, you should not bother pursuing a cure if you have cancer! You deserve the same opportunity to get well as any 20 or 30-year-old! God may not be through with you yet. He may still have work for you to do!

CHAPTER 11

The Miracle of pH Balance

****

I. Candida & Cancer – Oncology Physician Believes Cancer is a Fungus

Italian oncology physician, Dr. Tullio Simoncini, believes that cancer is actually a fungus. So convinced was he that he wrote a book entitled: *Cancer Is A Fungus* (281a). He suggests that cancer patients be given *sodium bicarbonate*, a non-poisonous substance, directly into the cancerous tissue (281a). If you are interested in more specifics on his treatment, see website: *http://www.cancerisafungus.com/cancer-fungus-content.html,* and this site as well: *http://www.cancerfungus.com* (281a). Dr. Simoncini believes that cancer is not caused by the genes that you inherit.

Is it any surprise that recent studies have shown that 80% of those with *Candida Yeast Infections* also have high levels of mercury in their bodies (107)?

You can order Dr. Simoncini's book at his website: *http://www.curenaturalicancro.com,* which also has a great deal more information on him and his treatment of cancer. Apparently, he has been very successful in using this therapy (281a). He has reports of patients "using sodium bicarbonate at five per cent solution" to heal *lung* cancers, cancers of the mouth, head and neck, *liver,* gastric and *intestinal, prostate, stomach, pancreas, spleen,* and many others (281a). If you go to website: *curenaturalicancro.com,* he has information and detailed *instructions* for using this *non-toxic, inexpensive* therapy (281a). He does recommend that you consult with your physician, rather than self-treating. You can also watch a video showing before and after cancer growths treated with soda bicarb at website:

http://articles.mercola.com/sites/articles/archive/2008/08/05/fungus-causing-cancer-a-novelapproach-to-the-most-common-form-of-death.aspx?source=nl.

Or just go to *mercola.com* and do a search for the article. Dr. Simoncini has a video of his "before-and-after footage of both bronchial cancer and colon cancer. Four days after his simple treatment on a bronchial cancer with a sodium bicarbonate and water flush, the tumors are gone" (26), and you can see this visually for yourself at the website above.

When you consider the SAD (Sad American Diet), which is so conducive to high acid levels and promoting fungal infections, Dr. Simoncini's approach makes a great deal of sense.

Dr. Simoncini says cancerous growths are usually white, the same color as most fungus and yeast. What does the soda bicarb do? It turns the entire cancerous area alkaline and allows more oxygen to get to the cancer cells and, as noted in other parts of this book and other books I have written, cancer cannot survive in a high oxygen, alkaline environment. Dr. Simoncini says that today's fungal drugs don't work because they only fight the top layer of the yeast, and besides that, the fungus simply adapts to the drug in just a few days (281a). He says that soda bicarb is absolutely the strongest anti-fungal substance you can use. He uses a port-a-cath to target tumors directly, going through a nearby vessel in, for example, reaching liver tumors or pancreatic tumors; however, in cavity tumors (those in the abdomen or peritoneal area), a peritoneal catheter can be used to deliver the sodium bicarb. In bladder cancers, he says that you can simply use a urethral catheter to deliver the soda bicarb (281a). The treatment is non-toxic and can be used to cure most solid cancers in days. He uses a soda bicarb wash for tumors in the colon. Dr. Simoncini also says that other disorders, such as MS, ALS, and psoriasis are caused by a fungus. (281a).

Is it possible that curing a disease so deadly can be this simple? How many alternative medicine physicians have been telling the public for years that cancer cannot thrive in an alkaline environment? Because of his exclusive non-toxic treatment of cancer, shunning chemo drugs, Dr. Simoncini has had his license revoked by the conventional medicine, pharmaceutical monopoly in his country. (Sound familiar?)

It is interesting that the very first patient Dr. Simoncini cured was an 11-year-old boy with leukemia who was already in a comatose state

(281a). For brain cancers, he uses *selective arteriography*, via the carotids. He says that the only cancer that isn't easily reached is that in the small bones found in the ribs and vertebrae due to the sparse arterial blood flow into these areas (281a). (See Dr. Sircus' opinion of this form of giving soda bicarb below and see other chapters in this book as well.)

For a complete list of individual protocols that Dr. Simoncini uses in his treatment of various cancers, see website *http://www.curenatural icancro.com,* and click on the tab that says: *Treatments with Sodium Bicarbonate* (281a). Dr. Simoncini has used his treatment on many types of cancer. He uses a 5% or 8.4% soda bicarbonate solution fed via a special catheter in order to make direct contact with the cancer. He says that the soda bicarb works so quickly that there is no time for the *fungi to adapt* and become resistant to treatment (281a), which is what happens many times in the world of chemo and antibiotic drugs.

Is cancer a fungus? Well if it isn't, then why do some children and adults with leukemia suddenly make a rapid recovery when they are given anti-fungals, and soda bicarb is a very **inexpensive** ANTI-FUNGAL (288)! Researchers have found that soda bicarb is even effective at killing green mold (fungus) on oranges (316).

Soda bicarb is useful in treating pancreatitis, autoimmune disorders, Type II diabetes, Parkinson's disease, HIV, SARS, osteoporosis, Alzheimer's, mucositis (mouth sores caused by chemo drugs), canker sores, and of course (as noted in this chapter), all forms of cancer.

As for side effects of this natural substance as used by Dr. Simoncini, they are few and generally mild, such as a feeling of thirst or *temporary tiredness*, and he says that some patients who have multiple tumors may experience a temperature rise after beginning treatment (281a); however, see the article below for taking soda bicarb by mouth.

If you want to read about a substance that promoters claim will destroy Candida in the body (THREELAC™), see website *www.ght health.com.* They also carry many other health products.

Dr. Theodore Baroody's Book, *Alkalize or Die*, describes how to alkalize the body by following an anti-fungal diet. You can find many websites that will tell you in great detail how to follow an anti-Candida diet. The article below also describes a cure for cancer using baking soda. Note that chlorophyll and products that contain it (e.g., chlorella), also fight Candida and are especially helpful if you are prone to yeast infections, and chlorophyll is rich in magnesium.

• Physician Says ORAL Soda Bicarb Just as Effective for Killing Cancer as Intravenous Soda Bicarb

Dr. Mark Sircus, author of *Sodium Bicarbonate Rich Man's Poor Man's Cancer Treatment*, says you don't need to travel to Europe for intravenous soda bicarb; because taking it by mouth is just as efficient at killing cancer, and you can find it at your local grocery store in the form of *Arm & Hammer*® baking soda, with directions right on their box for rapid alkalizing (288), though they do not promote their product for fighting cancer. He discusses the strange and bitter irony that is happening in the conventional cancer establishment—the fact that many chemo drugs are so toxic, soda bicarb must be hung alongside them to keep them from killing the patient, and he questions this: are physicians taking credit for healing cancer with toxic chemo drugs when what is really happening is that the soda bicarb is actually doing the healing (288)? Does the patient even need the chemo? Why not just give them the soda bicarb, which alkalizes the body? Alkalinity kills cancer. This is why cesium works so well, but cesium must be monitored very closely. It works extremely well at what it does, but it can rapidly remove potassium from the body. (See later in this chapter.)

Soda bicarb is non-toxic. How strange isn't it - that when cancer chemo victims develop mouth sores from chemo, doctors tell them to use a soda bicarb rinse to heal their mouth (288)!? THINK ABOUT THAT! Soda bicarb users should check with their doctors simply because it is so high in salt.

- **A "Country Doctor" Claims He Has Made an Amazing Substance that Will Cure Just About Any Cancer**

The 75-year-old former truck driver has no medical background but those loyal to him claim that he is a "miracle worker" (39). 64-year-old Ian Rodhouse with **lung cancer** was given *six months to live*. He used "Dr. Jim's" preparation. His cancer was gone *within two months* (39). "Dr. Jim," as his friends call him, has "dispensed his mixture to more than 200 patients diagnosed with terminal cancer" (39). He says "of that number, 185 lived at least 15 more years, and nearly half" went into complete remission" (39). Of course, state medical experts are already calling him a "quack" and threatening "to arrest him for practicing medicine without a license" (39). (Sound familiar? Remember Rene Caisse? See Chapter 13.) After all, should we not make sure that this terribly natural maple syrup and baking soda isn't HEALING anyone's cancer before they have first gone through the toxic chemo and radiation approved and recognized by the FDA?

Of course you may wish to consult with your doctor about any new regimen, but below is *Dr. Jim's recipe:*

> Add one part baking soda with three parts maple syrup in a small saucepan. Stir briskly. Heat for five minutes. Take one teaspoon daily, as needed. Be sure you use ALUMINUM-FREE baking soda and 100% organic maple syrup (377a). [Do not use an aluminum pan.]

This simple formula works on the premise that cancer cells thrive on sugar and suck it up rapidly, then the baking soda, which is very ALKALINE, is carried into the cells by "the maple syrup," and "removes the microbe inside the cancer cell" (377a). Remember that cancer cannot THRIVE in an alkaline-environment. (One person who uses this formula says you only need to heat it until it foams.)

According to Dr. Mark Sircus, you can substitute honey or blackstrap molasses and it does not necessarily need to be heated (288). You can use it with the maple syrup without heating, as well.

• Maple Syrup

Organic maple syrup can be found at most health food stores and grocery chains. Most other "maple" syrups that you find in grocery stores actually have no maple syrup at all in them. Check the label and you will find that they are full of corn syrup, maple *flavoring,* artificial sweeteners, and food dyes. Natural, organic maple syrup is slightly alkaline, but it is high in sugar, so should not be consumed in large quantities, especially by diabetics.

• Cesium

Cesium chloride has the highest alkaline level of any mineral. It is believed that it may kill cancer cells by preventing them from absorbing sugar, thus starving them to death, as well as raising the cells' alkalinity. Cesium goes inside the cancer cells only, and then destroys them, but beware, because taking large amounts of this mineral can lead to dangerous cardiac arrhythmias (28). The interesting thing is that normal cells won't absorb cesium, just the cancer cells. It is very effective for fast-growing cancers, especially those of the brain and bones and is often given along with DMSO (3).

You can get bottles of high dose ionic cesium chloride with rubidium at website: *http://www.thewolfeclinic.com/cesium.html*, or go to *http://www.thewolfeclinic.com*, their new website. You can also go to website: *http://www.liquid-cesium.com/products/buy-liquid-cesium-chloride.html.* Though cesium has been considered safe, do not take it unless you are under the guidance of your physician (29).

Symptoms you may experience from taking cesium include: "numbness in the face: lips, chin or nose; extreme muscle weakness, such as in the legs; very dry and scaly skin, which may split open or cause extreme itchiness; increased urination," but these symptoms can also mean excess levels of potassium in the body (29). The website above can give you plenty of information on how to use their product, details on dosing, and answer many of your questions about cesium. They also provide other health products.

In animal and human research studies done on cesium by A.K. Brewer, described by the U.S. National Library of Medicine, it was shown that "potassium, rubidium, and especially cesium are most efficiently taken up by cancer cells," and "This intake was enhanced by Vitamins A and C as well as salts of zinc and selenium" (179). The amount of "cesium taken up was sufficient to raise the cell to the 8 pH range." Tests on mice proved that "cesium and rubidium" could shrink "tumor masses" significantly "within 2 weeks," plus, "the mice showed none of the side effects of cancer" (179).

It is extremely interesting that testing was also done on more than *30 humans*, and "in each case the tumor masses disappeared" (179). Not only that, but "all pain and effects associated with cancer disappeared within 12 to 36 hrs; the more chemotherapy and morphine the patient had taken, the longer the withdrawal period" (179). With cesium working at raising cellular pH this rapidly, ever wonder WHY it isn't being used in oncology offices? Could it be because a bottle of cesium will run you about $100.00 - $140.00, rather than the $30,000 that the drug companies (and the oncologists charge) for two rounds of I.V. chemo drugs? (See Chapters 1 and 2.)

• Soda Bicarb for Every Day

Soda bicarb isn't just for a sour stomach and for alkalizing the body. It is often found in commercial mouthwashes, but is also used for treating *chronic renal failure, renal tubular acidosis, uric acid renal stones,* for *tricyclic antidepressant overdose,* and works great as a *topical paste* (*three parts baking soda to one part water* for *insect bites*) (155). It is a great *antiseptic* and can be used in a *paste* mixed with *3% hydrogen peroxide solution,* if you don't like using fluoride toothpaste (155). Website: *naturalhealing.cofah.com* says that it's best to take soda bicarb at night since that is when you have the most acid in your body (124). In spite of all of the great uses for hydrogen peroxide, you must keep it away from small children, who do not understand that it is a lethal poison when swallowed! Soda bicarb is non-toxic but is high in salt. Never leave containers of any type of chemical or medication around small children, or pets that might get into them.

• Arthritis, Gout, Rheumatic Diseases & Bicarb

Website *naturalhealing.cofah.com*, in their article on soda bicarb, says that the "usual dosage for sodium bicarbonate" for those with "arthritis, gout or any other rheumatic disease is 1 teaspoon mixed in an 8 ounce glass of water twice a day," and it's best to "take at least one dose before going to bed" (124), but no more than a total of "3 ½ teaspoons in a 24 hour period," and never more than two weeks at a time, then "take a one week break. Continue this routine until the pain completely goes away and you are cured" (124). Don't use water that contains chlorine and fluoride!

A word of caution, soda bicarb is high in SALT. You must check with your physician before undertaking a soda bicarb regimen, especially if you have high blood pressure, kidney problems, or other chronic disorders. (The amount of salt in 3.5 teaspoons of soda bicarb in a 24 hour period (described above) would require drinking a lot of water to flush the body and could cause a rapid potassium deficiency.) Always take extra potassium when using soda bicarb.

• Cancer Insanity

If it is true, as some scientists and physicians like Dr. Simoncini now believe, that cancer is indeed a FUNGUS, just consider the absurdity with which current conventional medicine treats these patients. Fungus thrives in a highly-acidifed, high-sugar environment. This overrun of fungus is the actual culprit that leads to cancer. Chemo and radiation INCREASE the body's acidity. As a matter-of-fact, some chemo drugs are so toxic; taking them into the body is like pouring acid into your cells. Physicians know this, so they often hang soda bicarb infusions to help neutralize the extreme acidity of the chemo drug. But consider this: if cancer is a fungus and chemo increases the acidity of the body, that means chemo makes an even more FAVORABLE environment for the further growth of fungus! Is this why chemo overall has such a high failure rate? Is this why some children with leukemia, who have a suppressed immune system, receive chemo, then succumb to fatal fungal infections, and the same reason why some children with leukemia, who are treated with anti-fungals, actually go into remission (288)? Are physicians NOT connecting-the-dots—not aware of the fact that cancer is a fungus and when anti-fungal drugs are given to treat secondary overgrowths of fungus in these patients, the angi-fungals are killing not just the new yeast overgrowths, but often the original cancer to begin with!?

- **Molasses Formula**

During the time before he was scheduled to start taking chemo, my relative, who was fighting stage IV bladder cancer (See Chapters 1 and 2), alkalized using the soda bicarb, blackstrap molasses formula, but he did not use as strong a dose of the bicarb as Vernon Johnston did that I discuss later (110) in Chapter 15; however, he kept a high urine pH for several days with smaller doses of the bicarb, and was also drinking at least 8 or more glasses of water every day (which included the water in the mixes).

- **Molasses**

Molasses, particularly blackstrap molasses, is being mentioned here because it is one of the few sweeteners richer in nutrients than it is in calories, and because of its anti-cancer properties. According to Cyril Scott and John Lust, Naturopath, in their book: *Crude Black Molasses, The Natural "Wonder Food,"* A physician known as Dr. Forbes Ross "drew attention to the value of Molasses in connection with cancer…" prior to WW I. It was he who noticed that "workers on sugar-cane plantations who were constantly sucking the crude sugar, seldom if ever were known to suffer from that dread disease [cancer]." He believed that it was due to the high level of "potassium salts in unrefined sugar-cane," and he believed that cancer was primarily due to a potash deficiency (280).

Authors Cyril Scott and John Lust also describe an account of James Persson, over sixty-years-old, from New Zealand, who was incapacitated with a bowel growth, heart disease, bronchial congestion, digestive problems, "pyorrhea, sinus trouble and weak nerves…" (280). He was also "losing weight, and his hair had turned white" (280). When he discovered that a neighbor of his had been sent home to die with a terminal colon cancer and cured himself completely by drinking crude black molasses, he decided to do the same. As a result, the bowel growth disappeared, along with his other health problems, and he claims that his hair regained its original color (280). The authors of the book also state that many other cases of cancer have been treated and "cured solely by Molasses-therapy," including "growths of the uterus…breast…intestinal growth…[and] numerous cases of growths of the tongue, diagnosed as malignant" (280). Another patient had been diagnosed with breast cancer and was told she was terminal. She began taking molasses and completely recovered, with no reoccurrences (280).

It is recommended that molasses be taken "before meals...one teaspoonful" dissolved in a few ounces of warm water, then add enough "cold water to equal a total of 2/3 cup. Drink it warm. For children, half the dosage" (280). For those with tumors, not only is the molasses taken "during the day [but] last thing at night and on rising," as well (280). There is night and day difference between processed white sugar and molasses. So much so, that processed white sugar is acid-forming, while crude black molasses is alkaline. Besides being high in potassium, this thick-syrupy liquid is high in several other minerals and vitamins (280).

Those who have decreased kidney function or other chronic illnesses will need to watch their salt and potassium consumption. If you use the soda bicarb/molasses formula several days for alkalizing (as described in Chapter 15 of this book), you will need extra potassium. Be aware that table salt isn't good for you because all it contains is sodium chloride. If you use sun-dried sea salt, Himalayan crystal salt or Celtic salt, they also contain vital trace minerals such as magnesium, potassium, silica, manganese, iodine and others.

II. Chlorophyll & Chlorophyllin for Cancer Prevention & Alkalinity

Scientists have discovered that eating green foods, which are high in natural chlorophyll, could protect from all cancers, but especially those of the colon and liver (30). Many animal studies have shown that natural chlorophyll and chlorophyllin (an extract made from chlorophyll) fight cancer. They discovered that this substance can also protect against a dangerous fungus that often affects nuts and cereals known as *aflatoxin*, a source of liver cancer, especially in nations that do not have adequate safety measures for storing their grains (30).

Chlorophyll and chlorophyllin also protect against the DNA damage from other cancer-causing substances, especially those found in *grilled meats* and *diesel exhaust* (30). Dr. George S. Bailey discussed the protective effects of this green substance in the LPI Research Newsletter "Chlorophylls and Cancer Prevention: passing the First

Hurdle" (30). He describes a human study using chlorophyllin, which was conducted in Eastern China for a group of people who were at risk for liver cancer from the *aflatoxin* mold (30). They were given the chlorophyllin three times a day in 100 mg pills for a total of 300 mg. The participants in the clinical trial experienced a 55% decrease in urinary output of the aflatoxin compounds, indicating that the chlorophyllin was neutralizing and destroying the toxins which are responsible for *DNA damage* (which causes liver cancer) (30).

A new 20-year clinical trial is being done in China to test chlorophyllin. They explained that eating a *moderate-to-high* amount *of green vegetables* would be necessary to obtain the *300 mg per day of chlorophyllin* given in the clinical trial (30). High amounts of chlorophyll in the diet via green vegetables could also help prevent the type of colon cancer caused by an iron found in red meats (30).

There is no toxicity in natural chlorophyll and chlorophyllin, however, do check with your physician or Naturopath before supplementing in large amounts, especially if you are taking prescription medications, such as blood thinners.

III. Rapid Alkalizers – Asparagus, Bicarb, Vinegar, Lemons & Limes

• Asparagus

I wrote about the healing properties of asparagus in my first two books, but wanted to give the tasty vegetable a little more recognition in this section, simply because it is probably one of the most alkalizing vegetables known to man. It is the only vegetable that retains its high alkalinity level even after it is cooked. Researchers knew this as far back as the late 70's, and the *Cancer News Journal* wrote at length about it in a Dec. 1979 article. Many people have no idea why it's such a healthy food.

Asparagus is high in folic acid, rutin, vitamin C, and may be the richest vegetable source you will ever find for glutathione, extremely important nutrients for fighting cancer and other illnesses (10a).

The article, written by an unnamed biochemist, gives several cases of people who were cured of various cancers by cooking asparagus and making a puree and taking "4 full tablesp. twice daily, morning and evening. Patients usually show some improvement in from 2—4 weeks," and it is noted that the dosage can be "diluted with water and used as a cold or hot drink" (10a). The article lists several cases of notable cancer cures using this formula:

- "A man with an almost hopeless case of **Hodgkin's disease**...who was completely incapacitated. Within 1 year of starting the asparagus therapy, his doctors were unable to detect any signs of cancer."
- A 68-year-old with **bladder cancer** who had not improved after conventional therapy. After using the asparagus puree for 3 months "his bladder tumour had disappeared and...his kidneys were normal."
- A patient with inoperable **lung cancer** who was considered "hopeless," started on the formula in early April and was totally cancer-free 4 months later, with clear x-rays.
- A woman cleared of **skin cancer** and **kidney disease** using the pureed formula (10a).

The writer says that you can use *Green Giant* and *Stokely* brand asparagus for this formula (10a). It is also an excellent vegetable to juice raw. One contributor from an internet site goes on to say "If I had cancer, I would eat as much asparagus as I could get down in any form, (cooked) preferably steamed) or raw, solid or liquid" (10a). You will have to check with your physician about using asparagus if you are taking blood thinners, because it also contains natural vitamin K. I would recommend using organic if available.

• Vinegar

Besides eating foods high in glutathione that also alkalize the body, bicarb, vinegar, lemons, and limes can quickly alkalize the cells. Apple cider vinegar is the only type of vinegar that has an alkalizing (rather than acidifying) effect on the body. Paul C. Bragg, N.D., Ph.D., and his wife, Patricia Bragg, N.D., Ph.D., wrote an entire book on *Apple Cider Vinegar Miracle Health System*. In this book, Paul and Patricia call apple cider vinegar "Nature's Healing Miracle," and they also say that most people succumb to disease because they violate "the natural laws that govern the physical body" (177). (Apple cider vinegar is more powerful at alkalizing the body than lemon juice.) Below is a three day detox regimen that I have used, which is based on apple cider vinegar:

• 3 Day Apple Cider Vinegar Detox

Use a mineral drink such as *Ola Loa®* or *Mineral Rich®* daily with any detox program to be sure that you are getting other essential minerals during the day. Be sure to spend time in prayer, worship, and Bible study every day.

Mix one teaspoon of apple cider vinegar in 8 ounces of fresh water and drink. Do this four to six times each day for three days, adding additional glasses of water during the day as desired. Never under any circumstances should you use water that contains chlorine or fluoride with this program. Doing so will just poison your body! And remember that every time you get a hot shower or bath, or drink a glass of chlorinated water, or clean with chlorine bleach, you lose valuable iodine from your body. If you mop your floors with chlorine water, then walk on them barefoot, some of the chlorine will evaporate, but you will also absorb some through your feet before it all evaporates. So will your pets and children.

If you already have cancer, drink 2 ounces of Essiac tea (as instructed and prepared on the brand you choose) when you first arise in the morning, then 2 ounces of the tea on retiring. Do not ever eat or drink anything else at least one hour before or one hour after you have ingested the Essiac Tea.

• Help for Autism

I read an article recently where a writer reported that her autistic child improved remarkably when she stopped bathing him in water that contained fluoride (53). Autistic children are usually deficient in sulfur and are often helped when their parents use **Epsom salts** in their bathwater (51). Epsom salts contain magnesium sulfate. This may also be helpful for those with "Alzheimer's disease, Parkinson's disease, rheumatoid arthritis, and chemical sensitivities" (51). According to Dr. Stephen M. Edelson, Ph.D., many autistic children and adults are helped by the addition of vitamin B6 and magnesium to their diets. The benefits include: "improvements in attention, learning, speech/ language, and eye contact," as well as "decreases in behavioral problems, improvements in appropriate behavior, and normalization of brain wave activity and urine biochemistry", and a reduction in "seizure activity" (197).

You can purchase a "flavored B6/magnesium formula," known as **Super Nuthera,** for autism patients at *www.kirkmanlabs.com*. They have been making the formula since 1968 (197). It is important to take B6 along with magnesium, because in order to work effectively, B6 needs *extra magnesium* (197). **NEVER** use the sweetener known as **Aspartame (*Nutra-Sweet*™, *Canderel*™, AminoSweet®, or *Equal*®)**, which is often found in children's candy, gum, vitamins, and desserts. It *can cause neurological damage* (197) and tumor growths. If the label has the above sweeteners in the list of ingredients, do not use them! Sometimes they are disguised and may be referred to in the label of ingredients as: *aspartyl-L-phenylalanine*, *APM, aspartic acid, methanol* (which is wood alcohol), or the label may tell you that there are *phenylalanines* in the product, or a word similar to this. AVOID them! Also, see website: *myaspartameexperiment.com*.

• Lemons & Limes

Though lemons and limes are very acidic, they have an amazing alkaline effect on the body (298). Concerned about yeast infections? Drink plenty of homemade lemonade without sugar. Use a natural herbal sweetener like Stevia® instead. If you love lemonade, but not the tartness, you can reduce the acidity of lemonade by adding a small amount of soda bicarb to it. Just put a teaspoon of soda bicarb in 2 quarts of lemonade and the tartness and acidity will be greatly reduced. Drink after it stops fizzing. This does add extra salt to your drink. Don't add sweetener until after you do this, because you won't need as much sweetener! You can also reduce the tartness of lime juice and grapefruit juice or fresh grapefruit in much the same way. I have seen people drown fresh grapefruit with sugar right before they eat it. Removing the tartness works much better with salt than sugar, or simply sprinkling with soda bicarb. Below is a rapid alkalizer for the body using lemons (you can also use limes).

• 7 Day Lemonade Detox

Use fresh-squeezed lemon juice (and/or lime juice) diluted in water to the concentration of your taste. Drink as often as you like with extra water as desired for seven days. This is a rapid alkalizer and detox. Use a mineral supplement such as *Ola Loa®* or *Mineral Rich®* once or twice daily on this detox program as with any fast you embark on. Remember to discontinue any detox such as this one gradually, and be sure to consult with your physician before beginning a strict detox or fasting program.

• 10 Day Lemonade Detox

Lemonade Diet by Stanley Burroughs: Mix 2 tablespoons of fresh-squeezed lemon juice, 2 tablespoons of maple syrup, and 1/10 tspn cayenne pepper into 8 oz of water. Drink as often as needed for energy. Follow for a ten day period, but eat and drink nothing else. (167). It is best to try this formula for about 2 or 3 days (167) to see how you are going to tolerate it, then wait a period of time before doing the full ten day program.

• Soda Bicarb

Next to cesium, as discussed earlier, the most powerful alkalizer of all is soda bicarb, also known as bicarbonate of soda or sodium bicarbonate. It is very high in salt and using large amounts can cause excess loss of **potassium** from the body. This is why it is very important to supplement with potassium if you are taking soda bicarb for rapidly alkalizing your body. You can check the label on the *Arm & Hammer®* soda bicarb you find in most grocery stores, and it will give you detailed instructions on how to use their product for a "sour stomach."

• The Biblical Saltines

Did you know that in the Bible Jesus said: "salt is good"? *(Mark 9:50.)* While we know that Jesus was using a metaphor to describe how Christians are to be the *salt of the earth*, perhaps he was also looking into the future when an overgrowth of yeast infections would plague the current generation of humanity on the earth. Modern science has certainly succeeded in convincing people that salt is bad. Well, not all salt is bad. Salt-laden fast food is bad. Natural salt in foods like celery is actually good for you, if not taken in excess and if you are not on a salt-restricted diet.

Italian physician, Dr. Tullio Simoncini, believes that cancer is a fungus. He has certainly been successful in curing many cancer patients in his own practice using an inexpensive soda bicarb solution and nothing more! For life-and-death cases of colon cancer, for example, he recommends one cup of soda bicarb in one quart of water for an enema for a large adult, otherwise, to use ¼ cup of soda bicarb in a quart of water for enema. See his website at: *http://www.cancerisafungus.com* (281a). It is interesting that you can use a product known as *Alka-Seltzer Gold®* for rapid alkalinity which not only has soda bicarb, but potassium bicarb as well. This is the only Alka-Seltzer® that I know of that does not contain aspirin. Do NOT use the Alka-Seltzer® that contains aspirin. Alka-Seltzer Gold® is a combination of "sodium and potassium bicarbonates with citric acid" (12).

• Ending the Detox Program or Extended Fast

Remember, you MUST go off any fast or prolonged detox program gradually. You cannot immediately begin eating solid and cooked foods in large amounts. It must be gradual, or you can end up in severe distress. You cannot break a detox program of 3, 7, 14, 21, or 40 days in ONE day, then go back to eating cooked foods and a regular diet. If you already have cancer, you may wish to keep taking Essiac every day until you have healed your immune system. Read the cancer-specific chapters in my last book, *Gentle Cures for Tough Cancers*, for the type cancer you have, to see what other supplements you may find helpful (e.g., if you have breast cancer, you will want to check the breast cancer chapter in that book), and discuss with your physician about working up to at least 390 mg/day or more of CoQ10, milk thistle, and many other nutrients that can help you recover. You will need a good multi-vitamin and multi-mineral. You will need sufficient calcium, selenium, zinc, B vitamins, iodine, magnesium, lycopene, omega-3s, and you may wish to take AHCC, B17, resveratrol, or PBs (which the liver converts into antineoplastons). You may wish to consider intravenous vitamin C injections, PSK injections, mushroom supplements, Life Mel Honey, liposome-encapsulated vitamin C, bee pollen, royal jelly, Jordan Rubin's RM-10 mushroom formula or HSO Primal Defense supplements, and any number of items to help boost your immunity, many of which I discussed in greater detail in *Gentle Cures for Tough Cancers*. I would highly recommend the three nutritional drinks that I developed and described in Chapter 2 of this book, especially the **Orange Wunder Formula** for anyone fighting cancer. Check with your physician, but be prepared, because some conventional medicine docs won't approve anything that does not come from a prescription pad.

IV. Is Your Water Making You Ill?

It is appalling that after using fluoridated water for five years, Kansas City's "infant mortality increased 36%..." (139). On the other hand of the spectrum, Japan does NOT use fluoride in most of their drinking water and they have a greater longevity than individuals in most other industrialized countries, and a lower "infant mortality" than the rest of the "industrialized world" (139). *The Journal of the American Medical Association* admitted at least fifty years ago that "Fluorine... tends to accumulate in the bones, leading to hypercalcifications and brittleness...loss of mobility of joints, easy fracture and pressure on the spinal cord...baldness in young men, anemia and decreased blood clotting power" (139). In women, fluorine causes "painful menstruation, lowered birth rate, high incidence of fracture, thyroid alterations and liver damage" (139).

An article at Environmental Working Group revealed that fluoride has been identified as a link to "osteosarcoma in young boys and teenagers less than 20 years of age..." most notably because their bones grow so fast (53).

• How Fluoride Kills

NEED PROOF? Well, all you need to do is look at the eruption of the *Eyjafjallajoekull* volcano in Iceland. Besides the dangers of ash and all the other poisons, fire, fumes and toxins associated with an erupting volcano, one very little talked about risk is the fact that erupting volcanoes cause FLUORIDE poisoning. That's right. The animals and people in the area are poisoned quite rapidly with fluoride. You won't see THIS story plastered all over the news media in the U.S. Why? Because, regardless of what you are told about fluoride being SAFE in your drinking water, it is a POISON and it is a killer! Writer Marilla Mulwane describes this volcanic toxicity and exactly what it does to living creatures:

> The volcanic ash contains fluoride, which is a corrosive substance. Yes, it is found in our toothpastes and mouthwashes, but haven't you been told many times not to swallow too much of it? **Fluoride is often considered as toxic and poisonous as lead or arsenic...** If the animals swallow or breathe in too much of the toxic volcanic ash, that contains lots of fluoride; it can cause a few health problems. The fluoride will corrode the stomach and intestines, causing hemorrhages...If the animals ingest large amounts of the volcanic ash in a short period of time **this will weaken their bones**, and possibly even make **them lose their teeth.** Fluoride doesn't sound like such a healthy substance now, does it? (259) [Emphasis mine.]

Another thing, you don't have to swallow fluoride. It is absorbed right through your gums and oral mucosa and the rich supply of blood vessels under your tongue every time you brush your teeth with it! Well, do the math. This chemical kills the animals in Iceland that can't escape from the onslaught of ash by CORRODING their stomach and intestines causing them to bleed to death. It will give them brittle, weak bones and cause tooth loss! (Hello?) And we are told its fine and dandy to drink fluoride (and chlorine) in our water supply every day and use it in toothpaste and mouthwash and give it to our children? Here's the problem, you can take your choice. Either take fluoride all at once and die rapidly, or ingest it in SMALLER amounts over a LONGER period of time and suffer the SAME consequences as the animals in Iceland: stomach ulcers, intestinal bleeding, osteoporosis, brittle bones, and tooth loss! How can the FDA be so monstrously stupid as to think that fluoride in drinking water for HUMANS is safe when it kills animals? They just die faster because they get bigger doses when the volcanco spits! Americans are getting bone cancers, osteoporosis, bladder cancers, gum disease (tooth loss), degenerating joints, and they just can't believe it could be coming from their DRINKING WATER! (YES, it is!)

Chlorine is no better! The almost unbelievable part about using chlorine in our drinking water isn't because it is a great disinfectant, but because it is "the cheapest" (31). It is no secret that people who drink chlorinated water have a "93% higher...risk for getting cancer," than for those who do not drink chlorinated water (31). In the 1960's, Dr. Joseph Price warned about increasing "atherosclerosis...heart attacks and stroke..." from drinking chlorinated water (31). How amazing, isn't it - that statistics for heart disease and stroke have been skyrocketing ever since, yet no one seems to be connecting-the-dots!?

Chlorinated water has been a contributor toward breast cancer in women because chlorine has a tendency to accumulate in "breast tissue" (31), and will nearly "double the risk of bladder cancer" (32). And don't think that your primary source of chlorine is in that glass of water you drink from your tap. Most of the chlorine that overwhelms your system comes from the amount you breathe in or absorb through your skin while bathing and showering (31)! For those of you who have chlorine in your water and you love to take long, hot showers, what you are doing, in essence, is creating a toxic cloud of chlorine steam that you absorb through your skin and inhale into your lungs for the entire time you are bathing or showering and long afterwards!

That chlorine shower you take can hold as much as "50 times the level of chemicals than tap water" (31), and every time your body takes in chlorine, you lose valuable iodine! A lack of iodine in itself causes many chronic diseases, including all forms of cancer, especially breast cancer! Is it any wonder that most Americans are iodine-deficient and so many women are fighting breast cancer? (My own relative finally quit drinking fluoridated and chlorinated water after he was diagnosed with bladder cancer, even though I had tried to get him to do so for years before he developed cancer!) See Chapters 1 and 2.

And don't think you are without risk in chlorinated swimming pools, because your body simply absorbs chlorine right through your skin. This is so dangerous because the detoxing filtration system in the liver gets bypassed, making the chlorine more deadly to your system (32). How many hours do you or your children spend in chlorinated pools every summer?

Remember that water is mostly composed of oxygen. When you rob your body of water, you are cutting off a major oxygen supply for your cells. If you don't have a water filtration system at home, use distilled water or a reputable spring water source. The reason a vegetarian diet promotes alkalinity is because most raw vegetables and fruits are alkaline and alkaline-forming, with a few exceptions. All MEATS, including raw meats and processed dairy are acidic. Processed, packaged foods, white sugar, and flour are also acid-forming. The only dairy I would recommend is for those who use the *Johanna Budwig Formula* (see Chapters 2 and 3), or the *Orange Wunder Formula* that I developed and discuss in Chapter 2, with organic yogurt.

• Heavy Metals in Your Water Supply

It isn't just prescription medications, fluoride and chlorine in drinking water that is making us sick as a population. Some cities have abnormally high levels of LEAD in their drinking water. A study in 2009 from the *Washington Post* admitted that 42,000 children in Washington, D.C. had toxic amounts of lead in their water supply, and that it had been a problem since 2001 (83). [That is an EIGHT year period of time!] What was the reaction of the state health officials? Well, they simply issued a statement that they could find "no evidence of negative health effects on the general public's health," from the high lead levels (83). Amazing, isn't it? How the health officials in the entire nation seem to be in denial!? Denial about chlorine and fluoride, denial about lead in drinking water, denial about the dangers of low levels of selenium in the soil, denial about the link between mercury and autism, and denial about the dangers of mercury in dental fillings. It is almost like a total and collective reality distortion has gripped the nation. We are being poisoned, and no one in the health department, or government officials will admit to it, let alone discuss it!

• LifeStraw®

Many people believe that iodine is an irrelevant trace mineral. Well, there is a new product on the market known as *LifeStraw®,* which is being used for water purification in third world countries and for disaster-infested areas where clean water makes the difference between life and death. You can read more about this remarkable little "straw" at website: *www.lifestraw.com,* though it is not yet available for sale in the U.S. It looks like a medium tubular suction device, but it purifies water on contact, using **IODINE** embedded within its walls to do so! One of these little devices will safely filter up to 18,000 liters of water (or 185 gallons), enough water to last a person for about one year. Their commercial videos show extremely dirty water (even some water polluted with cow manure) that is drinkable, thanks to the filtration cleaning power of LifeStraw®. The handy little contraptions cost around $5.00 (U.S.) each.

Iodine has proven such a reliable antibacterial agent that a PubMed research article reports that it outperformed Cipro and Gentamycin as a topical agent for fighting a form of staphylcocci in human eye (corneal) transplants (203). For "severe eye inflammation," the dosage of Nascent used is "Five to ten drops of nascent iodine into one ounce of water" as an *eye lotion* (74). Can you see why having iodine on hand during an emergency is so important?

V. Bacteria & the Raw Foods Diet - Which Foods Are Safer?

There are a lot of safety concerns regarding consumption of raw foods (fruits & vegetables), especially in light of the fact that the FDA has no risk-free guarantees on raw food in the U.S. marketplace. (They have no risk-free guarantees on anything.) There have been many outbreaks in the past few years from bacteria in raw food (spinach, tomatoes, peppers, salsa, lettuce, peanut butter), and in undercooked meats from fast-food restaurants that have sickened and killed many children and adults. So what is the FDA response? Now they are speaking of IRRADIATING all raw fruits and vegetables! Of course this would also kill all the vital nutrients, enzymes, and vitamins in the food so that it would be completely DEAD!

Even though organic is better because of lack of insecticide and herbicide use, this is no guarantee that organic raw foods will be safe from threats like salmonella, e-coli, and other dangers. You have no idea how many hands (clean or dirty) have touched the food you are bringing home. During the bubonic plague in Europe, many people saved their lives by soaking their food in wine before consumption. If you cannot get organic foods in your area, some of the non-organic foods that have the least amount of pesticides, herbicides, and other chemical sprays (the lowest amounts) were found by *foodnews.org* to be the following: (in order of lowest amount of pesticides to highest) "Onions (lowest pesticide load), Avocado, Frozen Sweet Corn, Pineapples, Mango, Frozen Sweet Peas, Asparagus, Kiwi, Bananas, Cabbage, [and] Broccoli..." (55)

Is it any wonder that health food grocers like **Whole Foods Market** stores (with all their organic produce) are usually elbow-to-elbow with customers eager to purchase their organically-grown, chemical-free products?

Some raw food proponents recommend filling a previously-scrubbed sink with cold water and putting in two ounces of regular 3% solution hydrogen peroxide, then letting (e.g., leafy greens, carrots) soak in the solution for twenty minutes (vegetables with thicker skins for 30-35 minutes), then rinsing them thoroughly before consuming or refrigerating. You can also make a spray with a few ounces of 3% hydrogen peroxide diluted in six to eight ounces of water for your countertops. Remember, this is NOT food grade peroxide you are using. It should not be ingested. You are only using it to kill germs. Always rinse thoroughly. Even this is not a total guarantee. I always recommend that people (especially if eating out) take with them either cinnamon, cloves, ginger, garlic capsules, oil of wild oregano capsules, or grapefruit-seed extract, and consume the capsules with their meals for added protection. Or you may want to consider carrying a small bottle of 2% *Magnascent©* iodine with you and putting about ten drops in your drinking water.

• Liver Protection

Milk thistle and alpha lipoic acid can protect the liver from toxins. These substances won't give 100% protection when eating out, but it is possible that they could save your life or the life of a loved one. Some people advocate sipping wine with meals as an added safety measure to help kill bacteria in food, however, even unfermented grape juice will kill bacteria. Alcohol will eventually harm the liver. Never consume raw seafood or raw, undercooked meat, fish, fowl, or eggs. You are taking a risk!

• The Future Farmer

I believe the day will come when people will be forced to have their own backyard gardens to grow their family's food in order to be safer about food consumption. With all the new free trade laws in effect (e.g. NAFTA, which basically bankrupted the farmers of Mexico), crops are being sent across international lines faster and more adamantly than ever before in the history of the world. There are times when you purchase vegetables in a local grocery store and you have no idea if they are from the U.S., Mexico, Thailand, Pakistan, Columbia, Peru, Egypt, Australia, or Kenya. Does anyone know the farming practices of all these countries? Even foods grown in the U.S. cannot be guaranteed safe for consumption. How can foods imported from foreign countries—where we have little intervention in growing standards—be guaranteed safe? Well, they can't.

• The Best Protection Against Germs

Realize that it won't do you one bit of good to practice scrupulous scrubbing and soaking of your fruits and vegetables to kill bacteria if your personal hygiene habits are poor. Human beings contain e-coli and other harmful germs in their intestines. The best way to prevent the spread of bacteria has always been proper hand washing. Teach your kids proper hand washing while they are young and let them know why it is so important. Also, be sure to use the little antiseptic wipes that some retail merchants are now providing to wipe off shopping cart handles to reduce your exposure to germs. Keep hand sanitizers in your home, your school, your car, and your workplace.

CHAPTER 12

God's Marvelous "Green Thumb"

****

I. The Power of Chlorophyll

• Alfalfa

Though not a *grass,* alfalfa has nutritive value comparable to *cereal grasses* because it contains many of the same minerals and vitamins. Alfalfa sprouts are especially nutritious. They are rich in minerals such as phosphorus, contain twice the calcium of lettuce, and are a great source of all the *essential amino acids* (209). Individuals with a diagnosis of **lupus** should **avoid alfalfa products**, as they may cause a flare-up.

• Barley Grass Used to Heal Carcinoma

The power of green grasses has been attributed mainly to their chlorophyll and magnesium content (196), as discussed earlier in this book. Chlorophyll is such a speed healer that D. H. Collings proved that wounds took less time to heal when patients were taking this nutrient, than when using sulfa drugs, *penicillin,* or nothing at all (196). It has also been used to treat G.I. conditions, such as ulcers and inflammation of the pancreas, and has been used for those with *endocarditis*.

Remember that wheat grass juice comes from the young green leaves of the wheat berry, so even those with *gluten allergies* can safely consume the juice (196). Chlorophyll thins the blood, and this helps to balance out the effects of vitamin K in green foods, which thicken the blood. The two complement each other; however, if you are on blood thinners, your physician will not want you taking green foods and drinks without their approval.

Researchers from Japan isolated a compound, *P4-D1,* from the juice of barley which appears to shield cells from the sun's radiation. Using chlorophyll (such as that found in barley grass) as therapy, has actually prevented people from having their limbs amputated (e.g., Ann Wigmore), and one of the greatest advantages to using chlorophyll, is that there are NO toxic side effects (196), and it contains MAGNESIUM.

Another example is that of a woman who was treated with a rare skin carcinoma by drinking a barley juice from Japan known as *bakuryokuso.* The woman opted out of chemo and radiation and instead mixed a teaspoon of the dried barley powder in water or her favorite juice, and took it with her meals. Her cancerous skin condition began clearing up in less than two months (196). Realize that surgery can often completely eliminate skin cancers before they spread to other sites. I would never hesitate to recommend surgery for those with skin cancer.

• Chlorella for All Cancers

Chlorella *(Chlorella vulgaris)* is an algae grown and harvested in fresh water. It is a one-celled organism containing more chlorophyll than any other green plant, including spirulina (209). This is reported by C. M. Hawken in *Green Foods: "Phyto-Foods" for Super Health.* Due to its high level of chlorophyll, chlorella is good for the body (209). Nutrient-dense foods, such as chlorella, as well as fresh fruits and vegetables, can counter-attack free radicals and their insidious effects, thus wiping them out before they can harm us. Chlorella can help remove dangerous heavy metals from the body, and many studies have been done to show that it can boost the immune system (209). Chlorella can also halt the formation of abnormal cells and restore them to normalcy, since it raises the body's levels of *interferon* (209), a natural substance that helps the immune system cells (the **T cells**) kill infections. There is even a special type of chlorella with extremely high levels of the **chlorella growth factor** that you can obtain from Swanson Health Products at *www.swansonvitamins.com,* which is said to be very powerful at detoxing heavy metals from the body.

Chlorella and other green grasses enable the body to maintain a state of alkalinity, rather than acidity. A high acid environment generates free radicals and causes the leaching of calcium out of the bones to de-acidify the blood. Keeping the body in a state of alkalinity fights free radicals and prevents this calcium leaching from the bones, thus preventing osteoporosis and other degenerative diseases. Chlorophyll—found in all green plants—soothes the colon and rebuilds damaged intestinal cells, prevents the build-up of harmful microbes in the intestines, helps heal gastro-intestinal problems (such as ulcer formation and colitis), purifies the liver, and keeps the colon healthy (209). Remember that there are many other "grasses" that are part of what we consider *green* foods, all of which are not discussed in detail here. Some of these include: sprouts, seaweed, the cruciferous vegetables, spinach, kale, mustard greens, other leafy greens, and many others (209). A benefit to chlorella is that you can carry the little green pills around with you and take them whenever you like.

• Chlorella & Protein in the Vegan Diet

Chlorella alga is vitamin and mineral-rich, and for those concerned about protein in a vegetarian diet (or vitamin B12), it is high in protein and vitamin B12. Also, realize that you don't need meat to get complete proteins in your diet. Combining grains and legumes (beans) gives complete proteins. In laboratory research with chlorella, tumor masses completely vanished in half the animals receiving chlorella. All of the animals not on the extract worsened as their cancers continued to grow. Unless they received chlorella—they all died—no exceptions and all of them had tumors. Some forms of chlorella do contain trace amounts of iodine. Most do not.

• Green Foods & Cholesterol

There are many natural ways to lower cholesterol without resorting to statin drugs with all their potentially disastrous side effects, but pharmaceutical companies make no money from natural substances, so they would rather you know nothing about them. The B vitamin, niacin, has been found to work just as well as pharmaceutical drugs at lowering cholesterol. **Do not take the timed-release** form of niacin.

You can use the flush-free if you do not like the flushing sensation that niacin can cause, but some physicians feel that the type of niacin that causes the body to flush indicates that it is working well. I usually tell people to start with a small dose, about 100 mg, and work up as you develop a tolerance for niacin. Taking niacin on an empty stomach will make it work more rapidly and you will feel a stronger effect than if you take it on a full stomach of food. Do not take niacin on an empty stomach, and then eat food while you are getting the flushing effect. It has a tendency to make the throat feel dry and it can cause you to choke, especially if you do not have any water nearby. This is because niacin dilates all the blood vessels, including the ones in the mouth and throat.

Other foods, treatments, and supplements that help lower harmful cholesterol and raise good cholesterol include: garlic, iodine, soya lecithin, exercise, omega-3 foods and supplements, policosanol, guggolipids, green tea, cayenne pepper, soluble fiber (such as oat bran or steel cut oats), fresh vegetable juices and fruit juices (that you juice yourself), krill oil, *Ecklonia Cava,* ginseng, ginger, barley, celery, red grapes, resveratrol, cernitin, Chinese red yeast rice with guggol, citrus pectin, flax, pomegranate, hibiscus tea, kombucha, olive oil, reishi mushroom, apple skins, fenugreek, cinnamon, rye bread, *Seanol*® (see website: *http://www.drsinatra.com* and go to the search box on the right-hand side of the page and type in the word Seanol), shiitake mushroom, spirulina, amla fruit, beta carotene, bilberry, Calcium D-Glucarate, magnesium, and many other natural substances. Sesame oil can help reduce high blood pressure. Note that if you do not have the time to get 3 or 4 servings of fresh vegetable juice every day, you may want to substitute a serving or two of **V8® Low Sodium Vegetable juice**, which may be helpful in lowering cholesterol and high blood pressure. It is low in salt (140 mg in 8 ounces) and contains several different types of vegetables (mostly tomatoes) and lycopene. Just be absolutely sure that what you purchase is the LOW SODIUM! V8® does market an organic juice, but the only one I have seen has 480 mg of salt per 8 ounce serving. I am not sure why their organic juice has more salt than the non-organic.

• Spirulina - Chelator & B12 Source

Spirulina is another green food that, when taken as a supplement, is still considered a *whole food* because the entire plant is used during production, not merely an extract of the plant (290). An ingredient in spirulina (known as *Phycocyanin)*, gives it that characteristic lovely, deep bluish-green color it is noted for. In animal testing, it had the ability to fend off viruses, cancer, and anemia by increasing the production of *red blood cells* in the body (290).

Spirulina can act like a chelator in removing heavy metals from the body, and has been used for helping diabetic patients, as well as those fighting high blood pressure and elevated blood fats (290). Spirulina is helpful in the intestines since it ensures survival of good *bacteria*, and it is given to children in third world countries for the prevention of *blindness* (290). There are no known adverse effects from ingesting this green wonder food. Even those with gout can take spirulina, and it is an excellent source of vitamin B12 (290). Spirulina can boost the immune system (209), and may be especially beneficial to those who are fighting blood disorders like leukemia, anemia, and multiple myelomas.

As described elsewhere in this book, you can also take vitamin B12 as a sublingual tablet that dissolves under the tongue, or injections from your physician. Another excellent source of B12 is chlorella. Just be sure to get the broken cell-wall chlorella. Chlorella has the highest concentration of chlorophyll of any green food.

You may want to check out Dr. Andrew W. Saul's recipe for a nasal delivery form of B12 at *http://www.doctoryourself.com/nasal.html* and Dr. Joseph Mercola's website for a new mist spray form of B12: *http://products.mercola.com/vitamin-B12-spray/?source=nl*.

• Spirulina & Mouth Cancer

Spirulina has also proven useful in the treatment of mouth cancer. When researchers gave *tobacco chewers,* who had abnormal pre-cancerous cells in their mouth, a gram of this green food every day for a year, nearly 50% of the participants receiving the spirulina had significant *improvement*, which did not happen in the control group. (290).

• Sprouts - Tiny Seeds that Pack a Punch

Ann Wigmore was so convinced of the high nutritional value of fresh sprouts that she not only grew them for her clients, she incorporated them into her meals on a daily basis and wrote a book called *The Sprouting Book.* She believed that sprouts were an excellent way of ridding the body of toxins (308). Sprouts are so nutritious and easily digestible; Ann Wigmore believed that when consumed, they are nearly capable of digesting themselves! They are very high in beneficial enzymes that aid digestion, amino acids (plant proteins), and many vitamins (308). The human body has the ability to manufacture 14 essential amino acids, but there are eight which must be obtained through outside sources, and sprouts have all eight of them (308). In *The Sprouting Book,* Ann Wigmore said that, unlike living foods, such as raw fruits and vegetables whose nutrient value begins going downhill as soon as they are picked or cut, sprouts keep their nutritional level until consumption (308), provided that you don't keep them refrigerated for days on end.

Ann Wigmore* also believed that you can triple the amount of vitamin E in your diet by relying on wheat berry sprouts, rather than wheat, since sprouting increases the vitamin E content, and this natural form of vitamin E has a tenfold greater absorption within the cells than the man-made E supplements (308). She reported that one of the highest sources of calcium is fresh sesame sprouts, which have more calcium than *cow's milk*. Other sprouts, such as those from *sunflower* seeds and *chick peas,* are also high in calcium (308). Sprouts are very high in chlorophyll, the benefits of which were discussed earlier in this chapter. They are so nutrient-dense that they enhance the immune system. Be sure that if you grow or purchase sprouts that you always buy organic seeds or sprouts. Sprouts can get contaminated with bacteria if not grown, handled, rinsed, and washed properly.

• **Wheat Grass & Alkalinity**

Wheat grass is very alkaline. Ann Wigmore said that it has been used to treat digestive problems, "ulcerative colitis...itchy or scaly scalp," sore throat, sore gums, sick pets, as an external poultice for skin problems, and a disinfectant, and for many other chronic health problems. It is high in chlorophyll (307). Did you know that most of the expensive mouth washes and breath fresheners sold in your dentist's office merely use chlorophyll to kill the bacteria that cause bad breath? Chlorophyll is one of the most important nutrients in fresh green juices like wheat grass.

Ann Wigmore advocated in her book, *The Hippocrates Diet And Health Program*, raw fresh foods, fruits, vegetables, and fresh juices, nothing cooked. (This was a total vegan diet—no meats—and no dairy products allowed) (307). Some cancer patients are so weak and debilitated that they cannot tolerate a totally raw diet. It is easier for them to gradually convert to a totally raw diet over a period of time; however, in most cases, the sooner they make this transition, the better off they are, though some simply cannot or will not make the transition. My own relative (see Chapter 1) ate the same diet he always eats when he was fighting bladder cancer and he is not much for raw foods. He did, however, ingest the nutritional formulas I developed (see Chapter 2). When facing a terminal illness, time suddenly becomes a very precious commodity that we often take for granted.

Stephen Blauer, author of *The Juicing Book*, considers chlorophyll an energizing blood *cleanser* and *tonic* (174). It is so much like the *hemoglobin molecule*, it has been discovered that animals can change "chlorophyll into hemoglobin…," and some scientists believe that we humans may have the same capacity (174).

What an amazing ability! Perhaps one day patients needing blood transfusions will simply be drinking chlorophyll products instead, thus eliminating all the potential complications related to receiving blood products. Is it any wonder that green drinks are so beneficial to leukemia patients and those with *anemia* and other blood disorders?

• Wheat Grass Has Antioxidants that Fight Many Types of Cancer

Website: *healingcancernaturally.com/barley-green-powder-medicine.html* has more information on the healing properties of wheat grass juice, which can be taken in fresh or powdered form (176). Wheat grass juice is not a panacea or *silver bullet* cure-all, though it may be close! Restoring health after a devastating illness depends on many factors, and nutritional juicing is just one of those factors. Wheat grass is an amazing boost for the immune system. Cancer and autoimmune disorders happen when the immune system is ill or suppressed. As many cancer patients described in this book and my other books have discovered, heal your immune system and it will get you well!

• Wheat Grass - Miracle Nutrient

Ann Wigmore was so impressed by the health effects of fresh wheat grass juice on her life that she not only wrote books about it, but she founded the *Hippocrates Health Institute* in Boston, where her guests were treated to a life of natural health living with a strict raw foods regimen. For years, many people came to the *Wigmore Mansion* as it was called, some with terminal illnesses. Many left totally cured, including Eydie Mae Hunsberger, who cured her breast cancer while on the Wigmore program. I discussed her case in more detail in my last book, *Gentle Cures for Tough Cancers.*

Ann Wigmore healed her own body of many ailments (caused, she said, by eating an American diet for two decades) after she began ingesting fresh wheat grass juice. She discovered that within *a few weeks* of starting on *wheat grass juice* (as well as using *sprouts and greens*), she was healed of *colitis* (309). Though she felt that a vegetarian diet of raw foods was very beneficial for health maintenance, she considered wheat grass juice the greatest healer for the *body's immunity* that exists (309). Wheat grass juice is very rapidly assimilated into the body when taken. It does not need 30-60 minutes to go through the digestive process, since the nutrients are almost immediately absorbed into your cells. If you are fighting a debilitating illness, you need nutrition that is immediately available and not taxing on your body.

• Wheat Grass Regimen Used Successfully to Treat Primary Peritoneal Cancer in 89-Year-Old Woman

For an amazing case study from Guisseppi A. Forgionne Ph.D., about an 89-year-old woman who experienced total remission from advanced peritoneal cancer using an alternative nutritional approach, see website: *http://www.cancerlynx.com/peritonealcase.html* (199). After having surgery, she refused chemo. According to the article, her nutritional regimen included *2 grams of wheat grass* per day (which she started taking a week after her surgery), then *100 mg of CoQ10* a week after that, and within 2 more weeks, the addition of *9 grams of bovine cartilage*/day. *Nine months* later, her CoQ10 was changed to *150 mg per day* (199). Her cancer completely disappeared. (The peritoneum is the lining that covers most of your abdominal organs.)

II. The Power of Grapes & Resveratrol

In her book, *The Grape Cure*, Johanna Brandt says that she came to America in 1927 to describe her amazing cure for cancer using common table grapes and a raw foods diet. She cured her own abdominal cancer when physicians had advised her that she would die without surgery. The story of her cleansing, fasting, raw diet is given in detail in a powerful little book known as *The Grape Cure,* which can be purchased at internet book stores and from Ehret Literature Publishing Co., Inc. (for $4.95), PO Box 24, Dobbs Ferry, N.Y. 10522. Their website is *www.arnoldehret.org.*

Johanna experienced a complete cure from her abdominal cancer by consuming fresh grapes and drinking fresh grape juice, as well as a total raw foods diet. It did not seem to matter what type of grape she consumed—the more the variety—the better. She healed herself completely without surgery, radiation, or chemotherapy (178). She stayed with the raw fruit and vegetable juices until her cancer had completely disappeared (178).

Grapes also contain another super antioxidant known as *caffeic acid*, and they are rich in ellagic acid, as are raspberries, pomegranates, strawberries, pecans, walnuts, cherries, cranberries, and other fruits. Ellagic acid helps boost the body's own immune system, giving it the ability to fight cells that are running amuck in the body and causing disease (253). Cranberries also cut the risk for ulcers and bladder infections, and help fight leukemia (8).

Johanna was a great believer in raw foods, and felt that a total raw food juicing diet was healthiest, especially for those already fighting cancer. We are living, electronically-functioning organisms. When you feed your body raw foods, you are giving your cells electrically-balanced food that can be recognized, processed, and used optimally. Once foods are cooked, the live enzymes within them are destroyed.

Johanna's book, though written more than 70 years ago, is still very relevant today.

Anti-angiogenesis foods and nutrients halt cancerous tumors from spreading by keeping them from growing blood vessels, without which they cannot obtain nutrition and they shrivel up and die. This isn't really new, because I first discussed it back in 2005 when my first book came out. Some of the items that have this remarkable property that I talked about are: Ukrain, bindweed, ellagic acid, shark cartilage, pawpaw, PRIMA-1 with 2aG4, Embolization Particle Therapy, Umbelliferae, **resveratrol**, the drug, Lodamin, and several others.

Dr. William Li says that red grapes prevent this blood vessel growth by 60% and the "ellagic acid found in strawberries," is even more powerful. He lists several other foods that starve cancer and fight obesity in much the same way (233a). A few of them are: "Green tea...Nutmeg, Garlic, Berries: strawberries, blackberries, raspberries, blueberries, Kale, Artichokes, Tomato, Cherries, Turmeric, Parsley [and] Maitake mushroom" (233a).

• Grapes Fight High Cholesterol & High Blood Pressure

Researchers at Madrid University took an extract of red grapes made, not from the juice, but its *byproducts*—the *skins and seeds*—(which many people discard) and made a *cocktail* from it that they referred to as *GADF* (*Grape Antioxidant Dietary Fibre*) (41). "Tests on human volunteers found the extract was extremely rich in both fibre and antioxidants which reduce the risks of cardiovascular disease - the world's biggest killer" (41). Red grapes also help fight high cholesterol and high blood pressure.

• Raw Food Diet & Oxalates

A note on the raw food diet—be aware that there are many raw foods, such as rhubarb, kiwi, berries, and spinach that are considered high-oxalate foods. They contain a form of acid that can aggregate to form kidney stones or gallstones (82). These foods should not be used in large amounts by those who may be prone to develop gallstones or kidney stones. These acid crystals can irritate joints, as in the case of gout or rheumatoid arthritis (82). Also, avoid taking calcium with high oxalate foods, since oxalates can inhibit calcium's use by the body. Wait a few hours in between (173). Many times, stone formation could be avoided by simply increasing fluid intake, and making sure that sufficient amounts of B vitamins and magnesium are taken daily; however, there will always be some folks who are prone to develop stones, regardless of what they do.

The majority of people have no problem with oxalate foods. There are many websites that give complete lists of all the foods that contain oxalates. If you are prone to develop stones, and are able to obtain one of them, have it analyzed by the hospital lab to find out the stone's composition. Depending on what the stone consists of, will tell you how to prevent a reoccurrence. For example, if you have stones that consist mostly of calcium phosphate or magnesium ammonium phosphate (sometimes called *struvite stones*), keeping your urine acidic with things like cranberry juice and/or ascorbic acid (vitamin C) will help prevent, and in some cases, even dissolve these type stones. If you have cystine stones or calcium oxalate stones, keeping your urine acidic will not help dissolve them, nor if you have uric acid stones. Even though vitamin C may increase oxalate formation, it won't cause you to form these type stones.

If you have a problem with gout caused by uric acid and purines, try eating sour cherries, increasing your intake of vitamin C, and decreasing meat, sugar, protein, and coffee intake. It is also important to maintain good water hydration and restrict the consumption of carbonated sodas to prevent stones. Be sure to get adequate B vitamins and alkalize your body. Most carbonated sodas are high in phosphorus. Drinking them over time will eventually damage your kidneys.

• Raw Food Vegan Diet & Vitamin B12 Concerns

Vegetarians are often told that they will suffer a vitamin B12 deficiency without consuming meats. B12 can be destroyed by gastric acid in the stomach, though some amounts of B12 are created by *friendly* bacteria in the intestines. For concern about gastric acid destruction of vitamin B12, this vitamin is available in **sublingual** tablets at most health food stores. You simply put the small tablet under your tongue and it is dissolved and absorbed directly into the rich supply of blood vessels there, completely bypassing the stomach acid. There is a vegetarian formula known as B-12 Dots® made by TwinLab®. They can be obtained at website: *http://www.twinlab.com/product/b-12-dots* and you can find them at most health food stores. Also, it is now possible to get B12 patches where the vitamin is absorbed directly into the skin.

• Grapes & Alkalinity

The healthiest state for the human body is one of moderate alkalinity. The ideal blood pH of the body is 7.35—7.45. The lower the number, the more acidic your body is; the higher the number, the more alkaline. If you keep your body in a state of alkalinity, rather than acidity, you will drastically slash your risks for getting cancer and other diseases, because diseases thrive when the body is kept in a state of acidity. A diet high in meat, dairy, and cooked food keeps the body in a state of constant acidity, increasing the risk for cancer and all chronic diseases. When the blood is acidic, it will try to alkalize on its own by pulling calcium and magnesium into the bloodstream. Where does it get these minerals? Well—usually from your BONES! This is why a cooked diet with excess meats, dairy, processed foods, and refined sugars causes joint pain, gout, heart disease, diabetes, osteoporosis, liver problems, stones, PVD, PAD, asthma, allergies, colon problems, inflammation, colds, viruses, flu, and other health ailments.

Raw fruits and vegetables contribute to the body's alkalinity. Any cooking of foods immediately reduces their alkalinity and makes them more acidic. Grapes alkalize the blood. Realize too that keeping the body acid-free has multiple benefits. Osteoporosis, osteopenia, joint pain, bone spurs, kidney stones, and fibromyalgia pains can all be caused by excess acid in the body. When acid builds up in the body, the blood removes calcium from the bones to reduce the acidity of the blood and raise its pH level. This also causes a loss of magnesium and other minerals from the bones, making them brittle and weak. This high acid level in the blood also lowers oxygen. Diseases like cancer flourish in a high-acid, low-oxygen environment, as do most fungi, viruses, bacteria, and parasites.

Diets that promote acidity also cause large amounts of free radicals to circulate in the human body. Free radicals are a type of aberrant electron, and though some are good for us, most are not. The harmful ones can cause chaos within the DNA, leading to mutations that result in cancer and chronic diseases.

Those who criticized Johanna Brandt during her lifetime did so out of ignorance. They knew nothing of free radicals, proanthocyanidins, carotenoids, or super antioxidants. As time goes by, more and more amazing properties of Johanna's miracle grapes are being discovered.

• Grape Power for pH Balance

During her day, many people adopted Johanna's grape cure, but others were critical, disbelieving that something this simple could affect disease so profoundly. Modern researchers, however, have isolated an amazing ingredient in grapes, known as ***resveratrol.*** It is a very powerful antioxidant that not only inhibits the growth of cancer cells, but contains healing and blood-thinning properties (165). Johanna Brandt's remarkable cure from abdominal cancer certainly proved that she was ahead of her time, and that there is something miraculous in the healing power of fasting, detoxification, and the lowly grape.

The reason white wine is white is because the resveratrol-rich grape skins are not used in white wine—only in red wines (196). For an excellent 58-page study on resveratrol's role in fighting cancer, which was conducted by M.D. Anderson Cancer Center and the UCLA Center for Human Nutrition, see website: *http://www.agrawal.org/PDF/ACR-Resveratrol1.pdf* (171). Resveratrol is also being touted as a way to fight obesity, since it keeps the body from storing fat. Studies at the University of Virginia Health System recently unraveled how resveratrol works at fighting cancer. Apparently, the resveratrol in red wine and grape skin blocks the effect of a very important protein that cancer cells can't live without; however, it only takes a small amount of wine (about 8 ounces a few times a week); too much, and the risk for cancer increases. Non-alcoholic wine works just as well (118) (119), can be used by children, and is safe for the liver. Better yet, use the grape skins in their original packaging as prepared by our Creator, or simply drink fresh grape juice!

Another very powerful antioxidant comes from the seeds and skins of grapes (as well as acai berries, raspberries, cranberries, strawberries, and other fruits) and the bark of the pine tree. It is pycnogenols (165).

Eat a variety of grapes and eat the skin and seeds as well! Choose red, purple, black, green, and white grapes. (165).

Most of us are familiar with recent health studies showing the lack of heart disease and lack of harmful cholesterol levels found in the French (known as the *French paradox*), yet they enjoy rich foods and consume wine with most of their meals. As mentioned in Reese Dubin's *Miracle Food Cures From the Bible*, this is because wine can raise good cholesterol levels, and also helps to scour harmful fats from the arteries (196). Grape extracts appear to strengthen the walls of blood vessels, thus preventing vein varicosities and degenerative diseases of the eye, such as diabetic retinopathy and others. When cholera broke out in the 18th century, many lives were saved when it was shown that wine killed bacteria. People used it to soak their foods, especially meat, fish, and fruits. During the 1970's when viruses were tested against grape extract, a day later, none of the viruses were alive (196), and this is the juice we are talking about, BEFORE it is fermented into wine!

Although wine kills harmful germs and bacteria, **you don't need alcohol-containing wine to do this**. Fasting, juicing, fresh grape juice, and a detox regimen can do the same thing. Try to use organic whenever possible. Many commercial grapes are heavily sprayed. Be aware that alcoholic drinks are harmful to the liver, not to mention what they do to the brain. Grape extract also kills viruses and bacteria without harming the liver or the brain, and it inhibits cancer rather than increasing its risks. No adverse side effects have been reported from taking grape seed extract. Just don't mix it with vitamin C supplements. Research suggests that taking them at the same time may raise blood pressure in some individuals. Grape extract has been useful in the treatment of many disorders, including those affecting the circulatory system.

- **Grapes Help Fight Lung Cancer, Colon, Breast, Prostate, Pancreatic, Liver Cancer & Leukemia**

This isn't the end of the miraculous grape and resveratrol. According to an article at website *CancerProject.org*, resveratrol can slow down the spread of many types of cancer, including those in the *breast, liver, colon, lungs,* and even *leukemia* (54). Grape seed extract can help kill colorectal cancer cells.

The University of Kentucky has just completed a lab study on grapeseed extract. Their findings (published in *Clinical Cancer Research*) showed that grape seed extract could kill more than two thirds of leukemia cells within just 24 hours! It's important when eating grapes, you must eat the seeds too (157a). You can now get resveratrol and grape seed supplements in natural health food stores and on the internet.

Is it any wonder that Johanna Brandt's *Grape Cure* was such a potent enemy against so many forms of cancer? She was considered a *genius* by some in her day, while others scoffed at her. It appears that where the scientific community is concerned, Johanna Brandt has had the last laugh. It is very unfortunate that her *Grape Cure* blessing never reached the majority of Americans for which it was intended. How many people have ever heard of it before now? **(Have you?)** When was the last time you or your children ate fresh grapes?

• Grapes & Resveratrol, the Super Flavenol

Research on this compound has shown that resveratrol can inhibit the cancer process in any of its three stages of development from beginning to end (191). It also has anti-inflammatory properties similar to some chemo drugs, but without the damaging affects that they cause. Even **concord grapes** have been shown to repress tumors as effectively as the common chemo drug *methotrexate* (191), and animal testing has shown a dramatic decrease in breast tumors in animals fed purple grape juice and **concord grapes** (58). All you have to do is look at the rich, blue-black color of concord grapes and you know instinctively that there is something powerful about those prized little orbs designed by our Creator!

According to website *http://www.mnwelldir.org/nw_current.htm,* "some call resveratrol the Fountain of Youth" (120). More and more studies continue to be done on this amazing antioxidant found in the "skin of grapes, berries and red wines" (120). As the website notes:

> Dr. Stuart Richer OD, PhD, Chief, Optometry Section at the Veterans Medical Center in North Chicago, speaking at the 111th annual American Academy of Optometry meeting in Seattle, says this may be the first time an intervention has been shown to reverse aging changes in the retina. The

patient, an 80-year-old male, came to the eye clinic complaining of loss of night vision. Commonly prescribed nutriceuticals, such as lutein, vitamin E and fish oil were employed with no positive result. After 5 months on the dietary supplement regimen [resveratrol], five measurable parameters of vision improved to varying but significant degrees including night (contrast) vision, visual acuity, color and side vision….it was also found the patient's mental capacity had improved (120).

Harvard studies have recently shown that resveratrol "Cleans your arteries of plaque making them smooth and youthful; gives you a boost of energy, helping to burn more calories; boosts the immune system, and might even reverse the damage from a lousy diet and lifestyle" (120).

Researchers even found, to their amazement, that they could feed half a group of aging mice a *high…trans fat, junk food diet*, and all of them "developed the same symptoms of humans who ate the same diet:" liver problems, "diabetes and cardiovascular issues…" (120). The rest of the mice ate the exact same diet, but were given resveratrol. They gained weight, were much healthier…functioned normally, looked healthier. All the rodents in the first "group died prematurely." Those in the "second group lived 15% longer than normal" and "…another related study showed that mice on resveratrol were able to run twice as fast as normal, healthy mice not taking resveratrol" (120).

More research keeps coming forth on the amazing rejuvenation powers of resveratrol. Dr. Robert Rowan's findings show that "rats who were given wine compounds for eight weeks maintained healthy blood pressure; one study shows resveratrol" outperformed "Pepto-Bismol in combating three strains of bacteria that cause diarrhea" (120). It is also an antifungal, offering some protection from pathogens, not just in the *grape plant*, but *in humans* as well and was shown to help prevent "cataracts (taken in the form of red wine)" (120).

• Other Health Benefits of Eating Grapes

Organically grown grapes should be purchased whenever possible. Grapes are often one of the most highly sprayed fruits in production. Organically grown grapes are certified to be free of pesticides and herbicides. Grapes are a rich source of quercetin, a potent antioxidant. They also contain the important anti-inflammatory, antioxidant—Pycnogenol®. Pycnogenol® helps fight debilitating disorders, such as cardiac and circulatory problems, arthritis, stress, and even inhibits allergies and cancerous growths.

A research group recently reported that resveratrol protects against both liver and breast cancer, but don't look for resveratrol in white wine, because it is found only in the pulp and seeds which are excluded when white wine is processed from the juice. It is found in red wine or red and purple grape juices; however, as stated earlier, alcohol consumption in itself can increase the risk of certain cancers. The cancer-fighting chemicals are found in grapes before they are ever fermented into wine. Why not consume them raw—the way our Creator God gave them to us—in their healthiest and most natural state? Resveratrol supplements are available in health food stores and many local supermarkets. If taking resveratrol, consult with your physician first, and don't hesitate to consult a Naturopathic physician. To locate one near you, see website: *http://altmedangel.com/physician_reference_list.htm,* or go to: *http://www.naturopathic.org.* Also, see Appendix II at the back of this book for other resources.

• Pterostilbene - Another Healing Ingredient Discovered in Grapes (& Blueberries)

In our annuals of modern medicine, every single day seems to bring more amazing discoveries about the healing properties of natural foods, such as grapes and their cancer-fighting nutrients. Yet another compound has recently been discovered in grapes that may not only fight cancer, but diabetes as well (37). The compound is known as *pterostilbene.* It is supposed to work much like resveratrol, but also lowers blood sugar (37). Blueberries are even higher in pterostilbene content than grapes (37), and researchers recently reported that blueberries can prevent and treat some forms of cancer in children. Pterostilbene also enhances memory and fights heart disease and harmful cholesterol (14).

One researcher noted that this compound could prevent cancer-causing changes in DNA, especially against malignant breast cells. This particular nutrient—though found in blue, red, and black grape skins—

is destroyed when the juice is made into wine; another reason to consume the grape in its natural, God-given, raw form—pulp, skin, seeds and all!

• Sources of Resveratrol

A very rich source of resveratrol is the root of the Japanese knotweed plant known as *hu zhang*. Some resveratrol supplements are taken from hu zhang, others use ground-up purple grape skin. Blueberries, peanuts, mulberry, cranberries, and many other food sources contain resveratrol. I am seeing more and more resveratrol supplements available in health food stores, pharmacies, and local supermarket shelves. This was rare when my first book came out in 2005. Everyone is now jumping on the resveratrol, acai berry, and Pycnogenol® bandwagon.

• Which Grapes Are Best?

I believe the best advice, as given by Johanna Brandt, is to eat a **variety**, because you will get more **resveratrol** in the red and purple grape skins, and, as noted by James F. Balch, M.D., author of *The Super Antioxidants,* there are more **OPCs** (super antioxidants, also known as *oligomeric proanthocyanidins),* in the "green and white grapes," and **you need both** (165). Remember that for OPCs, you need to eat the entire grape along with the seeds. (165). Red grapes also contain high OPC levels.

III. Juicing – Getting Started

• Benefits of Purchasing a Juicer

For those of you who are already ill, one of the first and most important things you can do is to purchase a juicer. Be sure that you obtain a juicer that has the capacity to juice not only fresh fruits and vegetables, but green foods like spinach, broccoli, wheat grass, celery, kale, and others. Some juicer manufacturers will claim that their juicers can juice wheat grass, but they do a very poor job of it. The juice will come out very foamy and warm, so that it has oxidized nearly all of its vital enzymes during the process.

• Types of Juicers

There are many good juicers on the market that will juice wheat grass as well as fresh vegetables and fruits. Four good choices that do this are: the *Samson* juicer, the *Green Star,* the *Green Power juicer,* and the *Omega 8003* juicer. These type juicers can sometimes be found at natural health food stores, or they can be ordered on the internet. If your local health food store does not have the model you desire, they can usually order it for you. The first large juicer I purchased was a *Champion*. I read on the internet that it did not do a good job of juicing grapes, but mine juiced grapes wonderfully. It juiced everything wonderfully, EXCEPT greens!

Some people like the large opening provided by the *Jack LaLanne Power Juicer™* and the *Juiceman®* juicer, while others argue that these type juicers pulverize the vegetables too quickly, causing oxidation. Regardless of the many opinions about which juicer is best, get one that you are comfortable using, with easy clean-up, and you will enjoy extraordinary benefits from ANY fresh organic juice that you make for yourself or your loved ones. Just remember this: if you use a juicer that will juice a whole apple without cutting it up, the center of the apple could have a large rotten place that you would never see unless you at least slice the apple one time before juicing it! Some juicers will allow you to juice bing cherries without even removing the seeds, others, like the *Jack LaLanne Power Juicer™,* will tell you to remove the seeds before juicing.

There are manual juicers that juice wheat grass only that are very economical, as well as electric juicers made just for juicing wheat grass; however, if you buy one of these, you will need another juicer for your fruits and vegetables. An excellent manual juicer is the *Miracle* manual wheat grass juicer. *Miracle* also makes electric wheat grass juicers, but as stated earlier, if you get this type, you will need a separate juicer for your fruits and vegetables. (See website: *http://www.sproutpeople.com/juicers/manual.html).*

If you juice citrus fruits (e.g., oranges and grapefruits) in your main juicer, you will need to peel them first, or you can obtain a very inexpensive citrus juicer for about twelve dollars just for oranges, grapefruits, lemons, and limes at your local department store, then your main juicer can be one that does vegetables, other fruits (such as berries, apples, grapes, cantaloupe, etc.) and greens. Good choices of juicers that do it all are the *Samson* juicer, the *Green Star,* the *Green Power juicer,* and the *Omega 8003* juicer. They will juice greens as well as veggies and fruits, and the *Omega 8003* is supposed to take just five minutes for cleanup. You can also find little hand-held, manual citrus juicers for lemons and limes that will cost about four or five dollars.

I received a *Jack Lalanne Power Juicer*™ as a gift, and I have no complaints about it, except that now I have to remove cherry pits before juicing fresh cherries and with my older machine I did not have to remove pits first. Also, while it is true that the motor runs very quietly—it does—until you start putting the vegetables or fruit in, then it gets very noisy and the machine shakes and shimmies a lot. You have to be sure and keep the plunger down on the fruit or vegetables, or the smaller vegetables (like pieces of broccoli) will jump right out of the machine and onto your floor or countertop. Clean-up is easy.

• Juicing Output

A good rule of thumb is that the softer the fruit you are juicing, the thicker the juice will be. You will get a much thicker juice from soft pears than hard pears. Strawberries, pineapples, and berries will give you a very thick, mushy-type juice. You can dilute it with water and other juices and drink it, or freeze it into popsicles. A general rule of thumb is that one pound of produce will usually give you approximately 6 - 8 ounces of juice. If you want an eight ounce glass of carrot juice, for example, be prepared to purchase about one pound of carrots; however, yield will also depend on the type juicer you choose as well. Some juicers extract more efficiently and you get more juice from your produce. The drier the pulp that comes out, the more juice you are getting. The 6-8 ounce rule does not apply to juicing greens. Yield depends on many variables, such as the type of greens you are juicing and the type juicer you are using.

The *Norwalk* juicer is said to give one of the best yields, but it is very expensive—more than $2,000. I have heard users complain that it takes 30 minutes to clean after each use, but it gives an excellent yield and quality of juice, possibly 50% higher yield than less expensive models. It is often used at health institutions, and you can order it on the internet.

• What to Juice

If you are seriously ill, purchasing a juicer that provides you with fresh wheat grass juice, vegetable, and fruit juices is one of the most important **first steps** you can take for your health. You can also use green powdered drinks. If you want to boost your immune system and prevent sickness in the first place, juicing is not an option, it is a lifestyle that you will need to incorporate, along with fresh air, exercise, reliance on God, adequate water, sunshine, and other tenets of health, as described in this book. You will soon find that investing in a juicer has priceless benefits that far outweigh your initial cost. Fresh wheat grass juice detoxifies the body so rapidly, only small amounts can be tolerated at a time. Start out consuming more than an ounce or two at a time and you will become nauseated or dizzy, simply because of the quick detox effect. You can gradually work up to larger amounts as needed. The same applies for beet root juice which detoxifies rapidly. Always mix it with another juice. Also, remember that raw foods (even those that are organic) must be washed thoroughly. You do not want to juice for health and end up with an e-coli or salmonella infection. If ever in doubt, put 8 or 10 drops of 2% *Magnascent©* iodine in your glass of juice.

Wheat grass and other green juices are excellent sources of calcium and chlorophyll. Many people have been led to believe that we must get our calcium from milk, dairy products, and supplements. This is not true. Even carrot juice is higher in calcium than milk! The best source of calcium is the SAME place that the cows and goats extract it. They get it from the soil—green plants in the soil. Your very best and most natural source of calcium is **green foods.** And you don't have to worry about whether or not your body is going to absorb the calcium when you ingest it in this format. The cells literally inhale it. (They know a good thing when they see it coming!) You can often purchase fresh wheat grass in trays at your health food store, or kits where you can try growing your own. It is also available in frozen cubes in some health food store freezers, that you simply thaw and use as needed.

Grasses, such as wheat grass, are rich in 17 amino acids (including the 8 *essential* amino acids), as well as dozens of different enzymes. They are also rich in many vitamins, minerals, trace minerals, and essential fatty acids (309). Because of this rich supply of nutrients, green foods and fresh juices are excellent for women who are pregnant; however, let your doctor know your dietary trends. It has been proven, in many cases, that cancer can be induced in laboratory animals by simply depriving them of specific minerals, vitamins or enzymes. Is it any wonder that fresh wheat grass juice with its wealth of nutrients is so good for the blood and immune system, as Ann Wigmore discovered?

• Green Powder Versus Fresh Green Juice

A word about green powders: there are some excellent green powders on the market. If you do not have the time to juice, powders are an acceptable alternative because you can easily take the powdered drinks with you and mix them during the day for a healthy alternative to coffee and soda. Dee Simmons' company, *Ultimate Living,* produces *Green Miracle*, an excellent green powder choice. Her green powder is advertised as *pharmaceutical grade pure,* containing 80 ingredients including: kamut, wheat grass, barley grass, spirulina, chlorella, flax seed, bee pollen, apple fiber, astragalus, reishi, papain, bromelain, curcumin, lutein, lycopene, carrot, beet, pepper powder and many others.

You can find Dee's popular health food products at her website: *www.ultimateliving.com*. Green *Kamut®* is a powdered wheat grass juice, while *Just Barley™* organic green juice, and *Barley Green™* contain barley only. Many green powdered drinks on the market, such as *Green Miracle*, not only contain green grasses, but medicinal mushrooms, minerals, spirulina, chlorella, vitamins, enzymes, herbs, and fibers that you would not get merely consuming powdered barley, algae, or alfalfa.

When possible, try to consume grasses (like wheat grass) in their most natural state immediately after they are cut. Doing this in combination with an excellent green powdered drink will boost the immune system and ensure optimal health. (Note that whole-leaf dried wheat grass actually has more chlorophyll than the fresh juice. This is because, once powdered, it is more concentrated.) A few of the health food stores in the area where I live have fresh juice bars. You can simply walk in and order an ounce or two (or six ounces if you want) of fresh-squeezed wheat grass, reasonably priced, and they will make it for you in minutes while you wait. They also juice fresh carrots, celery, beets, and smoothie mixes. Many people who cannot invest in the time and expense of a juicer, obtain their fresh juices at a juice bar, though after a period of time, you will spend enough at a juice bar to pay for a juicer.

When using fresh wheat grass juice, it is best to consume it within ten minutes of the time it is juiced. After that amount of time (unless it is frozen), the living enzymes begin to oxidize rapidly. The same is true of any fresh-squeezed juice. This is one reason why store-bought canned and bottled juices are no comparison to fresh-squeezed. By the time they are bottled, canned, packaged, homogenized, or pasteurized; all of the LIVING enzymes in them have been zapped. You may get a few benefits from the Vitamin C (if it hasn't all been killed by heat), but the syrups, sugars, food colorings, and preservatives that may also be added, provide empty calories and possible carcinogens. You can find bottled juices at health food stores that have no added sugars and preservatives. There are some brands that are *flash-pasteurized*, but you have to check the expiration date; they have a short shelf-life. There are a few commercial juicers that are finally getting the message that we don't want additives, food coloring, preservatives, and extra processed sugars (like fructose) put into our juices, no matter how pretty the color, and a few of them are coming out with better quality juices.

There is ONE exception when it comes to consuming wheat grass immediately after juicing. The late Dr. Virginia Livingston-Wheeler, who successfully cured many cancer patients at her clinic, used a "vaccine...based on abscisic acid" [an ingredient in wheat grass juice], and according to her, "the hormone abscisic acid (ABA) is 40 times more potent **4 hours** after cutting the wheat grass than it is at the time of cutting" (154). As *cancertutor.com* website asks: "what do you do, eat it immediately or 4 hours after you cut it? Perhaps both." They suggest that when juicing the wheat grass; consume most of it right away. Set the rest aside and drink it after 4 hours (154). In this manner, you are getting the benefit of live enzymes (as suggested by Ann

Wigmore) in consuming the juice within ten minutes of making it, and you are still getting large amounts of the abscisic acid 4 hours later. Fresh-squeezed juices are also excellent for children; however, before giving them to young children, check with their pediatrician. Infants and very young children do not have mature enough intestines to assimilate nutrients in raw juices that older children are capable of.

Never give honey and other bee products to children under two years of age. (Some pediatricians will let children over one-year-old take honey products.) The spores found in honey cannot be assimilated by young children and babies. The result can be the formation in a child's intestines of **infant botulism,** a deadly toxin.

Some of the sea vegetables recommended by Ann Wigmore were "arame, dulse, hiziki, kelp, kombu, nori [and] wakame" (307). She recommended covering and soaking sea veggies for twenty minutes in "warm water...until they are soft enough to slice," then to pitch the salty water when you are done (307). Because of the high iodine content of sea vegetables, if you have thyroid problems, check with your physician; however, realize too that most people have thyroid disorders to begin with because they have insufficient iodine in their diets.

Before you become concerned about overdosing on iodine, see Chapter 8 in this book. You should know that the Japanese are some of the healthiest people in the world and they consume about *13.8* **MILLIGRAMS** *of iodine* in their daily diets, mostly from ingesting seaweed, yet the US RDA for iodine for U.S. citizens is a paltry 150 **MICRO**GRAMS. How many people are aware that before the advent of all the "wonderful antibiotics" on the market, the primary killer used for the destruction of bacteria, viruses, and fungi was IODINE? When you have surgery and are about to get cut on, what does the surgeon do? They PAINT the surgical site with iodine because it kills GERMS! Many of the scrub sponges used in surgery suites are pre-filled with iodine. When I was a student nurse in my post-partum rotation, one of our daily tasks was scrubbing down all the little sitz-bathtubs with Betadine iodine for all our new moms. We didn't use chlorine, fluoride, alcohol, or any other germ killer. We used ONLY IODINE! Why? Because it kills just about any harmful critter that creeps, swims, wiggles, or crawls around with or without legs!

• Juice-Fasting

One of the best ways to restore your body's proper alkalinity is with a juice fast. While fasting is discussed in chapter 35 in my last book in greater detail, juice-fasting is being mentioned here simply because it is very important for establishing alkalinity and detoxifying the body.

Dr. Don Colbert in his book, *Toxic Relief,* explains that even though a total fast (taking in water only) will detoxify the body, using fruit and vegetable juices during a fast will help detoxify the body and result in alkalinity. Juice-fasting will help fortify the liver and maintain your energy level, something water-fasting will not do (188).

Remember too, that with any type of fasting, your body still needs water. I never recommend a total fast where even water is not permitted. You should never go for even one day without water. A total fast (without water) is very dangerous!

IV. How Raising pH Cured a Stage III Bladder Cancer

In *The pH Miracle*, Dr. Robert Young and Shelley Young related the story of a cancer patient diagnosed with advanced bladder cancer, who cured his cancer by reversing his body's acidity (315). The malignant bladder tumor had already cut off one of the patient's *ureters* (315). After he underwent chemo (which did nothing to decrease the size of the tumor), his physicians recommended complete surgical removal of his bladder. The patient came to see Dr. Young, who found his blood to be highly acidic, which the patient said was from years of eating the wrong foods (315). He refused surgery and completely changed his diet, beginning with a "ten-day fast, with vegetable juices and soups" (315). Within a *three month* period, the cancer had nearly disappeared. Though doctors still wanted to do a radical bladder removal, the patient chose minor surgery, which left all of his organs intact (315).

This may seem contrary, but it is possible for highly acidic foods to increase the body's alkalinity. Harald Tietze explains why in his book, *Papaya The Healing Fruit*. He says that limes are a good example (298). Though they are very acidic, with a pH of 1.9, consuming them has an *alkaline effect* on the body. The same is true of lemons. Not only is it important to know which foods are alkaline and acid-forming, but also to know how the body reacts to certain foods (298). See the recipe in Chapter 2 of this book on my ***Orange Wunder*** drink (and other formulas) for nutritional help with healing a Stage IV inoperable bladder cancer. The patient, a family member of mine, drank the nutritional formulas during the time he was undergoing chemo.

The best way to stay alkaline is with raw foods, juicing, and limiting cooked foods. Keeping your body in a state of alkalinity will increase oxygen at the cellular level. Cancer cells cannot survive in a highly oxygenated environment.

• Broccoli Sprouts Fight Bladder Cancer

Scientists found that they could slash the risk of *bladder cancer* in *half* simply by feeding test animals a substance from *broccoli sprouts* that had been *freeze dried* (making it more concentrated); further proof that cruciferous vegetables could save your life (18). The substance responsible is known as *ITC* or *isothyiocyanates,* powerful plant chemicals found in these vegetables that seem to target bladder cells. They found that *broccoli sprouts* "have approximately 30 times more" ITCs than broccoli that is fully-grown (18). The *freeze dried extract* that the researchers used in their study had **600 times as much ITC** as the sprouts (18). Cooking your broccoli and other cruciferous veggies destroys the ITC.

V. Bicarb for Healing the Kidneys

New research shows that sodium bicarbonate not only prevents kidney damage, but has been shown, in some cases, to reverse kidney damage, even to the point of getting some people off of dialysis! For greater details, see the full article at: *http://www.imva.info/news/sodiumbicarbonate-kidney-disease.html.*

CHAPTER 13

Other Life-Saving, Non-Toxic Cancer Killers

****

I. Burzynski's Antineoplastons

- **Antineoplastons - Miracle Non-Toxic Cures Used for Inoperable, "Terminal" Cancers**

No one will ever convince me that Dr. Stanislaw Burzynski, M.D., Ph.D., was not God-inspired when he devoted his life to the development of cancer-killing antineoplastons. They are still being used at his Houston, Texas, clinic. It is the only place in the country that the FDA allows his treatment, apart from the fact that they have finally approved the oral form of antineoplastons (PBs or sodium phenylbutrates) for off-label use.

Dr. Burzynski discovered that, secondary to the body's *immune system*, there is another defense system in the body (chemically) that is programmed to protect us from abnormal cells. He developed a group of peptides (he called *antineoplastons*) that were found to be effective against a variety of cancer cells in lab studies, yet they **were non-toxic to normal cells** (7). It is believed that antineoplastons work by causing cancer cells to revert or re-program back into normal cells. The compounds do occur naturally in humans, but for some unknown reason, at very **low levels in cancer patients**. Extensive **human** testing has been done with antineoplastons, so do not let your physician tell you that they are merely "experimental" or "untested"! More than **8000 people** have been treated with antineoplastons by Dr. Burzynski at his

Texas clinic. (Also, they are not the same thing as antineoplastics.) **Antineoplastics are very toxic to the body; antineoplastons are not!**

Dr. Burzynski's discovery has been used successfully in thousands of humans against "breast cancer, lymphoma, leukemia, and bone cancer," and many other cancers, and have been especially effective against malignant brain cancer cells. In 1988, he "treated twenty patients" diagnosed with a rapidly-advancing form of cancer growth known as *astrocytoma*. They were all in an advanced stage of the disease. This is a malignant type of brain tumor with a dismal chance of survival. (They can also occur in the spinal cord.) After diagnosis, very few patients live longer than two years. All the patients, several of them very young children, received the antineoplastons administered (outpatient intravenously) over a seven hour period during the night as they slept. As a result of the treatment, most of the patients had dramatic improvements (7). Within *six weeks*, all the children and most of the adults were able to return to school or *part-time work*. There was a positive response in *80 percent* of those tested. A checkup **four years later on all of them** revealed that many were still in total remission living a normal, active life (7).

This is remarkable when you consider that every one of these people had advanced, inoperable brain cancer, yet four years later, they are all still very much alive!

Dr. Burzynski presented diagnostic MRIs to the World Research Foundation Congress (1990) of a woman with a very *fast-growing astrocytoma*. Within 60 days of antineoplaston treatment, there was obvious *shrinkage* of the tumor, and six months later, no trace of the tumor. Not only that, but Dr. Burzynski revealed that the space where the tumor had once been—was **completely healed over with normal brain tissue**—there were no gaping holes or shadows showing scar tissue. Five years later, the patient, alive and well, still had no traces of cancer (7).

Have you or a loved one been told that you (or they) have an inoperable brain tumor, or that you are terminal, and the type tumor that you have cannot be cured? Do not let someone convince you of that—because there are many people who have been cured of "terminal" brain cancer without chemo, surgery, or radiation. This chapter will tell you about case histories of several of them, but they are not unique or isolated cases. They are routine cures for an alternative, non-toxic cancer therapy that most cancer patients are never told about! This is a blatant **cover-up,** and make no mistake about it, **it is very intentional.** There is one website, in particular, where you can read about the individual case histories of dozens of people who were told that their brain cancer was incurable, many of them children; people who are in complete remission today, living normal, healthy lives without brain tumors. See website: ***http://burzynskipatientgroup.org.*** Click on the section *"Our Stories"*. Some of the patients initially received chemo and/or radiation, but the tumors returned and they were cured with antineoplastons.

Many of the people you will read about at this website have included their email addresses, or home addresses where you can feel free to write to them. A few of those cases are described briefly in this chapter. Antineoplastons are often given intravenously; however, they can also be given in capsules that you simply swallow, known as sodium phenylbutrates or PBs. The FDA has finally approved the oral form of antineoplastons for off-label use, but you will need to ask your physician about prescribing them. Note that antineoplastons A10 and AS2-1 were recently given orphan drug status by the FDA for use on human brainstem gliomas. (*Orphan drugs* are drugs that can be used on rare cancers.) Some individuals can have mild side effects from antineoplastons, but they are quickly reversible, unlike toxic chemo drugs that often cause fatal, irreversible reactions.

• Astrocytoma Treated Successfully with Antineoplastons

Besides treating many other types of cancer with antineoplastons and PBs, Dr. Burzynski has successfully treated pilocytic astrocytoma. See website: *http://burzynskipatientgroup.org/jonathanc.html*, for the case of a young boy given two years to live (1997), who used antineoplastons to shrink a pilocytic astrocytoma. Seven years since being given a *terminal* diagnosis, he was planning a college degree and a real estate major.

- **Antineoplastons Cure Deadly Medulloblastoma in Children**

Case #1: When three-year-old little boy, Dustin K, was diagnosed with medulloblastoma his parents were given little hope. This is a rare and deadly form of cancer (20). He initially had surgery; however, doctors were not able to remove the entire tumor. They wanted to follow-up with chemo and radiation, to which the parents objected. Instead, they sought treatment at the Burzynski Clinic in Houston, Texas. Dustin was treated with antineoplastons and within months, his tumor had disappeared. When it returned a short while later, he was treated again with antineoplastons, and the tumor again disappeared and has not recurred (20). As of April 2008, he is 17-years-old, six feet tall, and is a *Certified Public Nurse!* He is cancer-free and living a normal, healthy life. His uncle is a practicing physician, who had advised his parents not to treat with Burzynski initially; however, in reading the case history of this child, it is his uncle who had a change of heart, and tells part of the story. You can read the details for yourself at *http://burzynskipatientgroup.org/dustink.htm* (20). What's more, this is NOT an isolated case!

Case #2: Roy H was only fifteen-months-old when he was diagnosed with this deadly brain cancer. After having a huge tumor surgically taken from his brain, his parents decided to treat the remaining two tumors (that had spread to the other side of his brain) with Dr. Burzynski's antineoplastons, rather than the chemo and radiation which Roy's pediatrician had recommended. The antineoplastons totally cured the little boy. At last update, he was eight-years-old, enjoying school, and has had no reoccurrence of the cancer. For details on his case, see website: *http://www.burzynskipatientgroup.org/royh.htm* (22).

- **Atypical Teratoid/Rhabdoid Tumors of the Central Nervous System (CNS) in Children**

For a study using antineoplastons on this type of rare tumor, see the Burzynski Research Institute article at *http://www.burzynskiclinic.com/ph/media-corner-publications.html.*

- **Malignant Rhabdoid Brain Tumor**

This same website describes the story of a four-year-old little girl who was diagnosed with a rhabdoid brain tumor, Crystin S, whose parents were advised that the tumor was incurable, and all they could hope for was to possibly extend her life briefly by giving both chemo and radiation at the same time, which they agreed to. The tumor initially shrank, and then returned. Her parents took her to Burzynski's Clinic in Houston, Texas, for antineoplaston treatment, which ultimately resulted in a complete cure. For several months, the little girl seemed fine; however, her parents were later to find out that something dreadful had happened to her (19). The physician, certain that Crystin was going to die anyway, had given double the radiation dosage that she should have received. After being completely cured of brain cancer on Burzynski's antineoplastons, the little girl died several months later. Upon autopsy, her parents were told that her death was caused by the massive doses of chemo and radiotherapy she had been given, which had resulted in irreversible injury to her brain (19). Had the child never received chemo and radiation to begin with, she would probably still be alive today.

- **Inoperable Brain Stem Tumor Cured With Antineoplastons**

Jason Merkle was only thirteen-years-old when he was first diagnosed with a benign inoperable brain stem tumor in 1994. Because of hydrocephalus, a shunt was inserted and he did fine until July of 2001, when the tumor had transformed into a high-grade brain stem glioma (248). When his parents were offered BBBD (a form of "intra-arterial platinum therapy," a therapy that most patients don't even live through), they opted instead to go to the Burzynski clinic in August of that year (248).

As described by Jason's mother, Patty:

> We sought opinions from several major cancer centers. John Hopkins, Brigham and Women's, Henry Ford Brain Tumor Center, University of Michigan and MD Anderson. The consensus was the same from all the doctors. Jason's

condition was terminal. Radiation and chemotherapy were the recommended forms of treatment, both of which are non-curative. Success, by these doctors standards, with radiation and chemo is determined if the patient lives 3 months after the treatment. The side effects of radiation in the brain stem are devastating, plus there is the risk of radiation necrosis. Chemotherapy does not penetrate the blood brain barrier. It is accepted, but not effective in brain tumors. None of the doctors could give us a success story. Jason's local neurosurgeon told us if he were in our position, he would not radiate or do chemo because of the devastating side effects they create in terms of quality and length of life. Just "let him die" (248) [they were told].

Though none of their physicians supported the decision, Jason's parents forged ahead with non-toxic antineoplastons at Dr. Burzynski's Texas clinic (248). Jason was able to live a normal lifestyle while on the antineoplastons, even having the ability to go on a safari, as told by his mom:

In July 2002, Jason, his dad and I were sent to South Africa for a hunting safari. Jason was able to go hunting, and shot a warthog, an impala, a kudu and a zebra. He also darted a white rhino and implanted microchips in its horns to guard against poachers. All of this was done while he was on the antineoplaston. We transported the medicine to Africa with us and continued on with the daily routine. This was a dream come true. God brought some very gracious and generous people into our lives because of this tragedy (248).

Patty describes the difficult months that lay ahead of them:

For four months the tumor continued to grow. We spent a lot of time in prayer. There were people all around the country praying for Jason and our family. Jason was beginning to have some neurological problems because of the size of the tumor. He couldn't hear very well, his eyes were only partly open and he had a very difficult time staying awake. The FDA wanted to pull Jason out of the trial, but the doctors at the Burzynski Clinic convinced them to give Jason a little more time. Finally in December 2001, the tumor quit growing. For three months there was no change. In February the tumor started to respond. It was 20% smaller. Jason's hearing came back, his eyes opened and he was able to stay awake all day. The tumor continued to shrink. Not rapidly, but nonetheless it was getting smaller. The side effects of the antineoplastons are minimal. Watching sodium intake, drinking lots of water and taking supplements to keep the electrolytes in balance became part of the daily routine. Once the tumor began to shrink, Jason was able to resume a fairly normal life style...December 4, 2002 the MRI showed no tumor. Jason had a PET scan in January which showed no active cancer cells. Jason continued on the infusion treatment and the next three MRI's showed no cancer. On April 21, 2003 we returned to the Burzynski Clinic. Jason is in remission (248).

By December of 2002, Jason's brain tumor had completely disappeared. He had also made several dietary changes, including the elimination of all "sugars, white flour, rice, simple carbs, dairy..." and ate "vegetables and meat." He also incorporated routine exercise into his schedule (248).

As of the most recent communication I have received (June 2010) from both Jason Merkle and his mom, Patty, his cancer has never returned, he has graduated from college and has a full-time job. I have seen Jason's chart. I have seen the diagnostic tests that were done on him before and AFTER he was treated with antineoplastons. He truly is a miracle case, and fortunately for him and his parents, he was not forced against his will by the FDA to accept toxic chemo drugs with all their dismal (and potentially deadly) side-effects.

- ## Stage III Inoperable Anaplastic Astrocytoma Cured Without Chemo or Radiation

See the amazing story of Jodi G, who was completely cured of an inoperable, stage III Anaplastic Astrocytoma (brain tumor), using only Burzynski's antineoplastons (21). She was diagnosed in May 2000. Jodi refused chemo and radiation because doctors never talked *cure*, to her. They gave her *6 – 18 months to live*. All they discussed was possibly extending her life. Details of her story are posted at website: *http://*

burzynskipatientgroup.org/jodig.htm. As of her most recent update (March of 2009), Jodi remains cancer-free and doing well after having just given birth to a beautiful baby boy (21)!

- ## Myxopapillary Ependymoma Treated Successfully With Antineoplastons

For details on a little boy who was diagnosed with myxopapillary ependymoma and successfully treated with non-toxic antineoplastons, see website: *http://burzynskipatientgroup.org/kylel.htm.*

- ## Antineoplastons for Glioblastoma

Glioblastoma is another very deadly and difficult-to-treat type of brain tumor. Most people survive less than a year from the time that they are diagnosed. When Dr. Burzynski realized that this type of cancer was not responding to his overnight *IV drip,* he created *a small pump* device that the patient could attach to their clothes so that the antineoplastons could be given in continuous infusion over a 24-hour period, rather than just at night (7). One of his first patients to try the pump was a child with "a brain stem glioblastoma..." an inoperable location. He underwent radiation first and the tumor shrank initially, but then began **growing again a short time later** (7). Dr. Burzynski started the child on the pump he developed. **The brain tumor disappeared completely within 4 weeks, replaced by *normal, brain tissue.*** Dr. Burzynski revealed diagnostic pictures of this case in 1990 from the child's MRI results. A follow-up (three years later) showed that the child was still cancer-free. The new pump delivery system has had "favorable results in approximately 60 percent of the patients who have been treated with it" (7). This is particularly remarkable when you realize that most of the patients receiving this treatment are **terminal cases of inoperable brain cancer.** (As noted earlier, antineoplastons A10 and AS2-1 were recently given orphan drug status for use on human brainstem gliomas. Orphan drugs are drugs that can be used for rare cancers.)

• Antineoplastons Cure Child's Pineoblastoma

When Sophia G was ten-and-a-half months old, she was diagnosed with pineoblastoma (a brain tumor). Surgeons removed the tumor, but it returned—and her parents were told that the only treatment available was chemo and radiation—there was nothing else available for her. The parents knew that most children treated for brain tumors with chemo and radiation suffer irreversible brain damage, and many never recover. When they asked the oncologist if their little girl would ever get on a bus for school, the response was "no" (23). They refused the chemo and radiation, took Sophia home, contacted Hospice, and expected to watch her die. Instead, relatives who were looking out for them discovered the amazing story behind antineoplastons. Sophia was treated by Dr. Burzynski with antineoplastons and cured! That was many years ago. As of her most recent update (March 2009), she remains cancer-free and is living a normal, healthy life enjoying middle school. She proved the doctors wrong and got on that school bus after all! For details on her case history, see website: *http://burzynskipatientgroup.org/Sophiag.htm,* or *http://www.burzynskipatientgroup.org/stories.html,* and look under pinoblastoma (23).

• Antineoplastons & the FDA

It is noteworthy that Dr. Burzynski has had great success at curing some of the most aggressive, deadly cancers, especially "terminal" patients having malignant brain cancers. I wonder how many patients in the U.S. (and other countries) diagnosed with *hopeless,* inoperable brain tumors are ever told about antineoplastons by the oncologists treating them. Do YOU know someone recently diagnosed with an inoperable brain tumor or another deadly cancer? Has their physician mentioned this non-toxic, alternative treatment? You may run into the same type opposition I did when I asked my own relative's oncologist about antineoplastons (see Chapter 1). Three of his other family members were furious with me for even questioning the chemo protocol that his oncologist was planning for him.

Some insurance companies are **finally** getting around to covering antineoplastons. Be prepared, however, to butt heads with the FDA if you try to pursue antineoplastons. Only those with lymphomas or malignant brain tumors can use them. Any other type of cancer and the FDA will usually tell you that you must first use chemotherapy or radiation before trying I.V. antineoplastons, even though chemo and radiation are toxic treatments, and **antineoplastons are NON-TOXIC.**

The FDA has vigorously attacked Burzynski from day one of his discovery. They charged that one of his patients died of blood-poisoning (from an intravenous infusion), yet the report never gave any specifics, and not at any time did Dr. Burzynski ever receive documentation of a patient of his having fatal septicemia. All studies ever done on these compounds have shown them to be safe. They are *natural products,* accepted into the cells, "even in high doses, without any of the serious side effects" found in chemotherapy agents (19). The trumped-up attack by the FDA was just one more attempt to try to find something negative, in their desperate plan to discredit this very successful alternative cancer therapy and the hard-working physician behind it! Their tactics over the years haven't changed in the least. How upset do they get when 500 chemo patients die as a result of adverse reactions from chemo drugs? On the other hand, they will abruptly remove an herb from every shelf in America if three people have an allergic reaction to it, and leave a deadly drug (like Vioxx®) on the market for years even AFTER it kills thousands of people! Their hypocrisy is totally amazing!

A new movie has come out that describes antineoplastons and the 14 year struggle that Dr. Burzynski has been through in fighting with the FDA, Texas State Medical Board and others, to keep his treatment available for cancer-sufferers. You can read about this new movie at their website: *http://www.burzynskipatientgroup.org,* or *www.burzynski movie.com* and watch several trailers. It is called: ***Burzynski, The Movie.*** When describing the movie, the latter website had this to say:

> As with anything that changes current-day paradigms, Burzynski's ability to successfully treat incurable cancer with such consistency has baffled the industry. However this fact has prompted numerous investigations by the Texas Medical Board, who relentlessly took Dr. Burzynski as high as the state supreme court in their failed attempt to halt his practices. Likewise, **the Food and Drug Administration engaged in four Federal Grand Juries spanning over a decade attempting to indict Dr. Burzynski, all of which ended in no finding of fault on his behalf.** Finally, Dr. Burzynski was

indicted in their 5th Grand Jury in 1995, resulting in two federal trials and two sets of jurors finding him not guilty of any wrongdoing. If convicted, Dr. Burzynski would have faced a maximum of 290 years in a federal prison and $18.5 million in fines. However, what was revealed a few years after Dr. Burzynski won his freedom, helps to paint a more coherent picture regarding the true motivation of the United States government's relentless persecution of Stanislaw Burzysnki, M.D., Ph.D. (23a). [Emphasis mine.]

Dr. Burzynski's story has been mainly a *fight to survive* since he has had to spend a great deal of his own time and finances fighting legal and political battles "brought against him by the FDA, the American Cancer Society, National Cancer Institute, large insurance companies [and], the medical board and health department of Texas..." However, during this same period of time, he has gained global fame for his work. Clinical trials are still being conducted around the world with his discovery (7). Dr. Burzynski's story is an interesting one and it has finally been made into a movie! He has had a great deal of success in curing cancer patients, many of them initially diagnosed as *terminal*, but he has also spent a good portion of his life fighting constant harassment by the modern medical establishment in much the same way that Rene Caisse, Joseph Gold, Harry Hoxsey, and Emmanuel Revici did. Apparently, their success rates against cancer makes those who are promoting and selling toxic treatments uncomfortable.

Antineoplastons are given intravenously and PBs are taken orally. PBs are converted by the liver into antineoplastons. See Burzynski's Clinic website at: *www.burzynskiclinic.com*. Additional information can also be found at: *www.curezone.com*. At Burzynski Patient Group website: *http://burzynskipatientgroup.org/stories.html*, you can also read the case histories of dozens of people who had brain tumors, glioblastomas, astrocytoma, astrocytoma III, anaplastic astrocytoma, brain stem gliomas, ependymoma, pineoblastoma, and neuroblastoma, brought into remission with antineoplastons and PBs. There are also case histories of remarkable remissions in many other cancers at this website including: multiple myeloma, lymphocytic lymphoma, non-Hodgkins lymphoma, prostate cancer, breast cancer, ovarian cancer, and esophageal cancer. There is even a case history of a patient who has had good results using antineoplastons with a rare type of lymphocytic lymphoma known as ***Waldenstrom's macroglobulinemia*** (see website *http://burzynskipatientgroup.org/margaretl.htm*), and a patient whose **lupus** was brought into remission (see website: *http://burzynskipatientgroup.org/darlenen.html).* **Dr. Burzynski has treated more than 8000 cancer patients.** A small sampling of those case histories is at the website: *http://www.burzynskipatientgroup.org/.*

Dr. Burzynski also treats other autoimmune disorders. What I find most disturbing about so many of these cases, including those involving young children, is that when (the parents) were given a poor prognosis and asked their oncologist if there was anything available that could offer hope, apart from devastating chemo and radiation, they were told ***no.*** In one case in particular, a doctor knew the history of a patient who had been cured of an aggressive brain tumor at the Burzynski Clinic, and still never revealed this information to the parents of his brain cancer patient, pushing them instead to put their child through chemo and radiation. You have read what happened in Chapter 1 of this book when I asked my own family member's oncologist about using antineoplastons for his Stage IV inoperable bladder cancer. I don't think he even knew what I was talking about (or pretended not to if he did), because I received an evasive reply and a very angry reaction from three of his other close family members who thought it was simply unforgivable of me to even question the oncologist's protocol!

Many cancer patients were also told that the only thing chemo or radiation could do was *possibly* gain them a few more months of life at the most, yet they were never told about antineoplastons. The Burzynski Clinic also treats multiple other cancers and disorders including: CLL and CML (leukemias), fibrous histiocytoma, mesothelioma, neuro-endocrine tumors, Wilm's tumor, mantle zone lymphoma, Hodgkins & non-Hodgkins lymphoma, mycosis-fungoides-sezary syndrome, choroid plexus neoplasm, craniopharyngioma, mixed olioma, high-grade gliomas, visual pathway gliomas, and many others, too numerous to mention here. The main webpage for the Burzynski Clinic is: ***www.burzynskiclinic.com.***

- **Burzynski Therapy for Neuroblastoma & Optic Pathway Gliomas**

See website *http://burzynskipatientgroup.org/tavism.htm,* for the case of a little boy cured of neuroblastoma using Dr. Burzynski's antineoplaston (ANP) therapy. He first received surgery, radiation, and chemo—all of which failed to shrink his tumor.

Note that neuroblastoma cancers usually form in the *nerve tissues* found in the *adrenal gland, neck, chest, or spinal cord*, and are more common in children (164). It is believed that if the cancer is due to faulty DNA (*Unb11qLOH and 1p36LOH* chromosomes), survival chances are less likely than victims who do not have these genetic defects. Their treatment choices may be more aggressive than those not having the chromosomal abnormality (164). (The issue of genetics in cancer is still being debated worldwide.)

For Burzynski Research Institute studies on optic pathway gliomas and treatment with antineoplastons, see the article at site: *http://www.tradingmarkets.com/print.site/news/Stock%20News/2038966.* Also, see information at the Burzynski Research Institute website: *http://www.burzynskiclinic.com,* as well as clinical trial reports at website: *http://www.burzynskiclinic.com/ph/media-corner-publications.html.*

- **How to Prevent Neuroblastoma, Brain Tumors & Leukemia in Your Child Before They Are Born**

Seven studies by researchers at the University of Toronto from 1960-2005, looking at how a mother's vitamin intake could affect her child's later development of cancer, had some surprising results (202). As noted by *CancerConsultants.com*, all vitamins were studied, including *folic acid*. Mothers who took vitamin supplements (that included folic acid) had children with *36%* fewer cases of *pediatric leukemia; 18% reduction in pediatric brain tumors*, and *47% reduction in neuroblastoma* in their children. Authors of the study theorized that folic acid might have been the most important of the vitamins (202), and it is already a well known fact that women who take folic acid can help prevent neural tube birth defects in their babies.

This study is described in the Journal *Clinical Pharmacology and Therapeutics* (retrieved from website article: "Vitamins During

Pregnancy Decrease Childhood Cancer Risk" at *http://patient.cancer consultants.com/CancerNews_Neuroblastoma.aspx?DocumentId=39373)* (202); more proof that nutrition plays a critical role in disease prevention, even in the womb! Did you know that for YEARS, the FDA fought bitterly to keep vitamin manufacturers from telling pregnant women on their vitamin labels that folic acid could help prevent spinal cord defects in their babies? They did an about-face when the vitamin manufacturers were proven right, but only after thousands of babies were born with the defect, a defect that could have been prevented had the moms knew about folic acid!

- ## Non-Toxic Alternative Treatment for Curing Glioblastoma Multiforme

BEFORE you choose conventional treatment for glioblastoma multiforme, please see the case of Susan H at Dr. Burzynski's patient group website: *http://www.burzynskipatientgroup.org/susanhale.htm* (129). Susan's brain tumor returned after radiation (Gamma Knife®). She then went to the Burzynski Clinic and received antineoplaston therapy. She was completely cured of glioblastoma multiforme using Dr. Burzynski's antineoplastons (129). You can call the Burzynski Clinic and ask for her dad (his name is at the end of the article), and he will give you more details about his daughter's amazing recovery.

- ## Antineoplastons Cure Bladder Cancers

When Dr. Burzynski gave more than a dozen patients with cancer of the bladder his antineoplastons, the results were amazing. They were all treated, and then studied over the next decade. At the study's completion, the following results were reported: out of the original 19 participants, *thirteen* were in complete "remission…two [in] partial remission…one [had] stable disease [and] three" were advancing in the disease. Antineoplastons have been found to be safe and non-toxic, even in large doses (257). Note that they are **not** the same as antineoplastics. Do not confuse the two.

• Burzynski's Antineoplastons for Curing Lymphomas & Other Cancers WITHOUT Toxic Side Effects

Maryjo Siegel was diagnosed with a fatal non-Hodgkin's lymphoma in 1991. She was completely cured using non-toxic antineoplastons developed by Dr. Stanislaw Burzynski in Houston, Texas. She is still alive and well (as of my most recent emails from her in June 2010), living a normal life, and has never had a reoccurrence of cancer). You can send her an email at *maryjo@siegel.net,* and she will tell you about her experience with antineoplastons. She testified before a government committee on February 4, 1998. Below is that amazing testimony:

Testimony before the US House of Representatives Government Reform and Oversight Committee on February 4, 1998:

> Seven years ago, I was stricken with a fatal cancer, non-Hodgkin's lymphoma, for which no conventional cure yet exists. This disease is treatable for periods of time with chemotherapy and/or radiation, but the outcome is always death. My relative Steve and I were devastated by my prognosis, but determined to find a cure. Our research took us to top lymphoma specialists at esteemed medical institutions like UCLA, USC, Stanford, and the Dana Farber Cancer Institute in Boston. All the experts confirmed our worst fears: with existing therapies, my disease was incurable.
>
> At Dana Farber, a ray of hope emerged with the recommendation that I undergo an autologous bone marrow transplant. This highly controversial procedure would require that I receive extremely high-dose chemotherapy and as much radiation as people who were within 1 mile of 'ground zero' at Hiroshima. I would lose my hair, experience severe nausea and vomiting, and the threat of bacterial and viral infection would keep me in complete isolation for 6 weeks. My quality of life after treatment would be drastically

diminished. From the chemotherapy, I would become sterile. There would be damage to my heart, lungs, liver, kidneys, and bladder. Collateral radiation damage would affect my eyes, salivary glands and thyroid, with a greater than 50% chance that I would develop leukemia if I were lucky enough to survive just 10 years. I was frightened and suspicious because only a handful of patients had survived this procedure with good long-term results. One such person was the late Senator Paul Tsongas, who eventually died of complications caused by the procedure.

Fortunately, we discovered the work of Stanislaw Burzynski MD, PhD, who was treating patients who have advanced cancer with a gentle, nontoxic therapy he had discovered. As I began Dr. Burzynski's antineoplaston treatment, my lymphoma had progressed to a stage IV (there is no stage V). Malignant tumors were growing throughout my body. My bone marrow was infiltrated, and there was a large tumor growing on the side of my neck. After only 3 weeks on this medicine, that tumor disappeared! Subsequent scans performed at UCLA showed continued reduction in tumor size.

During antineoplaston treatment, my quality of life was excellent, virtually free of side effects. I was an active and involved mother, an absolute necessity when you are raising three teenagers. More importantly, the drug stopped my supposedly terminal cancer. Within 12 months I was pronounced in remission, not by Dr. Burzynski, but by the same lymphoma expert at UCLA who had originally diagnosed me and told me I faced certain death from this disease. I went off treatment and remained in remission for 2 years, when a follow-up scan revealed a possible return of the disease. Immediately, Dr. Burzynski prescribed a regimen of antineoplaston capsules. Within 5 months, I was once again in remission and have remained cancer-free to this day.

That's the end of the good news. The tragedy is that our government, namely the FDA, has been keeping what author [of The Burzynski Breakthrough] Tom Elias calls 'the century's most promising cancer treatment' from becoming widely available to cancer patients. The agency has spent untold millions of taxpayer dollars in a systematic attempt to harass, discredit, stonewall, and even imprison Dr. Burzynski.

As incredible as it sounds, in November 1995, the FDA indicted Dr. Burzynski on 75 criminal counts, most having to do with alleged technical violations of the Interstate Commerce Act and none having to do with his practice of medicine or the effectiveness of his drug. Dr. Burzynski had been legally treating patients under Texas State law for some 20 years, and not one patient in all that time had ever filed a complaint. If Dr. Burzynski had been convicted on all 75 counts, he could have been sentenced to 290 years in a federal prison.

Are antineoplastons effective? Ask the FDA. Apparently, the FDA believes the answer is "Yes," because it fought tenaciously to keep the question of the effectiveness of antineoplastons out of the trial. Dr. Burzynski tried to make it a part of the trial. Apparently, both the FDA and Dr. Burzynski believed he could prove the drug works. The FDA also fought to keep the full truth from the jury by preventing Dr. Burzynski's patients from testifying, while Burzynski asked the judge to allow the patients to tell their stories.

In the end, Dr. Burzynski was acquitted on all counts. But I ask you in Congress, and particularly my representative, Mr. Waxman, how you can allow the FDA to squander taxpayer money in an idiotic prosecution, the success of which would mean the deaths of hundreds of cancer patients? The FDA was unable to find even a single patient to testify against Dr. Burzynski!

Peter Barton Hutt, a former FDA Chief Counsel, has said 'If you beat the FDA in court, you have an angry FDA that is willing to slit your throat.' Indeed, although the FDA lost the courtroom battle against Dr. Burzynski, it continues to wage war against him and his patients. The agency interferes in his practice by telling him whom he can and cannot treat. With many types of cancer, the FDA requires patients to have failed not one but two rounds of chemotherapy before they can be treated with antineoplastons. In many cases the chemo has so ravaged their immune systems that they literally have nothing left to fight with, and they die. The FDA forbids the use of steroids in the treatment of Dr. Burzynski's lymphoma patients, even when they are needed to temporarily shrink tumors and relieve pain, as in my own case. Because I was on treatment prior to the FDA taking over his practice of medicine, Dr. Burzynski was able to inject me with Medrol to relieve the pain and tightness in my neck caused by the tumor. Now, however, the FDA is not concerned with patient comfort, rather, their twisted logic dictates that good data collection outweighs humane medical treatment.

The FDA demands that Dr. Burzynski's patients with lymphoma stop treatment if they have not achieved 50% tumor reduction within 6 months. The absurdity of this typically arbitrary FDA requirement became clear when one Burzynski patient — Frances Langham — was to be forced off treatment because she had only a 44% reduction after 6 months! She is lucky to be from Arkansas and politically connected. She received a 'special dispensation,' allowing her to continue treatment. But the FDA removed her from the clinical trial, meaning that even if cured in the future, the FDA will count her as a 'treatment failure' in determining how effective antineoplastons are! These treatment 'restrictions' are only applied to Dr. Burzynski's clinical trials, whereas lymphoma patients involved in Idec Pharmaceutical's C2B8 and Elan Pharmaceutical's phenyl acetate trials, do not have to meet these same treatment criteria. Is it possible that [the] FDA has a bias against Dr. Burzynski and his patients have to suffer as a result?

Who gave the FDA the right to play God? Was it the intent of Congress to give the FDA the kind of power it exercises over life and death decisions with no accountability? By denying terminally ill patients with cancer access to antineoplastons, this agency literally decides 'who shall live and who shall die.'

I have had to watch as children and adults suffer and die as a result of FDA intransigence. Patients plead to be allowed into antineoplaston clinical trials; however, the FDA says 'No. You don't qualify.' Shouldn't it be the doctor, in concert with the patient, making these important medical treatment decisions, rather than an FDA official who does not even know the case? Clearly, the FDA is denying these patients their freedom of medical choice. Because conventional FDA-approved remedies have failed to work for the majority of Dr. Burzynski's patients, often their only choice is antineoplastons or death!

It has been 26 years since President Nixon declared the War on Cancer. Public expenditures now exceed $30 billion, and private research and development funds must total at least 10 times that amount, yet the death rate continues its relentless climb. It is time for a new approach to treating cancer. The only way this will become a reality is by allowing patients with cancer expanded access to new, experimental, and innovative treatments. Until we have a cure, all treatments, conventional and alternative, are experimental!

Dr. Nicolas Patronas, Chief of Neuroradiology at the National Cancer Institute, testified under oath that antineoplastons are the most effective treatment for brain tumors he has ever seen. [Emphasis, mine.] Top oncologists have lauded Dr. Burzynski's work, including those at the University of Washington and Georgetown University. Doctors and scientists around the world eagerly await the approval of antineoplastons. [In 1991] Dr. Michael Friedman, [past] commissioner of the FDA, wrote that 'Antineoplastons deserve a closer look...the human brain tumor responses are real.' So why is the FDA so determined to impede the progress of a drug with such promising results?

Congressmen, we implore you to restore the right to choose our own health care. You have the power to give us back our freedom. Mr. Waxman, as your constituent I know you staunchly support both the FDA and a woman's right to an abortion. But can you really condone a government policy which grants a mother the right to choose death for her fetus, while denying a dying cancer patient one last hope for life?

In his March 29, 1996, press conference, President Clinton announced new initiatives to expedite the approval process for innovative new cancer drugs like antineoplastons. Since then, the FDA has bluntly stated that the President's initiative has changed nothing. It is time for congressional oversight to ensure that this mandate is carried out. Patients with terminal illnesses deserve the chance to win their personal War on Cancer, and it is up to Congress to ensure they have the weaponry with which to fight.
Thank you (281).

Submitted by Mary Jo Siegel to the Burzynski Patient Group website (281).

See chapter 14 in my last book, *Gentle Cures for Tough Cancers*, for more information on the non-toxic therapy of antineoplastons, which have brought many hopeless, inoperable cancer patients into total remission, even those with lymphomas and so-called *terminal* brain cancers, many of them children! Maryjo also sent a letter to Ted Kennedy about antineoplastons after he was diagnosed with a brain tumor. She was basically ignored. The Burzynski Clinic website is at *www.burzynskiclinic.com*. See the story of another woman with Stage IV non-Hodgkins lymphoma who was cured with antineoplastons at:

http://burzynskipatientgroup.org/rebeccas.htm and
http://burzynskipatientgroup.org/karolr.htm.

• Burzynski's Antineoplastons Cure Nurse With Non-Hodgkin's Lymphoma

For another case of a patient (an RN) who was completely cured of non-Hodgkin's lymphoma through Dr. Burzynski's clinic, see website: *http://burzynskipatientgroup.org/melodyc.htm*.

• Burzynski's Antineoplastons & Mantle-Cell Non-Hodgkin's Lymphoma

For the case of a 53-year-old woman treated with antincoplastons after being told she had mantle-cell, non-Hodgkin's lymphoma, see website: *http://burzynskipatientgroup.org/margaretm.htm*.

• Burzynski's Antineoplastons Cure Stage IV Melanoma in Child

Jessica K was only three-years-old when she was diagnosed with stage IV melanoma. It started on her foot in 1984, and it was removed, but returned in 1985, and had spread as a large malignant tumor in her groin and into nearby lymph nodes. Not wishing to subject their daughter to chemo and radiation, her parents took her to Dr. Burzynski in Houston, Texas (223). She was put on antineoplastons and completely cured. As of September 2009 (her most recent update—nearly twenty-five years after being diagnosed), she is still cancer-free and leading a normal life. She is now a *Certified Behavior Analyst*, working with kids that have developmental needs, and is a wife and mother of two children. See her complete report at website: *http://burzynskipatient group.org/Jessicak.htm* (223).

- ## Antineoplastons & Mesothelioma

Mesothelioma is a very rare cancer caused by asbestos exposure. It usually affects the thoracic cavity where the heart and lungs are located, but can affect other areas of the body. Non-toxic antineoplastons (discussed above) have been used at Burzynski's Clinic in Houston, Texas, for treating this disease. See their website at: *www.burzynskiclinic.com.* The FDA has finally approved the oral form of antineoplastons (PBs) for off-label use, but you will need to ask your physician about prescribing them.

- ## Burzynski's Antineoplastons for Curing Colon Cancer

June H was diagnosed at age 78 with *adenocarcinoma* of the colon that had spread to her lymph nodes. This was in June of 2002. She chose not to have the chemo and radiation her physician recommended and instead, went to see Dr. Burzynski and underwent his PB (oral antineoplaston) non-toxic cancer treatment. By April of 2003, her cancer had disappeared and she is now considered cancer-free. For details about her case, see website: *http://burzynskipatientgroup.org/ juneh.htm.*

For the main Burzynski website, go to: *http://www. burzynskiclinic.com.* Their INFOLINE is 800-714-7181. For International calls: +1 713.335.5697.

The FDA has finally approved the use of PBs (sodium phenylbutrates), which you can obtain by prescription from your physician, and the use of antineoplastons as *orphan drug status* for gliomas. (PBs, taken orally, are converted by the liver into antineoplastons.) Unfortunately, you still cannot get intravenous antineoplastons from your local oncologist, not unless you travel to Houston, Texas and visit the Burzynski Clinic. Chances are, your local oncologist will NEVER tell you about them, and why should they? What incentive do they have? Why should they broadcast this safe, non-toxic, very effective treatment as long as they are milking the current chemo system and charging their patients $30,000.00 for two rounds of chemo drugs? If they treat only 30 patients a month (and most of them are seeing 8 to 15 patients a DAY or more), that comes to nearly a million dollars. You can see what a conservative estimate this is! How many other professions do you know that make that kind of money? Do you honestly think the drug makers want to see those profits go up in smoke? Is it any wonder that Dr. Burzynski has been fighting them most of his life?

- ## Antineoplastons for Pancreatic Cancer & Undifferentiated Connective Tissue Disease (UCTD)

Antineoplastons are also used for pancreatic cancers, UCTD, and nearly every other cancer imaginable. See their main website at: *www.burzynskiclinic.com,* and read some of the many testimonials of patients who have successfully used antineoplastons to cure their cancers at: *http://burzynskipatientgroup.org/stories.html.*

- ## Antineoplastons & Prostate Cancer

For an amazing account of a man who had been diagnosed with "untreatable prostate cancer," who was still cancer-free six years later after being treated with Burzynski's antineoplastons, see website: *http://burzynskipatientgroup.org/kenb.html* (168). The patient received absolutely no other treatment for his cancer before checking into the Burzynski treatment center in Texas. At that time, his PSA was 50.8 and the cancer had gone into his "ribs, shoulder bones, spine, and hips," and he was in "excruciating pain." 14 days after starting on antineoplastons, his PSA was 1.3, and his only side effect was mild stomach acidity (168). For other testimonies of prostate cancer survivors using antineoplastons see website testimonials at: *http://burzynski*

patientgroup.org. There are case studies of other prostate cancer survivors using antineoplastons at these sites:

- *http://burzynskipatientgroup.org/john.htm,*
- *http://burzynskipatientgroup.org/ronaldm.htm,*
- *http://burzynskipatientgroup.org/robertm.htm,*
- *http://burzynskipatientgroup.org/ronldg.htm,*
- *http://burzynskipatientgroup.org/carle.htm,*
- *http://burzynskipatientgroup.org/isaiahc.htm* (168).

If you have problems pulling up any of the individual cases under these URLs, just go to *http://burzynskipatientgroup.org/stories.html,* or to: *http://burzynskipatientgroup.org* and click on the link that says **Our Stories** at the very top left side of the page.

II. Curing With Tea Power

I discussed several teas with healing, curative powers in my last book, *Gentle Cures for Tough Cancers*, in great detail. In this chapter, I am only including a few of what I consider the premier teas for fighting cancer. There are so many other teas that can be important in boosting immunity and fighting cancer, but they cannot all be discussed in a book of this length. Sometimes you will be told that the NCI, or some other institution, has tested compounds (for example those in pau d'arco), and flatly announced that they do not help cancer; however, what you sometimes are not told is that when a tea is tested, it isn't always the entire tea with ALL of its components that are tested by them. They will extract one or two compounds from the tea and use that extract to test it, then claim that the tea is ineffective. This does not always work because teas (e.g., Essiac, pau d'arco, green tea) usually need to be taken as a whole, without breaking them up into ten different compounds, using only one or two of their main ingredients for the test. There are times, however, when individual extracts taken from teas DO kill cancer cells. Just realize that before you begin any tea regimen, let your physician know, since teas are considered herbs and as such, may be incompatible with some treatments and prescription medications.

Black Tea—Cancer Fighter & Anthrax Fighter

For years scientists have agreed that tea, green and black, help boost the body's natural immune system. A new study from Cardiff University and the University of Maryland has revealed that black tea (and it has to be black tea) could be important in warding off anthrax; however, don't be too quick to add a dash of milk to that *cup of tea,* because the milk eliminates the *antibacterial* effect against the anthrax (40).

• Chaparral Tea

Dr. Ralph W. Moss in his book, *Cancer Therapy,* describes an ingredient in chaparral tea known as *NDGA (nordihydroguaiaretic acid),* which prevented abnormal colon growths in animal tests. It also stopped the formation of cancers in the breast. Lab testing of NDGA blocked leukemia, as well as a type of brain tumor known as *glioma* (256).

In a **human** study done by scientists in the western U.S., Dr. Ralph Moss tells of a patient with melanoma who enjoyed a near total remission after taking chaparral tea. Research conducted by the NCI revealed chaparral tea to be very helpful in fighting cancer (256).

In another remarkable case, an elderly man with skin cancer on his face, who had opted out of surgery, began self-treating with chaparral tea. The patient came back to his physician after several months, having had remarkable reduction in the melanoma (256). I would never advise someone with melanoma not to have surgery, because sometimes surgical removal alone will cure skin cancer, depending on how far it has advanced.

There was one report, from Canada, of a consumer harming her liver many weeks after she began ingesting a product known as *Chaparral Leaf* (256). The FDA reported a total of four cases of liver toxicity from this tea. It was taken off the market, but many people still make their own chaparral tea, as it grows wild in some states. Amazing, isn't it? How fast the FDA moved to strip this tea from every store shelf in the U.S., but managed to leave Vioxx® on the market long after it had killed thousands of people!?

• Essiac Tea & The Canadian Nurse Who Cured Hundreds, Perhaps Thousands of Cancer Patients, with Four Herbs

• How It All Began

In 1924 Rene Caisse's aunt was diagnosed with advanced cancer of the stomach and liver and told that she was terminal. Rene, a Canadian nurse, asked her aunt's physician about using an herbal formula that she had obtained from another patient who used the tea to cure her breast cancer. The story is described in Reese Dubin's book, *Miracle Food Cures From the Bible* (196). The patient told Rene that she had been given the tea recipe by an Indian friend of her relative's. The physician approved for Rene's aunt to try the same herbal blend. It contained four herbs: *slippery-elm bark, sheep sorrel, Turkish rhubarb, and burdock root* (196). Rene's aunt used the herbal remedy for only 60 days. She was completely cured and outlived her ordeal by more than 20 *years* (196).

• More Amazing Cures!

When Dr. A.F. Bastedo of Bracebridge, Ontario, allowed Rene to use her formula on a terminally ill bowel cancer patient of his, the patient's recovery was so dramatic that he talked the authorities into letting Rene use one of their hotels as a cancer clinic, to which they agreed (296). Shortly thereafter, Rene's 72-year-old mother was discovered to have terminal liver cancer and given just days to live. Rene treated her own mother with the formula she named *Essiac*. Her mother not only recovered, but she lived a normal life for another 18 years, dying at the age of 90 from cardiac problems (296).

One patient in particular, Herbert Rawson, was pushing fifty when two physicians diagnosed him with rectal cancer. He declined surgery and came to Rene Caisse with a note from his physician giving Rene the green light to allow him to use her formula (263). He started Essiac and received the *last of 30* treatments slightly more than a year later. At this time, Rene was giving an injectable form of the herbal remedy. Examinations shortly thereafter revealed no cancer whatsoever, and he outlived his ordeal another 25 years. His cancer never returned (263).

• The Word Gets Out

Another physician, R.O. Fisher, M.D., was so completely amazed with the results of the remedy; he began working with Rene on researching with animals, and then used the concoction on several of his own terminal cancer patients with excellent results (196). Other physicians began referring their terminally ill patients to Rene. A short while later, a physician asked Rene to use her herbal tea remedy on a diabetic colon cancer patient. To their astonishment, not only did the tea and the injections made from the tea cure the bowel cancer, but the diabetes as well. Only three of the herbs were used in the injections. The exact *injectable* formula that was developed was said to have been lost (196); however, long before Rene's death, Dr. Brusch, who worked closely with Rene, found that the injectable form of the tea was no longer needed, because the drinkable form was just as effective (296).

• Rene's Popularity Grows

For an excellent book describing the effectiveness of this tea and how it was suppressed by the health industry in Canada see: *The Essiac Report Canada's Remarkable Unknown Cancer Remedy,* by Richard Thomas. He claims that Flor-Essence® is the original (drinkable) formula that Rene Caisse used and shared with Dr. Brusch (296). Mr. Thomas' book contains several pages of documentation from physicians and patients who successfully used the Flor-Essence® tea to cure their cancers, in spite of the incessant, underhanded attempts by the Canadian government's Health Department to discredit and destroy the formula. I highly recommend this book to those interested in Essiac.

Richard Thomas' book will show you many of the original letters written by physicians and patients who used this amazing tea. Unbelievable as it sounds, the only way that the tea was finally able to make it into health food stores was to change the label and remove all claims, so that it could not be considered a drug. Mr. Thomas, in one chapter of his book, refers to Rene as *St. Rene* (296), simply because she saved so many lives. Rene was probably the closest thing to a Nurse Practitioner before that profession ever came about.

• Competing Tea Brands

Note that there is some competition between the tea produced by Resperin Canada Essiac® and Flor-Essence® Essiac tea. Both companies claim that they have the original Essiac formula (the drinkable formula, not the injectable) that Rene Caisse gave her patients. You can find Resperin Canada Essiac® tea at this website: *http://www.billybest.net/index.htm,* along with Billy's testimony of how this tea helped cure his cancer. I also discussed Billy's fight with Hodgkin's lymphoma in my book, *Gentle Cures for Tough Cancers,* in the lymphoma chapter. You can find Essiac in other brands. As noted above, the two major competing brands are Flor-Essence® and Resperin Canada Essiac®. You can obtain Flor-Essence® at many natural health food stores in an already prepared drinkable form, or a powdered form that you brew yourself.

- **Prominent Physicians Join Rene**

Dr. J. A. Faulkner, who was provincial Minister of Health in Canada at the time Rene was treating patients, was supportive of the Essiac formula. He discussed the formula with Sr. Frederick Banting, M.D., who is considered a co-discoverer of insulin and who at that time, was one of the most highly acclaimed doctors in the world (296). He was so impressed with the formula that he tried to talk Rene into coming to work with him at the Banting Institute in Toronto. She refused, because she had already tested her formula many times on mice and felt that her human patients needed her more (296), besides, she already knew her formula worked on humans!

- **Government Beaurocrats Close In**

Several Canadian physicians were so amazed at the results of Essiac tea, that in 1926, they petitioned the Canadian government to let Rene conduct further studies on the formula, insisting that she be allowed the proper equipment for doing so (196). Instead, Ottawa officials came to arrest her for practicing medicine. When it was discovered that she was working under the supervision of several very distinguished Canadian physicians, they backed down (196). Over many decades, Rene ultimately went on to treat multiple hundreds of terminally ill cancer patients with her herbal tea remedy, many of whom recovered completely. She did not charge for her services and always worked with prominent physicians. She accepted countless Canadian and American patients (196).

Cynthia Olsen, in her book, *Essiac A Native Herbal Cancer Remedy,* said that in 1932 a story in the *Toronto Star* credited Rene with a "Notable Discovery Against Cancer," but because of this article, Rene Caisse was again threatened with legal action, including prison (263). Ms. Olson further explains that in 1938, Rene's supporters, including many physicians, again petitioned the government of Ontario to pass a bill giving Rene permission to use her formula for cancer patients unharrassed (263). Thousands of people signed the petition, but it fell three votes short of being passed, mostly because the Cancer Commission and the CMA (Canadian Medical Association) were in bed together (263). A few months later, 387 of Rene's patients came forward to testify in her behalf. For some never revealed reason, the Cancer Commission allowed just 49 to testify (263).

- **Rene Does Not Give Up**

Because of continual threats of arrest, Rene finally shut her clinic doors, but covertly continued to see patients over the next three decades; however, she was constantly observed and faced years of imprisonment if it was found that she was using her formula (263). Imagine that! A beaurocratic bunch of thugs trying to shut her down when there was irrefutable proof that she was saving lives! Sound familiar? She must have been putting a real crunch to the pharmaceutical industry! Rene's fame came to the attention of publishing editor, Ralph Daigh, who was suspicious of the medical establishment. Daigh's support of Rene and her herbal formula resulted in her being able to work with then President John F. Kennedy's private doctor, Charles Brusch, M.D; however, the president was killed before he was able to influence any change in the way Rene Caisse and her formula were treated by the Canadian health system (263).

- **Rene Passes the Formula**

Dr. Brusch gave Essiac tea his total endorsement, firmly stating that Essiac was curing cancer patients. He admitted that the formula had been tested in several laboratories and said (in 1990) that he had even cured his own colon cancer using only Essiac (296). He had been diagnosed in 1984. He said that before Rene died in 1978, she *confided* to him the Essiac formula (296).

Rene wanted nothing more than to selflessly help cancer patients with her herbal tea remedy, yet she endured years of incessant and needless harassment from the Canadian Ministry of Health. She died from problems related to hip surgery when she was 90-years-old, but she had credited her own lifetime of excellent health and lack of illness to the fact that she had taken Essiac tea for half a century (196). She shared the formula with Dr. Brusch, with whom she had worked for years.

Do not use the tea if you are nursing, pregnant, or taking medications that could be incompatible. Check with your physician. Richard Thomas, as noted above, says that the formula given to Dr. Brusch is still available today as *Flor-Essence®* Essiac Tea.

• Green Tea

Drinking several cups of green tea a day may be one of the most important things you can do to prevent and fight cancer.

In a human research study described by Dr. James F. Balch in his book: *The Super Antioxidants*, this tea was able to reduce pancreatic cancer by 50% in participants consuming the tea. More and more data is supporting the use of green tea as a major preventative in all forms of cancer, including those of the G.I. tract and liver (165). Research also showed that this tea could help kill certain types of leukemia, such as myeloblastic (165). In fact, green tea could be one of the most important developments in fighting leukemia. In the research, it caused premature death in abnormal cells (165). An excellent green tea, which is usually caffeine-free, is **Tulsi** tea. If you see *Golden Green Tea* at your local health food store, it is merely green tea combined with the herb, *lemon grass*.

Research shows that green tea can prevent dental caries and halitosis (115). I would recommend decaffeinated green tea since caffeine can be dehydrating, however, some believe that it does not fight arterial plaque as well as caffeinated tea. There are many pros and cons to using caffeine. I believe there are more advantages in NOT using caffeine. There are other natural ways of fighting arterial plaque, some of which are discussed in this book and my prior writings.

• Green Tea & Leukemia

A study reported at *foodnavigator.com* reveals that green tea, in laboratory testing, could interfere with the production of "B-cell chronic lymphocytic leukemia (CLL)," common in people in their sixties, and for which there is no known cure (60).

• Green Tea & Reishi Mushrooms Kill Sarcoma

Scientists in Beijing, China, recently made an amazing discovery during animal testing with sarcoma cancer. They discovered that they could combine nutrients from the reishi mushroom and green tea and dramatically slow the growth of sarcoma tumors, as well as increase the life span in the animals receiving the treatment (52).

• Green Tea Protects Against Stomach Cancer, Bladder Cancer & Regenerates Brain Cells

Researchers have known for many years of the anti-cancer properties of green tea. Studies show that stomach cancer rates dropped dramatically in humans drinking *7 cups or more a day* (83). Scientists in China found that regularly drinking green tea cuts stomach cancer risk by as much as 50%. Green tea has also been found, in animal testing by Israeli researchers, to actually regenerate brain cells, something hitherto thought impossible (79). A **human** study (from Japan) shows that this tea can reduce a woman's risk for getting stomach cancer by a whopping *75%* (61).

• Hoxsey's Famous Tea

Harry Hoxsey developed an herbal tea that he used in fighting cancer; however, he was very much against the cancer establishment and even had his own radio program where he boldly proclaimed a very "anti-AMA message" at every opportunity. He successfully operated several *clinics* until the federal government moved in and closed them (256). The Hoxsey Formula is still being used at his Mexico clinic, and a Hoxsey tincture list of ingredients can be found at website *www.natural opinion.com* (99), as well as other internet sites.

Hoxsey was ridiculed, made to look like a *snake oil salesman*, harassed, and finally run out of the country when he claimed that his formula was curing cancer patients. This is nothing new and often happens when someone uses a cancer remedy that defies the golden calf of the cancer industry (chemo and radiation). They do not take kindly to physicians and nurses that buck their system. In the years that followed his death, research into Hoxsey's herbal formula revealed that many of the compounds Hoxsey used have powerful anti-cancer effects (256). Some of the herbs (e.g., the pokeweed root and the burdock) can be dangerous if taken in excess amounts or improperly prepared. Burdock contains a substance that, as reported by WHO (*the World Health Organization*), can fight HIV, and another Hoxsey tea compound, known as barberry, can help fight cancer (256).

The treatment that Harry Hoxsey received at the hands of the AMA was nothing short of criminal, and is described as a 25-year-battle between the AMA's Morris Fishbein and Hoxsey, with Hoxsey winning, though the FDA, with all its beaurocratic clout, eventually moved in and closed his U.S. clinics (269).

The Hoxsey formula is still available at their clinic in Tijuana, Mexico. They can be reached at: Bio-Medical center 615 General Ferreira, Colonia Juarez Tijuana, B.C. Mexico. Tel: 011-52-664-684-9011/Fax: 011-52-664-684-9744.

• Kombucha Tea

Kombucha tea *(Fungus Japonicus)* is derived from a popular fungus that resembles a mushroom. According to Marie Nadine Antol in *Healing Teas,* kombucha can help boost the immunity, attacking the HIV virus and abnormal cancer cells. It helps normalize blood lipids, neutralize toxins, stabilize *blood pressure*, attack acne, reduce wrinkling, promote hair growth, relieve arthritis, energize the body, and it has been said to help restore hair color in some individuals (162).

• Parsley Tea

Marie Nadine Antol describes parsley as a natural diuretic, overall cleanser, important antioxidant, and health promoter (162). Scientists have recently discovered a substance in parsley that fights cancer. If you buy it dried, be sure to find out if it came from the **leaf or roots.** Tea made from the roots will be much more potent than leaf tea. Parsley tea can help the body in prevention and dissolving of stones (e.g., gallstones), provided that they are small enough. Once they enlarge, it may be too late (162). It can also cause uterine contractions, so should not be used during pregnancy, nor during nursing. It should not be used during any type of infectious process, says Ms. Antol, "especially if the kidneys are involved" (162).

• Sir Jason Winters' Tea

Sir Jason Winters was diagnosed in 1977 with a huge, visible neck tumor. He went the conventional medicine route, but refused major surgery. Nothing happened to the growth. He was sent home with a diagnosis of *terminal* and given a few months of life at the most (313). As described at his website, *www.sirjasonwinters.com*, what happened next is nothing less than miraculous! He traveled to three different continents and developed a tea blend containing red clover, herbalene (a Chinese spice), and Indian sage, that he combined and began drinking religiously. The cancer began shrinking, until it disappeared completely (313). The tea that he used is now called his *Classic Blend Tea*. When it "was tested by Dr. Ian Pierce of England, it was said that the Herbalene acted as a catalyst to make the other two herbs in the tea 27 times stronger" (313). According to their website above, "Hashimoto, the former Prime Minister of Japan, considers Jason Winters Tea to be THE HEALTHIEST DRINK IN THE WORLD" (313). Jason Winters' book, *Killing Cancer,* is available at his website, along with his *Classic Blend Tea*, and several other teas that he offers. His website reports that he has "won awards from six foreign governments and the U.S...for his work in the health field" (313). I would certainly recommend *Jason Winters Tea* for anyone fighting cancer, should they choose to do so. He has since passed, but not from cancer.

III. Mushrooms – The Good Fungi

Some mushroom varieties have already been discussed in this book. There are many others, barely mentioned, with amazing healing properties. This section is devoted to some of those.

• Agaricus Blazeil Murill (ABM)

Agaricus mushroom (also known as the *himematsutake* mushroom) is described at website: *www.mnwelldir.org/docs/Newsletters/01_Aug.htm* as "The most powerful chemotherapy in Japan today." According to them, the healing properties of this Brazilian mushroom are amazing and known for curing many deadly cancers (1). One health provider in Brazil was so impressed with the healing results of the agaricus, that he invited people from anywhere in the world to come stay with him, at his expense, and witness for themselves the curing properties of this mushroom (1). He had very few people who took him up on his offer. When researchers visited the province where this mushroom grew, they found that the people who lived in the area were free of disease, many of them living over a century. Since that time, it has been discovered that a substance found in this mushroom is "effective against Ehrlich's ascites carcinoma, sigmoid colonic cancer, ovarian cancer, breast cancer, lung cancer and liver cancer as well as against solid cancers" (2).

The School of Medicine at Ehime University in Japan discovered, in animal testing, that ABM (Agaricus Blazei Murill) mushroom can help prevent and fight cancer even when the animals were given *Lewis Lung Carcinoma* (LLC) cells (224). Not only did the mushroom prevent the growth of tumors, but metastases as well. The report also showed that the mushroom increased *natural killer cells* in the immune system (224). The substance that was extracted from the Agaricus mushroom was *sodium pyroglutamate* (224).

There are many websites that provide agaricus or ABM mushroom—some in dried form—some fresh. If you need these mushrooms fast, at the very best prices, check website: *www.mitobi.com*. This mushroom is introduced into cooking much like any other type of mushroom. *Wellness Directory of Minnesota's*™ website recommends taking vitamin C with your mushroom supplements for better absorption (2). Also included in fighting cancer are the reishi, mesima, chaga, tinder polypore, split-gill mushroom, and many others (5).

- **AHCC—Mushroom Combo Enhances Immunity**

AHCC (*Active hexose correlated compound*) is a substance composed of the mycelia of many mushrooms. In **human** testing, it was found (when given to patients in doses of *3g/day orally for 2-6 months*) to significantly increase the body's natural immunity, thus enabling the immune cells to kill multiple myeloma cells and several other types of cancer cells (113). This compound is found at many natural health food stores and online supplement providers, such as *www.discount-vitamins-herbs.net*. New Chapter® is a company that also makes many important mushroom supplements and other nutritional supplements. Their website is: *http://www.newchapter.com/product-categories/life shield-mushrooms*. You can find their supplements in most health food stores.

- **Cordyceps Sinensis**

Cordyceps sinensis is considered by Chinese medicine experts as their most valuable, powerful mushroom (300). Kate Gilbert Udall in her book, *Cordyceps Sinensis,* says of this mushroom: "It has been helpful in curing asthma and other respiratory ailments" (300). An extract from this fungi, known as *cordycepin* (in a 1989 study), was helpful at fighting HIV. Cordyceps sinensis, says Ms. Udall, can help stop the division of cancer cells and strengthen the immunity (300). New research is showing that this potent mushroom helps fight cancer aggressively, keeps cancer cells from spreading, and prevents them from growing and dividing (157).

Note that the common table spice, turmeric, also inhibits HIV. It has also been used in treating autistic children and topically for eczema and psoriasis. (Use organic turmeric rather than curry. You will get more curcumin in turmeric than you will in curry powder.)

Topical applications of soda bicarb and magnesium are also helpful for psoriasis and eczema (85) (287).

- **Coriolus Versicolor (Karawatake) Mushroom**

An important cancer-fighting extract comes from this mushroom, called *PSK*. This derivative may help extend the lives of those fighting gastric, intestinal, and lung cancers (111). Also, lab studies show that coriolus versicolor can help fight HIV, but further testing is needed to see if it will function the same way in humans with the disease. When these mushrooms were used to fight cancer in humans, there was no toxicity whatsoever (111). Be sure, if using coriolus, you use the heat-extracted form. (However, as noted earlier, agaricus appears to be more potent than PSK – you may wish to try both.)

• Enoki

Research from Japan showed that people consuming enoki mushrooms could reduce cancer risk by 40% (143). You can often purchase fresh enoki in health food stores.

• Hoelen

This mushroom, known as *hoelen (Poria cocos)*, can be found underneath some types of tree roots. According to an article at *herbs2000.com*, they are sometimes used in a form of bread known as *tuckahoe bread* (68). They are high in potassium and have been used for the regulation of *blood sugar*, hydrochloric acid, and *kidney* problems (68). An ingredient in this mushroom (*poriatrin*) appears to be helpful for patients struggling with *kidney disease* caused by *lupus*. Best results are obtained from actually ingesting the mushroom, rather than relying on extracts (68).

• Maitake

Dr. Ralph Moss, author of *Cancer Therapy*, says that maitake mushrooms have successfully halted cancers in animal tests. In one study in particular, ten mice were fed the powdered form of the mushroom for "one month after tumors had been implanted," and 40% of the mice were cured. For the others on the mushroom, tumors decreased *86.3%* (256).

In his book, *Alternative Cures*, Bill Gottlieb says forget the *chicken soup* because these mushrooms outperform the soup when it comes to combating the common cold (204)!

Maitake D-fraction and *beta-glucan* are discussed in other cancer-specific chapters of my last book for their ability at reducing the size of tumors in animal tests, and human usage. Most nutritionists recommend cooking mushrooms, because, as noted by Selene Yeager in *Doctors Book of FOOD REMEDIES,* there are *toxins* in the raw fungi that are destroyed at high temperatures (314). Maitake should not be taken by those with *multiple sclerosis*. It can increase a substance that destroys nerve tissue in people with MS (97). New research is showing that MS may be caused by severe vitamin D deficiencies! Also, insufficient vitamin D levels will set you up for the development of diabetes, since vitamin D lowers insulin resistance at the cellular level. **Human** studies prove that this vitamin also boosts the immunity, preventing colds and flu viruses. Another reason that winter is called the *flu season*, and people get sick in the winter is because they do not get sufficient sunshine, a primary source of natural vitamin D.

When I was giving my family member my **Orange Wunder Formula** (see Chapters 1 and 2), at first I used Maitake D-Fraction drops in the formula, but I had to discontinue using the Maitake because the type cancer he had caused leg clots. He was placed on blood thinners and Maitake can thin the blood. I also wanted him to be on Essiac, but since it contains 4 herbs that could be incompatible with blood-thinners, that too was not an option.

• Polyporus Umbellatus Mushroom

For Recurrent Bladder Cancer & For Ovarian Cancer

This immune-boosting mushroom is one of ten mushrooms found in *Garden of Life's® RM-10* product developed by Jordan Rubin (153). His 80-year-old grandmother used the product to heal her advanced ovarian cancer (see more info in below paragraph). See Chapter **7** in my book *Gentle Cures for Tough Cancers* for her testimonial, as well as website: *http://www.crohns.net/Miva/education/testimonial_rosemenlowe.shtml* (13). It has also been helpful for those with urinary tract infections, and may help the immune system in stopping the spread of leukemia (153). You can find RM-10 at this website: *http://www.crohns.net/Miva/productinfo/whatsinRM10.shtml* (153). It has also been helpful in cutting in half the reoccurrence of **bladder cancer** in a test involving 146 **human** participants (153).

• RM-10 Mushroom Formula & Advanced Ovarian Cancer

When Jordan Rubin (author of The *Maker's Diet* and other health books) found that his own 80-year-old grandmother had an advanced form of ovarian cancer, he began to look at ways that her immune system could be activated to kill the cancer cells (13). He studied *polysaccharides* or *glyconutrients,* as well as mushrooms, cat's claw, and aloe vera. He used a *fermentation process* with many of the *homeostatic soil organisms (that* had gotten him well from Crohn's Disease) to *predigest the 10 mushrooms, aloe vera and cat's claw* in a compound that would enable his grandmother to easily absorb the nutrients (13). His formula, known as *RM-10,* is sold through *Garden of Life®* products. Using RM-10, Rubin's grandmother completely recovered from ovarian cancer, and it also healed a *fatty liver* (13).

• Reishi Mushroom

According to Deanne Tenney, author of *Medicinal Mushrooms*, the reishi mushroom *(Ganoderma lucidum)* comes in several types, each one being a different color. They are "Akashiba (red reishi), Kuroshiba (black reishi), Aoshiba (blue reishi), Shiroshiba (white reishi), Kishiba (yellow reishi), and Murasakishiba (purple reishi)" (295). Studies from Moscow's *Cancer Research Center* prove that this mushroom can enhance immunity and halt tumor progression (295).

Dr. Earl Mindell, popular nutrition author, says that Reishi in Japan is known as *kisshotake* or the *lucky fungus*, and that compounds in reishi boost the immune system, fight dangerous fats and clots in the blood, and act as *antihistamines* (254). As discovered by one researcher, you can greatly enhance the *cancer-fighting* properties of this mushroom by taking it with *vitamin C* (227). Be aware that reishi has blood-thinning abilities. Some people are allergic to mushrooms. and could have severe reactions to matsuka mushroom and others.

• Shiitake & Immunity

Shiitake mushroom increases *interferon* in the body and helps the body fight cancer. **Human testing** has been done in China on those with leukemia and in Japan on *breast cancer,* using shiitake. The mushroom can also lower harmful blood cholesterol (182). An extract from shiitake, *lentinan,* has been very popular in fighting cancer (314). Scientists discovered that this shiitake extract, in animal testing, halted tumors by *67%* (314). It was during the 1980's that researchers from Japan discovered, in animal testing, that shiitake could stop liver cancer (256). Lentinan injections are often given by alternative health physicians and are discussed in more detail in cancer-specific chapters of my last book, *Gentle Cures for Tough Cancers.*

New Chapter® makes several nutritional supplements, including mushroom supplements, such as Host Defense®, which contains 17 different mushrooms. You can find them in many health food stores and at their site: *http://www.newchapter.com/products/hostdefense.*

IV. Vitamin A & Zinc for Leukemia

Research shows that the lifespan of *chronic myeloid leukemia* patients could be extended by minimal supplementation with vitamin A (277). It appears that Vitamin A also plays an important role in tumor prevention. Even a synthetic form of vitamin A caused remission in dozens of APL (*acute promyelocytic leukemia*) sufferers. A study from Italy involving dozens of patients revealed that deficiencies in *zinc and thymulin* could throw *acute lymphoblastic leukemia* patients into relapse (277).

Yourhealthbase.com reports that researchers in Houston, Texas, have found that *retinoic acid* and *retinal* (synthetic forms of vitamin A) could inhibit and fight cancers of the prostate, as well as *acute promyelocyte leukemias* (146).

Dr. Abram Hoffer, M.D., Ph.D., in his book, *Healing Cancer— Complementary Vitamin & Drug Treatment,* says that it is very common for cancer patients to have excessive levels of copper in their body, possibly caused by a lack of zinc (213).

V. Zinc, Riboflavin (B-2), Chinese Herbs, Vitamin A & Selenium Help Prevent Mouth & Esophageal Cancer

Experiments done in China to see if vitamins could stop the high rate of esophageal cancers, rampant in some parts of the country, had remarkable results. In his book, *Cancer Therapy*, Dr. Ralph Moss says that in one area, out of thousands of people, more than half already had signs of cancer of the esophagus with significant abnormal cell growth (256). Over two thousand had precancerous cells. Patients were given either *riboflavin or a placebo*, or a specially prepared herbal mix called *anti-tumor B*, or vitamin A (retinamide), depending on how extensive the dysplasia was. When the participants were checked 36 months later, the group receiving the herbal formula had more than fifty-percent **fewer cancers** than the placebo group. Those receiving vitamin A and riboflavin had *33.7 and 19 percent* fewer esophageal cancers (256). Anti-tumor B is a Chinese herbal remedy that you can find described in a study at: *http://www.nature.com/onc/journal/v23/n21/full/1207496a.html*.

The combined nutrients, *zinc, vitamin A...riboflavin, and selenium*, can reduce the incidence of oral cancer (255). In 1995, researchers from India discovered that using a combo of these 4 items decreased damaged DNA by *72 to 95 percent* in a group of volunteers receiving it (255). Out of hundreds of *heavy smokers* that were tested, Dr. Moss says that 150 were given the vitamin-mineral combo and the other half, a placebo. Of those participants given the nutritional regimen, more than half experienced a total remission from their oral cancer; however, in those not receiving the vitamins and minerals, *only 8 percent* enjoyed remission (255).

Research has proven that oral doses of zinc, taken by those with increased susceptibility to cancer, can decrease their incidence of mouth and throat cancer. In lab studies, scientists were able to reverse abnormal cell growth (potentially cancerous) in animals by merely feeding them zinc.

CHAPTER 14

Immune System Killers: The Worst Offenders

****

I. The Mercury Poisoning Tragedy

Without a doubt, the main mercury contaminant that has caused the most chronic illness and disease is the mercury placed into **millions of people's mouths** in the form of dental mercury amalgam fillings! Though mercury is undoubtedly the second most toxic substance known to man (with radiation being first), the FDA has declared it safe to put into the mouths of millions of people, children included! They will tell you that it is safe a few inches from your brain, but once removed from your mouth, legally it must be placed into a hazardous waste container so as not to poison the environment! This is the type absurd reasoning that has been going on with the FDA and the ADA (American Dental Association) for more than 60 years! Want to give your children a fighting chance in life? Never, ever allow a dentist to put an amalgam mercury filling in their mouth and never, ever allow them to undergo a root canal filling, EVER!

Even the World Health Organization (WHO), in combination with the International Program on Chemical Safety, admitted in 1991 that (apart from *certain occupations*), the "largest single source of human mercury exposure," is *dental amalgam*, the mercury fillings that are put into the mouths of millions of dental patients every year (317)!

Some wary dentists are now coming forth and admitting the dangers of amalgam fillings. When Dr. Richard D. Fischer, DDS, testified in front of *The Subcommittee on Human Rights & Wellness* on

September 8, 2004 at the U.S. House of Representatives, he had this to say about dental amalgam fillings:

> Scrap amalgam, that unused portion of the filling material remaining after the filling is placed into a patient's tooth, must be handled as a toxic waste disposal hazard. It cannot be thrown in the trash, buried in the ground or incinerated. It must be stored in an airtight vessel until properly disposed of. How can we justify storing this same mixture inches from a child's brainstem and declare it harmless (103)?

• Health Crisis With Mercury

Dr. Hulda Clark also linked many of our health issues, such as arthritis, cancer, and autoimmune diseases, to the metal dentistry that we allow in our mouths. Have you ever noticed that if you have a mercury filling removed from your mouth, your dentist will very carefully put it in a *hazardous* materials waste box, yet tell you that when it was inside your mouth, not to worry, that it won't harm you? (186). All polymers and metals eventually deteriorate and begin seeping. Dental ingredients and appliances are no exception. Not only that, but clostridium bacteria may get into dental fillings and caps (186). If you don't believe this, the next time a cap comes loose from a tooth and you take it back to have it replaced, before you do, have it cultured at a local laboratory. It may be swarming with clostridium bacteria.

Because of all the dangerous chemicals that can leach into our bodies from plastic and metal dental fillings in teeth, Dr. Clark believed that we are giving ourselves diseases (like cancer) due to the way that these chemicals suppress our immune system. She suggested that, for anyone who is bound in a wheelchair for disability that has no *reliable diagnosis*, try this: get a dentist who knows what he or she is doing and have all the metal taken out of your mouth (186), and have any root canal fillings removed and reamed out thoroughly.

Some of the staunchest advocates against amalgam fillings have become the dentists themselves! If you are interested in the dangers of metal in dentistry, a very good book on the subject is by Dr. Frank J. Jerome, D.D.S., *Tooth Truth—If You Want to be Healthy Don't Metal With Your Mouth.* Other good books are: *Root Canal Cover-up* by George E. Meinig; *Elements of Danger: Protect Yourself Against the*

Hazards of Modern Dentistry, by Morton Walker; and *Dentistry Without Mercury*, by Sam Ziff and Michael F. Ziff, D.D.S. If you ask your dentist not to put a mercury (amalgam) filling in your mouth, he or she will usually tell you that it is perfectly safe and harmless, that the mercury is bound up with other chemicals which cannot be broken down, exactly what the dentistry profession has been telling us for years. There are some dentists; however, who are now speaking out and telling the truth about these hazards (see the article below).

For those of you still not convinced of the dangers of mercury in modern dentistry, documentation at this website could very well change your mind: *http://pollutioncontrol.suite101.com/article.cfm/dental_amalgam_and_mercury_bans,* especially when you see that both Norway and Sweden have banned all amalgam fillings in their population (311). As noted in their article on having these fillings removed:

> The more fillings people have that contain mercury the higher the mercury levels are in their blood. Once the fillings are removed, the mercury levels decrease. Some people who have had reactions to dental amalgam report improved health after removal. The removals need to be done carefully so that neither the dentist nor the patient is exposed to mercury vapors (311).

How does this mercury constantly seep into the bloodstream? Well according to website: *http://www.encognitive.com/node/4750:*

> "…activity such as chewing, drinking hot liquids, polishing or brushing the teeth increase mercury vapors as much as fifteen times (for up to 90 minutes after). In this vapor form, it is inhaled and absorbed through the lungs into the bloodstream…Autopsy reports of accident victims show that as few as five fillings can raise the level of mercury in the brain 300 percent and confirm the mercury residue is distributed to tissues and organs throughout the body. The main points of accumulation are the brain and kidneys; other common storage sites include the thyroid, pituitary, liver, heart and blood…First of all, let's establish one fact. Mercury is more toxic than arsenic or lead… no level of mercury can logically be considered safe (10).

It is also a proven fact that dentists and dental hygienists with all their mercury exposure are at high risk for neurotoxicity, as the website explains:

> OSHA has found that approximately 10% of all dental offices are **severely mercury-contaminated**. Most dental offices have inadequate mercury decontamination systems. The results of a study presented to the Society of Toxicology earlier this year showed reduced fertility in dental assistants who are occupationally exposed to mercury vapor from amalgam. The high incidence of suicide among dental professionals may also point to the 'neurotoxic' effects of mercury accumulated in the brain (10).

When homes of dentists were analyzed, it was found that many of their homes contain unsafe amounts of mercury. How did it get there? By the dentists themselves "bringing mercury home on shoes and clothes" (105). When studies from Sweden (during autopsies) revealed that "the pituitary glands of dentists hold **800 times more mercury** than people who were not in dentistry" [emphasis mine] (104), did anyone take notice?

Not only that, but per Dr. Mark Sircus, Ac., OMD, "Dental workers show 50-300% more mercury in hair and fingernails than the average population" (287). Many dentists are denying that amalgam fillings present any sort of danger. Perhaps the sad irony is that while in denial, they are even poisoning themselves and their families with mercury.

Even the ADA will tell dentists and dental workers not to touch mercury fillings because they are so toxic and mercury is absorbed right through the skin, yet they think nothing of sticking them into the mouths of more than 100 million people!

Elevated levels of mercury in your body (which happens with amalgam fillings and other environmental sources) causes the probiotics or "friendly bacteria" in your gut to *"convert the mercury into methyl mercury, which is at least 100 times more toxic than ordinary mercury"* (104). It is strange but true that Candida binds with mercury. People who go through a detox regimen and initially experience the *Herxheimer's reaction*, where they actually feel worse at the beginning of the regimen, is because the detox program itself will kill off Candida, releasing all that mercury that has been stored along with it (104), another good reason to include selenium, chlorella and cilantro as part of your detox program. You want to kill the Candida, but rid your body of mercury at the same time! Is this another reason cancer is a yeast overgrowth—its MERCURY content which is so deadly?

Website *http://tuberose.com/Mercury.html,* recommends a detox supplement that contains "cell wall broken probiotics" to help drive out the yeast "without breaking their cells walls," thus keeping the mercury bound up. This product is known as NDF (*Nanocolloidal Detox Factors*), and it can be found at their website above, as well as many other nutritional supplements (104).

- **FDA Finally Admits That Amalgam (Mercury) Fillings Could Be Harmful—AFTER They Have Been Put Into the Mouths of Millions of People!**

After decades of denying that mercury fillings were potentially harmful, the FDA has finally admitted (in 2008) that mercury fillings could be hazardous to your health! In response to a *legal settlement*, the FDA *agreed to release* a statement to alert consumers about *potential related hazards* of mercury fillings (106). They are finally admitting that amalgam (mercury) fillings not only *release mercury vapour* into the mouth, but that *mercury vapour* is also released *during chewing*, and these fillings could have "neurotoxic effects on the nervous systems of developing children and fetuses…" (106).

Why has it taken them this long? Why did they drag their feet in admitting that folic acid prevents neural tube birth defects, while they were persecuting vitamin manufacturers from trying to warn the public?! How do you think that all the baby-boomers with a mouth full of amalgam fillings feel about this ruling? They have admitted that these fillings can give off mercury, which can cause problems for those women who are *pregnant* and people with *kidney disease* (106). How many people are aware that amalgam fillings have already been banned in *Sweden and Norway* (106)? This issue has become so volatile in Canada that it has resulted "in a class action lawsuit representing millions of Canadians who claim that they were not warned of the potential health risks of their mercury" [fillings] (279).

It is mercury that causes some bacteria to "mutate for self-preservation," and this is one reason we have many "new strains of bacteria" that current antibiotics won't kill (279). For more details, you can google "FDA and amalgam fillings" on the internet to see many related articles, such as the one found at website: *http://www.cbc.ca/consumer/story/2008/06/05/dentalamalgam.html* (106).

• Research on Thousands of Humans Verifies Danger

Though some dentists still claim that the mercury in amalgam fillings is in a *dead* state where it cannot *escape* into your mouth or into the environment, thousands of studies have been done on **human** saliva, showing that those people who have more mercury fillings in their mouth have correlating higher amounts of mercury in their saliva (319). In their book *Dentistry Without Mercury*, Doctors Sam Ziff and Michael F. Ziff, D.D.S., discuss 1995 German research involving **more than 17,000 people**, which showed that saliva levels of mercury in those people with amalgam fillings was anywhere from 10-100 times the "acceptable" level (319) [emphasis mine], yet many dentists will still argue that mercury is bound in a non-toxic compound when it is used for fillings. They will insist that no large human studies have proven otherwise. Well, you can feel free to point out the 1995 German study above which DOES prove otherwise and involved **17,000 human beings,** not lab rats!

Dr. Gary Null, PhD., and Dr. Martin Feldman, MD, have issued a study pointing out irrefutable *evidence that mercury* is constantly being leached out of *amalgam fillings,* and it is no secret that mercury kills **white blood cells** and harms the normal functioning of our kidneys (261). It has also been proven that the T-cells of our immune system decrease *when amalgam fillings are placed in the mouth,* then levels again rise when *the fillings are removed* (261). When the Karolinska Institute of Sweden did autopsies, they discovered that "people with amalgam fillings had three times more mercury in the brain and nine times more in the kidneys" than those without the fillings (261), yet your dentist will insist that these fillings are harmless!

The University of Calgary researched on the effects of putting mercury fillings in the teeth of sheep about ten years ago. As noted by *www.rense.com,* "They used a very minor amount [of radioactive mercury] as a trace element...so that it would be distinguishable from any other mercury that might already be present in the sheep" (131). [What they discovered was shocking. The mercury did not stay in the mouth like your dentist will tell you it does!] Within just "28 to 29 days the mercury went through the entire system of the animal, including crossing the placental membrane and going into the fetus," and when the sheep were put to sleep and "tested using a radioscope...they found mercury literally everywhere in the body" (131). It was found "massively in the gastrointestinal area. It goes everywhere very rapidly." Just to be sure there were no errors, they repeated the research with monkeys, but the results were the same. The mercury "went throughout the entire system in" the same *time period* (131). Still feel that all that mercury in your mouth is safe?

Other governments outside the U.S. are finally warning their citizens about the dangers of amalgam fillings. The Canadians and several European countries have issued warnings to dentists telling them to avoid either inserting or extracting *amalgam fillings in pregnant women* (261). After they determined "that at least 250,000 Swedes have immune and other health disorders directly related to the mercury in their teeth...Denmark" placed a "ban on amalgams beginning in January 1999" (108). Other research they had done revealed that "MS [multiple sclerosis] patients had eight times higher levels of mercury in their cerebrospinal fluid" over those tested without MS (108). As noted by *naturallifemagazine.com*, Dr. Hal Huggins is a Colorado Springs dentist who also suffers from MS. He helps his patients with chronic diseases like MS and others by extracting their "mercury amalgam fillings," and with a special dietary and detox program he puts them through. He says that they have an *80 to 85 percent* improvement rate (108).

While Dr. Murray Vinney believes "that every time you chew, brush, or grind your teeth you absorb mercury," he advises people that they should replace their mercury fillings "with non-mercury materials like resin composites, porcelain, or gold, as needed," and says that "There is some risk that mass replacements could expose the patient to more mercury than if old fillings were left alone" (108). This is especially true if you let a dentist remove the fillings who is not experienced in proper removal of mercury amalgam from the mouth. Many precautions have to be taken and several fillings cannot and should not be removed at one time. Doing so can cause severe heart damage, as well as damage to the entire body and could even kill you! Mercury is so toxic that it only takes very small amounts to kill you.

In 1991 "German's Health Ministry recommended to the German Dental Association that no further amalgam fillings be placed in children, pregnant women, or people with kidney disease" (108). In 1993 the Germans expanded this advice "to include all women of child-bearing age, pregnant or not," and "Austria is also phasing out mercury fillings" (108). But not here! Not in the USA! Of course not! Dentists are still purchasing tons of mercury every year and packing it into the mouths of unwary patients just a few inches from their brains!

The American Dental Association (ADA) insists that "replacing amalgam fillings…for the purpose of removing toxic substances from the body is 'improper and unethical" (108). [For WHOM, I wonder, and now they are talking ethics? After years of putting toxins in people's mouth without a conscience?] Dr. Sandra Denton, MD, whose specialty is in treating people with "chronic mercury toxicity, asks 'What is it about the mouth that makes the same stuff non-toxic?'" (108)

• Mercury Warning Signs – Too Little, Too Late?

International Health News reported that beginning in November of 2000 everyone practicing dentistry in the State of *California* had to put *the following sign* on display for their patients to see:

> 'WARNING – Amalgam fillings contain a chemical element known to the State of California to cause birth defects or other reproductive harm,' though the California Dental Association apparently lobbied successfully to ensure that the word **mercury** did not appear in the warning (261) [emphasis mine].

Realize too, that consuming acidic foods, which interacts with amalgam, has been linked to the pain associated with trigeminal neuralgia (261), and also increases the leaching of mercury from fillings.

According to Sam Ziff and Michael F. Ziff, D.D.S., in their book, *Dentistry Without Mercury,* it takes very little mercury to make you seriously ill. Microscopic amounts can adversely affect every single vital organ in your body, including damage to the blood, hormones, and immune system (319).

These dentists have a survey that was done showing 221 patients who had all their mercury fillings removed, and as a result, the majority of them were cured of many ailments, including: allergies, blood pressure problems, fatigue, migraines, multiple sclerosis, insomnia, memory loss, skin disorders, and thyroid problems, to name a few (319). Even Alzheimer's has been linked to mercury fillings.

Researchers in Saudi Arabia recently finished a human study that showed that "amalgam fillings and skin-lightening creams...contain significant amounts of mercury," and this mercury may be causing significant loss of *kidney function* (261). Beware of purchasing minerals harvested from the Great Salt Lake. This lake is said to be full of very *toxic mercury* (126)!

• Mercury & Parasites

Dr. Hulda Clark not only blamed parasites on dentistry metal (as well as pets), but isopropyl alcohol. She recommended that once you rid yourself of parasites, stay away from isopropyl alcohol, because once it gets into the body, it enables flukes to multiply in some people. For those fighting cancer and other illnesses, it is also advised to get all toxic chemicals and cleaners out of the home environment; because we are often inundated with toxins in the everyday cleaners, shampoos, soaps, sprays, and even toothpastes that we use (186). Each item alone may have little effect on your health, but if your immune system is already compromised, the combination of all of them can be overwhelming, especially for those already fighting a chronic illness or a disease like cancer. Realize that exposure to chemicals such as benzene, hexane, toluene, and many others, can cause leukemia and other illnesses. Many of these toxins are absorbed right through your skin or are inhaled into your lungs. Why do you think so many people have died from mesothelioma? Because their employers convinced them that working around asbestos was harmless! People were once convinced that inhaling tobacco smoke was safe and inhaling coal dust was harmless. Why? Because someone they trusted lied to them! I have long advocated against the excessive use of heavily scented perfumes, deodorizers, scented candles, and room air fresheners. These items are full of thousands of chemicals, and you have no idea what they are doing to your body! Some have been known to cause kidney and blood disorders, yet people think nothing of spraying themselves with them and saturating their homes with them, inhaling them, breathing their fumes, and exposing their children to them 24 hours a day! Do you know what you are inhaling in them? Have you ever read the list of ingredients in a scented candle, air freshener, or a bottle of perfume from any retail store shelf? Take each ingredient, list it on a piece of paper and look it up on the internet. What country is your air freshener made in? China? The same country that was shipping thousands of lead-laden toys to American consumers to give their children?

For information on using a form of *calcium bentonite clay* to detox your body from mercury (and other toxins), see the article: "New Safe Detox for Mercury Amalgam Fillings" at website: *http://www.naturalnews.com/023652.html*. This clay has also been discussed in my book *Gentle Cures for Tough Cancers* for its ability at killing MRSA. Also, those with painful skin after having radiation treatments, chicken pox or measles, shingles, herpes sores, poison oak, bed sores, infected sores, dermatitis or poison ivy, may find this clay helpful. It works like a magnet, drawing poisons out of the body, and gives relief to children suffering from unbearably itchy skin rashes and chicken pox.

• Children & Mercury Fillings

Want to give your children a fighting chance in a world of toxins and pollutants? Never, ever allow a dentist to put a mercury amalgam filling in their mouth and never allow them to undergo a root canal filling, not for any reason! This plague of amalgam mercury is causing not only gum disease, CAD, atherosclerosis, and strokes, but increased oral cancers and all other forms of cancer because of its depressive effect on the body's natural immunity.

• How Did This Happen?

What happened with mercury fillings? How did they end up in the mouths of millions of people? Well, according to website: *http://www.myyogaonline.com/healthy_living_203_MERCURY_FILLINGS:_THE_ENEMY_WITHIN.html*, this was not always the case:

> Soon after in the 1840's North American dentistry turned away from its use [mercury] largely due to concerns about the toxic nature of mercury. In fact, as a requirement of membership in the American Society of Dental Surgeons, **members had to sign a document that stated they would not use mercury amalgam in their practice.** However, this progressive, health-oriented stance was to be short-lived. In 1859 the organization we now know as the American Dental Association was formed and **chose to endorse the use of mercury amalgam, declaring it safe for use in the human body.** This puzzling about-turn became less so when it was revealed some years later [SURPRISE! SURPRISE!] that **some members of the ADA held patents on the mercury amalgam 'recipe'** (301) [emphasis mine].

Can you see what it is all about? It is greed and money! How do you feel knowing that you have these deadly toxins in your mouth just inches from your brain? How many of them are in the mouths of your children or grandchildren?

• Kicking the Mercury Out

Good chelators (removers) of mercury are the antioxidants selenium, glutathione, chlorella, vitamin C and E, cilantro, onions, garlic, hyaluronic acid, iodine, magnesium, and zinc. Also, for those wanting a great way to eliminate heavy metals from your body, try ***HMD*™** (Heavy Metal Detox), which you can obtain from website: *http://www.vnfnutrition.com/index.html*. HMD™ contains chlorella growth factor, organic coriander sativum leaf tincture and homaacord of cell-decimated, energized chlorella. This website also contains one of the best forms of easily absorbed selenium (L-selenomethionine) you can find:
http://www.vnfnutrition.com/phpshop/ /index.php?page=shop/flypage&product_id=23609&category_id=

Also, if you are looking to remove amalgam fillings from your mouth, check this site out first: *http://www.ehow.com/how_5086941_replace-mercury-fillings.html*. And for a dentist in your area, who will remove mercury fillings from your mouth, check the list by state given at website: *http://www.dentalwellness4u.com/freeservices/find_dentists.ht*

ml. Also, see website *mercuryfreenow.com*. If you wish to detox your body from lead, see the product **Detoxamin**® at *http://www.detoxamin.com*.

Dr. Joseph Mercola has a detox program at his website: *http://www.mercola.com/article/mercury/detox_protocol.htm*, which you may want to consider. He uses many products, including probiotics, whey protein, garlic, MSM, chlorella, cilantro, and others.

You can find a wealth of information on using *bentonite (clay), bladderwrack, blue green algae, burdock (root), cilantro, garlic, glutathione, onion, selenium, and Zeolite* for removing heavy metals from your body at *Natural News Network* website: *http://www.naturalnews.com/026885_zeolite_heavy_metals_cilantro.html*, in an article by Kirk Patrick (265).

You can purchase Zeolite at many websites including: *http://zeoliteliquid.com, http://www.liquidzeolitecompany.com*, and *http://www.globalhealingcenter.com/zeotrex.php*. You can find bentonite clay (and many other health ingredients) at: *http://www.magneticclay.com/benefits.php* (261).

Another item, mentioned earlier, that is supposed to get these toxic heavy metals out of your body is HMD™ (Heavy Metal Detox), a solution available at: *http://www.heavymetaldetox.net*, and *http://www.vnfnutrition.com/index.html*, and you can also do so by using selenium, glutathione, cysteine, cilantro, and chlorella (concentrated chlorophyll foods). While you can remove these toxins from your body on a daily basis, if you have a mouth full of amalgam fillings, mercury will keep seeping from them every single day as long as they remain in your mouth. The worst pollutant for mercury is amalgam mercury fillings.

For a cilantro chelation **pesto** recipe (for those of you who love pesto) to remove heavy metals from your body, see this website: *http://proliberty.com/observer/20080201.htm* (183).

As described in an earlier chapter, Dr. Dietrich Klinghardt, MD, says that according to his research findings, "one of the best" ways of ridding toxic mercury from your brain is by ingesting "5 grams (teaspoonful[s]) a day" as "the minimum dose" of cilantro (35). Do not cook it in metal pans or use metal utensils. "Use only Pyrex or Corning ware!" Chop up "eight or more heaping teaspoons" and steep in about "one quart" of water that has just been boiled. It should be "covered for twenty minutes" (35).

One study in particular revealed that cilantro (often called *Chinese parsley*), not only rids mercury from cells, it "protects the body from pre-cancerous lesions" (101). Be sure you are using organically-grown cilantro.

• Periodontal Disease Increases Cancer Risk

A good treatment for periodontal disease is to rinse and gargle with a half cup of water that has about 10 drops of 2% *Magnascent©* iodine stirred into it. You can swish the formula, then gargle with it and swallow it. This is also a good sore throat remedy. Just be aware that using iodine on a regular basis as a mouth cleanser can stain your teeth. Brushing with soda bicarb will help remove stains. Iodine also helps in the removal of toxic heavy metals from the body. It is possible that HMD™ (Heavy Metal Detox at website: *http://www.vnfnutrition.com/index.html)*, iodine, selenium, and glutathione could help improve the lives of autistic children. (If using *Magnascent©* iodine during the day as a supplement, take it on an empty stomach mixed into water that does not contain fluoride or chlorine.)

Be aware that having periodontal disease can increase your risk for certain cancers, including those of the pancreas. A human study showed that men with this gum disease have a **"63 percent higher risk of developing pancreatic cancer compared to those reporting no periodontal disease"** (268). They also adjusted for other factors such as "age, smoking, diabetes, body mass," and other *factors;* however, even people who had never smoked cigarettes, were twice as likely to get pancreatic cancer if they had periodontal disease (268).

II. Toxic Chemo – Immune Destroyer, Cancer Culprit

Most people, even those who undertake chemo, have no idea how toxic most chemo drugs really are. So toxic, in fact, that the physicians, pharmacists, and nurses who handle them must wear safety gloves to keep from absorbing the chemicals through their own skin, chemicals that can cause them to develop cancer themselves! I can recall working between med/surg floors and orthopedic floors in a hospital where we were having a discussion late one night between all the nurses; a middle-of-the-shift discussion about the perplexity of why so many nurses who worked with cancer patients were themselves getting cancer. The statistics were incredible, but no one seemed to be following them. We wondered if perhaps the disease was caused by a virus and these particular nurses were succumbing to the viruses their patients carried. What we didn't say, perhaps because it seemed too unbelievable and frightening to contemplate, was that perhaps just handling the toxic drugs and caring for patients who were saturated with the drugs, was increasing the nurses' risk for the disease. That was more than 25 years ago.

Well, just recently, articles have come out noting the vigorous efforts OSHA has taken to protect workers from secondhand cigarette smoke, asbestos exposure, and other dangerous chemicals, but they have been strangely silent about the secondhand dangers caused by toxic chemo chemicals (157b). WHY? When was the last time you saw a news article researching how many nurses and pharmacists handling chemo drugs end up with cancer themselves from the drugs being absorbed into their skin? Such an article exists at Mike Adams' *www.naturalnews.com* website:

> …hundreds of thousands of people are killed each year around the world by chemotherapy drugs. Now you can add pharmacists to that statistic. For decades, they simply looked the other way, pretending they were playing a valuable role in our system of 'modern' medicine, not admitting they were actually dolling out chemicals that killed people…They are in the business of death, and it is killing them off, one by one. *The Seattle Times* now reports the story of…a veteran pharmacist of two decades who spent much of her time dispensing chemotherapy drugs….[she] died last September of pancreatic cancer, and one of her dying wishes was that the truth would be told about how her on-the-job exposure to chemotherapy chemicals contributed to her own cancer (157b).

Is OSHA ignoring the dangers to physicians, nurses, and pharmacists of secondhand chemo drugs? The *Natural News* article adds that OSHA "has only issued one citation in the last decade to a hospital for inadequate safety handling of toxic chemotherapy drugs" (157b). *The Seattle Times* noted that not only do these drugs "contaminate the work spaces" where they are used, but "in some cases **[are] being found in the urine of those who handle it**" (157b). [Emphasis mine.] Mike Adams asks, "if nurses can become violently ill after merely *spilling* chemotherapy chemicals on themselves (it's true), then what effect do you suppose these chemicals have when *injected* into patients? (157b). Danish studies on oncology nurses found that they have an "increased risk of leukemia," while "another Danish study...last year" involving "more than 92,000 nurses" revealed that they had an "elevated risk for breast, thyroid, nervous-system and brain cancers" (157b). Pretty scary findings for those health care professionals who handle these toxic drugs day-after-day for months and years! What about all the nurses in cancer clinics that handle, splash on their skin, drop, or infuse bags of chemo drugs by the dozens every day in their workplace? They are supposed to use gloves, some don't.

III. Vaccines – Deadly Deception

Are you aware that there are many health issues related to vaccinations? Childhood vaccinations have been suspected in Crohn's Disease, autism, juvenile diabetes, other autoimmune disorders, brain tumors in children, and many other illnesses, yet your school officials will tell you that you MUST have your child vaccinated. The reality is that you can always request a *waiver* from your school to opt out of the vaccination. For one of the most amazing and informative articles (and videos) on the vaccine-autism-bowel-disease-connection you will ever witness, see website: *http://articles.mercola.com/sites/articles/archive/ 2010/04/10/wakefield-interview.aspx*. You may wish to read the book by Neil Z. Miller, *Vaccines: Are They Really Safe & Effective?* before you take that next flu shot or pneumonia shot, or take your child for their next vaccination.

For a website that has a great deal of information that is helpful to parents of autistic children, see *http://www.child-autism-parent-café. com/autism-treatment.html.* This website warns parents of autistic children about giving them even more vaccines which "could push their immune system further over the edge," and to be very careful about giving their siblings vaccines, because "if one of your children has autism, there is a greater than average chance that your other children are genetically or physically more susceptible to damage from vaccines" (12).

There are many news articles circulating regarding a preservative in vaccines (thimerosal or mercury) causing autism in children, and many websites have information about the dangers associated with flu shots. A Hollywood celebrity recently came out and admitted that she believed her young child's autism was caused by a recent vaccination. Though this is all being ignored by the CDC, T.V. news abounds with the Gestapo-like tactics the U.S. government has resorted to in order to force vaccinations (and chemo drugs) on children!

Horrific as it sounds, there are many over-the-counter products that continue to include thimerosal in them, all approved by the FDA! This includes some "medications...steroids and injected collagen" (222). Vaccines with this dangerous product continue to be shipped overseas to other countries, "some of which are now experiencing a sudden explosion in autism rates" (222). Autism is now widespread in places like Argentina, India, and Nicaragua where the U.S. has shipped mercury-containing vaccines (222). In the meantime, the World Health Organization refuses to address the issue (222). In a report from "Deadly Immunity—Autism," by Robert F. Kennedy, Jr., environmental lawyer, dated June 16, 2005, he stated that: "If, as the evidence suggests, our public-health authorities knowingly allowed the pharmaceutical industry to poison an entire generation of American children, their actions arguably constitute one of the biggest scandals in the annals of American medicine" (222). Well, isn't this exactly what they have done?

Kennedy states that "More than 500,000 kids currently suffer from autism, and pediatricians diagnose more than 40,000 new cases every year...The disease was unknown until 1943, when it was identified and diagnosed among 11 children born in the months after thimerosal was first added to baby vaccines" (306). Kennedy adds that "federal officials covered up proven scientific links between thimerosal and a 15-fold increase in autism cases since 1991" (306). Because of the public outcry, thimerosal is being phased out of vaccines; however, vaccine makers continue to export thimerosal-containing vaccines to other countries (306), and it is well documented that Eli Lilly knew as far back as the 1930's that mercury-based (thimerosal) vaccines were implicated in "causing neurological injury to infants" (45).

• Autism Statistics

It is also a well known fact that one out of every 150 babies will end up with autism (142)! How many people stop and think about the fact that by the time a child in America is two years old, they have received "237 micrograms of mercury through vaccines alone, which far exceeds current EPA 'safe' levels of .1 mcg/kg per day. That's one-tenth of a microgram, not one microgram" (142). Also, the mandated (1991) hepatitis B shot for newborns contains 250 mcg of aluminum (145), right along with that toxic mercury, and by the time a baby gets that "first big round of shots," he or she could be getting between "295 mcg to a whopping 1225 mcg" of aluminum, then the same dosage at "four and six months" of age, even though the FDA says that premies and "anyone with impaired kidney function, receive no more than 10 to 25 mcg of injected aluminum at any one time" (145). The question is this – WHY INJECT ANYONE WITH ALUMINUM—especially a baby?! WHY? For what possible reason? Why put aluminum or mercury in any vaccines, or anything ELSE for that matter?

Well, our kids may not have measles or mumps, but there's a trade-off, because too many of them are fighting for their lives with asthma, Crohn's, autism, leukemia, lymphoma, other cancers, diabetes, autoimmune disorders, meningitis, muscular dystrophy, cystic fibrosis, degenerative diseases, bi-polar disorders, and a host of other ailments, many of which have been linked to mercury and aluminum toxicity, and things like recombinant monkey viruses, pigs blood, and other disgusting items used in making vaccines that should never, ever be introduced into a child's bloodstream! Scientists know next to nothing about what these foreign invaders will do once mixed in with the genetic DNA of human cells. Many children today, because of these pharmaceutical blunders, are possibly facing worse disasters than had they simply fought measles, mumps, or rubella instead! Which is the lesser of two evils?

And for those who still have doubts about the connection between mercury in vaccines and autism, statistics show that after "the introduction of the hepatitis B vaccine in 1990" [in California], there was a *"900 percent* increase in *autism rates in less than a generation"* (220). The rate in the rest of the nation rose *714 percent* (220). In California, during the "first three quarters of 2004 – five years after thimerosal was removed from vaccines – the data showed a decline in the incidence of autism in California for the first time" (220). (Do the math! Something is rotten about this, especially when the government comes out with a report telling us that there is NO connection between vaccines and autism!) As reported by Dr. Mark Hyman, M.D:

> What is even more alarming is that **vaccine strains of measles virus seem to migrate into the brains of children with autism.** That means it may not be only gut related inflammation that is causing the problems, but the measles virus may take root in the brain itself...Vaccine measles strains have been isolated from the spinal fluid of autistic children [and]...the 4 to 1 ratio of autism in males to females may, in part, be due to the effects of testosterone on mercury excretion. Antibiotics also prevent excretion of mercury, and antibiotic use is higher among autistic children (220). [Emphasis mine.]

Dr. Hyman also points out that the EPA has said that "the 'safe' daily level of mercury exposure for a five kilogram, two-month-old infant is 0.5 micrograms or 0.1 micrograms per kg," however these levels are only for the mercury that is commonly found in certain fish, not the mercury contained in vaccines (220). The actual *vaccination schedule* that most two-month old babies receive, gives them a total of *62.5 micrograms of mercury* (220)! And keep in mind that this is just the ones they receive at 2 months of age!

A study from JAMA (*the Journal of the American Medical Association)* claimed that there was "no increased risk of autism with thimerosal..." *the problem,* however, "was that **the authors were affiliated with the state-run Statens Serum Institute," and "Eighty percent of the Institute's profits are from vaccines!"** (220). A rather awkward conflict-of-interest here, ya think? [How stupid do they think the public really is? Emphasis mine.]

- ## Vaccine Deaths

Michael Belkin's five week old daughter, Lyla Rose, died "shortly after" she was given a "Hepatitis B vaccine booster shot" in 1998 (65). The drug company that makes this vaccine in the US is Merck. You remember Merck, don't you? They are the same drug company who made Vioxx® and intentionally hid some of the dangerous side effects from the public. This is the drug that was responsible for the injury and deaths of thousands of people, some directly and some indirectly. But, not to worry, they are STILL IN BUSINESS! Yes, operating every day, business as usual! Who else would we have to thank for all those Hep B sticks in all our newborns, had they been shut down a long time ago after that Vioxx® disaster!?

Mr. Belkin testified before "The Advisory Committee on Immunization Practices – Centers for Disease Control and Prevention (February 17, 1999) – Atlanta, Georgia" (65). He said that his little girl had never been sick before she was given the Hepatitis B shot on the afternoon of the day that she died. She simply went to sleep that night and never woke up. Of course, he got the usual pat answer from physicians he spoke to after an autopsy showed that she had a "swollen brain," that it must have been SIDS. He wasn't convinced and began investigating other cases of "disturbing evidence of adverse reactions" that others had had to this same vaccine (65).

The type of hepatitis that his little girl was vaccinated against usually affects "drug users, homosexuals, prostitutes and promiscuous heterosexuals," and gets "transmitted by "blood, through sex or dirty needles." He asked himself, since his wife had already "tested negative," how in the world was his newborn baby supposed to get this disease? Well, it would be next to impossible! So why are babies even given this vaccination (65)? The only reason he could see that this vaccine was mandated for U.S. babies at birth is:

> An unrestrained health bureaucracy decided it couldn't get junkies, gays, prostitutes and promiscuous heterosexuals to take the Hepatitis B vaccine so they mandated that all babies must be vaccinated at birth. Drug companies such as Merck (reaching for new markets) were instrumental in pushing government scientists to adopt an at-birth Hepatitis B vaccination policy although the vaccine was never tested in newborns and no vaccines had ever been mandated at birth before. It is widely recognized that newborns have underdeveloped immune systems, which can be overwhelmed or shocked (65).

This precious little girl should never have lost her life and the parents have every right to be angry! You will often hear the CDC talk about all the "good" that vaccines do. They don't seem to mind sacrificing 3000 children to give 100,000 of them vaccines. Do you remember the old movies where a ship wrecked and the survivors all clung to a single lifeboat? Well, they had no idea how long they would be floating at sea. They calculated that they only had enough food and water to get about one-third of the people in the lifeboat to shore. What did they do? They began dumping the older, less fit lifeboat victims into the water telling them that it was for the good of all that they be sacrificed so a few could make it to shore alive! That is a perfect picture of what is happening with vaccinations and is probably exactly what will happen under government-run healthcare in the U.S! Their rationale says it is okay if 3,000 children die (or get autism or some other disease) from vaccines as long as you save the other 300,000 who don't get autism! The only thing is—in the movie—a huge ship came along within a short period of time and rescued the "survivors" in the lifeboat. It was not necessary that anyone be sacrificed! All of them would have been saved, but it was too late for the ones tossed into the ocean. They had already drowned or become shark bait. Communism, Socialism, and Marxism at their very best, coming to a happy little town near you!

- **Gardasil® - Deadly Statistics**

Many parents have been lulled into believing that they MUST have their pre-teen and teen daughters vaccinated against cervical cancer with the new vaccine, Gardasil®, but this vaccine is already suspect in the maiming and deaths of several young girls. Be sure you read up on the stories of young girls who have suffered irreversible, declining health after they received this new "promising" vaccine, including many cases of Gullain-Barré syndrome and many who have died after taking the vaccine. (See website: *http://truthaboutgardasil.org*) (25). **The website also reports the suspension of the Gardasil® vaccination program in India after four girls died and 120 suffered "complications…" after taking the vaccine** (25) [Emphasis mine]. See this article about a young teen who developed total paralysis shortly after being vaccinated with Gardasil®:

http://articles.mercola.com/sites/articles/archive/2008/08/02/hpv-vaccine-blamed-for-teen-paralysis.as px?source=nl

And this documented report of three young girls who also say that they were paralyzed by the Gardasil® vaccine and are now seeking damages from the drug manufacturer:

http://www.theoneclickgroup.co.uk/news.php?start=2300&end=2320&view=yes&id=2816#newspost.

And this dreadful news article about **twelve babies that died** in Argentina after receiving an experimental pneumonia vaccine:

http://www.theoneclickgroup.co.uk/news.php?start=2300&end=2320&view=yes&id=2819#newspost

Realize that there is already some government scrubbing taking place of website articles that are unfavorable (to them), so I have no idea how long these articles will be available.

Some pediatricians are demanding that childhood vaccines be spread out over a longer period of time, with children receiving fewer vaccines at any given time to reduce the risk of overwhelming their young immune systems. Why are they not being heard?

• More Big Pharma & FDA Hypocrisy

Compare the rapid and drastic action by the FDA against the makers of an herbal tea when they quickly moved to get Chaparral off U.S. shelves (when FOUR cases of liver toxicity were reported), to the FDA dragging its feet to remove drugs like Baycol, Rezulin, and Vioxx® from the market when they already knew that the drugs were killing people! Many people are totally unaware of the depth of depravity that Merck had reached in trying to keep Vioxx® on the market.

Dr. Joseph Mercola says that: "The company is alleged to have used intimidation tactics against researchers, including dropping hints that the company would stop funding their institutions, and possibly even interfering with academic appointments" (243). He added that: "The international drug company Merck had a **hit list of doctors who had to be 'neutralized' or discredited because they had criticized the painkiller Vioxx®**, a now-withdrawn drug that the pharmaceutical giant produced. **'We may need to seek them out and destroy them**

where they live,' a Merck employee wrote, according to an email excerpt read to the court'" (243) [emphasis mine]. Did you read that last sentence? Seeking out doctors who were critical of Vioxx® and "destroying them where they live..." (243)?! Dr. Mercola himself was wondering exactly "how FAR" this drug company "would have gone...had Vioxx® not been pulled from the market" (243). What did they mean by **"neutralizing" their opposition?** Did you hear anything ANYWHERE about all the people involved in this cover-up that were given prison terms? No, because they are still walking the streets! And this company is STILL IN BUSINESS!? Business as usual—when internal records said that they were speaking of **destroying doctors who speak out against their drug?**

Merck isn't the only questionable pharmaceutical maker out there. CBS and AP News did a report on June 9, 2010, about the drug-maker Pfizer concealing "serious injuries" to patients caused by their drugs Lipitor, Lyrica, and Viagra (52a). In some cases, the drug manufacturer was late in reporting the side effects—in other cases—they completely omitted reporting them at all (52a), and as recently as July 2010, many news reports are circulating the world about the maker's of the diabetic drug, *Avandia,* leaving the drug on the market long AFTER it knew it was causing heart disease in users—facts that were intentionally hidden from the public. How awful though, isn't it? I mean, the drug company was making $3 BILLION a year on this drug! Do you really think they are concerned about human life when they stand to lose so much in profits? Apparently not! Will this be the next big drug recall, or will doctors and patients simply be told *the benefits outweigh the risks* – uh, yeah – right. The BENEFITS to the company making the $3 billion a year that they don't want to see go down the drain!? They don't care that the drug might kill YOU! To them, you are just a number.

• More Drug Recalls

There was a recent recall of Tylenol® products for children after complaints from many parents that the products had black flecks in them. The company actually dragged their feet in recalling the Tylenol®! The products were finally recalled, but there is no way to estimate how many children ingested these defective products, nor how to determine what kind of harm may have been done to them as a result. The news media was actually telling the public to use GENERIC products instead. These are CHILDREN'S medicines we are talking about! How could any company drag their feet in recalling a defective product being ingested by children? Do you have any idea what would have happened had this been a VITAMIN or herbal manufacturer instead of a multi-billion dollar drug conglomerate with powerful drug lobbyists behind them? We would still be seeing the herbal manufacturer being maligned and crucified on the nightly national news media, their doors shut down, and the owners facing prison terms!

• Mercury & Neurological Disorders

Those who suffer from neurological disorders such as *Alzheimer's, Parkinson's, and Lou Gehrig's Disease,* have also been discovered to have high levels of mercury in their *brain, blood or spinal fluid* (102). In light of this, it should come as no surprise to you that "elderly people who get annual flu vaccines for five years," have a "10-times increase in Alzheimer's disease" (102). How much more at risk are those who get these yearly flu shots for 10, 15, and 20 years (if they live that long)?

If you are a user of solutions for contact lens, read the label on the brand you use, because many of these solutions contain mercury (101). Other products that are famous for containing mercury include: "many over-the-counter drugs and cosmetics: e.g. mascara…[and] hemorrhoid preparations, etc." (104). Even some ear drops and nasal drops used for babies contain mercury! But beware, because the industry won't ADMIT that their products actually contain deadly MERCURY in them! Of course not! What they do is DISGUISE it under a name that most consumers won't even recognize! Read the label and if the product contains: *"thimerosal, phenylmercuric acetate, phenylmercuric nitrate, mercuric acetate, mercuric nitrate, MB for merbromin, and mercuric oxide yellow,"* its got mercury; and pitch any item in your first aid kit that has mercurochrome or methiolate, both of which contain mercury (104). Avoid it like the plague! Be a label reader. The label may tell you that their product only contains "trace" amounts of these items, but remember this: mercury is so toxic that it only takes "trace" amounts to make you sick enough to kill you! Why does the FDA allow ANY AMOUNT of mercury to be put near a human being?

Instead of the Food & Drug Administration (FDA), they should be re-labeled the *Federal Death Agency!*

• The FDA Hearing

On July 18, 2000, the House Committee on Government Reform held *a hearing entitled:* "'Mercury in Medicine: Are We Taking Unnecessary Risks?'" And *during* this *hearing,* "the FDA admitted that children are being exposed to unsafe levels of mercury through vaccines containing Thimerosal," and they "also determined that symptoms of mercury poisoning mimic symptoms of autism..." (101), yet the most absurd part of all is that the FDA even admits on their own website that "lead, cadmium, and mercury are examples of elements that are toxic when present at relatively low levels"...(101) What was their reaction to this hearing? Did the FDA recall all mercury-containing vaccines? Of course not! They simply allowed the "pharmaceutical companies to merely phase out their use of Thimerosal, leaving mercury-containing vaccines at public and private health facilities" (101). It is just one big YAWN to them!

• Where Many Diseases Originate

Much of the chronic illness and disease we are now facing as a population comes from the indiscriminate use of poisons (like mercury in dental fillings and other health products our children are using) and chlorine, fluoride, and lead in drinking water.

Scientific studies have shown that levels of mercury can be as much as "20,000 [times] higher in those with cardiac abnormalities" (101), and since this heavy metal is so toxic to the body's entire nervous system, it has also been linked to many other health problems including: "insomnia, polyneuropathy [an illness that attacks several nerves at the same time], paresthesias [numbness]... irritability, personality changes, headaches, weakness, blurred vision, dysarthria [a speech disorder], slowed mental response and unsteady gait" [difficulty walking normally] (101).

• Vaccine Horrors

The FDA just recently "recommended" that a vaccine commonly given to U.S. kids be halted. Why? Because it has been discovered that it is contaminated with pig DNA! Of course the makers of the vaccine claim that they have absolutely NO IDEA how this could have happened and are just as dumbfounded as the rest of us (246). The big **Oooops!?** Well, it's a little too late, because more than a million children have already received it, not to mention more than 30,000 children in other nations (246). It is the GlaxoSmithKline Rotarix vaccine. (I wonder how many of THEIR kids got the vaccine.) That's not the worst part. No, unfortunately, there's more. Two other vaccines were also found to be contaminated. "A measles vaccine...found [with] low levels of the retrovirus avian leukosis virus," and the "Rotateq" vaccine made by Merck discovered to be contaminated with "a virus similar to simian (monkey) retrovirus" (246). (Well, there is Merck again. Aren't they popular?) Of the vaccines tested, it was not a little bitty batch that was contaminated. On the contrary, it was 40% (246)! Well, of course, both the FDA and the vaccine makers are insisting that "no safety risk has been uncovered from the contamination..." (246) and if there is, I'm sure that WE will be the first to know, right?

Folks, do you realize what "avian leukosis virus" is? That is the **BIRD FLU** virus! While the FDA itself and the feds, and everyone in Asia, is yelling and screaming about the dangers of the BIRD FLU and how many people it can kill—and here we are giving it to our kids in VACCINATION shots—and no one knows how this happened or where it came from, and we are supposed to believe THAT?!

Well, as of May 20, 2010, now we know that the FDA has decided NOT to recall the vaccines infected with the pig virus. Yes, you guessed it; they are leaving it on the market! Per an article at Mike Adams' website:

> Think about that for a moment: The discovery that a vaccine being injected into children is contaminated with a virus from a pig doesn't even result in a product recall! It doesn't raise any red flags! It's just *business as usual* in the vaccine industry, where DNA from any number of diseased animals is often used in the vaccine formulas. Last year, rotavirus vaccines earned nearly a billion dollars in revenues for Big

Pharma. The risk of a child in the United States actually dying from a rotavirus infection is ridiculously small. [So WHY is this vaccine even needed?] What these kids need is good nutrition and vitamin D, not an injection of a questionable vaccine made with pig virus DNA (157c).

Remember the people in the lifeboat story? What about YOU? Are you willing to gamble that your child won't get autism, hoping that they also will not get polio, measles, mumps, or some other infectious disease, or is it okay if it's just someone else's child that gets sacrificed?

How many of the people on that committee have kids with autism, do you suppose? Hmmm....sacrificing a few for the good of all? Where have I heard that lofty philosophy before? Communism? Socialism? Marxism? Remember when all the dangerous side effects were reported about HRT and birth control pills—blood clots, heart attacks, strokes? What was the rationale of the drug companies? Their pat answer for everything that looks shady: "The benefits outweigh the risks." I guess they are trying to apply that philosophy to vaccines. The benefit of saving 80,000 kids from polio and measles, outweighs the risks of condemning 8,000 children to a life of autism, SIDS death, or total paralysis, not to mention their families!? They never read the research of Dr. Frederick Klenner who CURED all of his polio patients by giving them megadoses of vitamin C. (See website: *http://www.doctoryourself.com/klennerbio.html.*) The Salk vaccine had just been developed, so was not even available in some areas yet. I said all that to say this: how many of you are beginning to smell a rat yet? A really BIG rat? Does it not yet appear that there is statistical evidence that some of these so-called *errors* are in fact deliberate? We are playing a form of Russian roulette with the lives of our children. The question is—if it's YOUR child—are you willing to play the game?

Here is what Dr. J. W. Hodge, M.D. said of the AMA:

> The medical monopoly or medical trust, euphemistically called the American Medical Association, is not merely the meanest monopoly ever organized, but the most arrogant, dangerous and despotic organisation which ever managed a free people in this or any other age. Any and all methods of healing the sick by means of safe, simple and natural

> remedies are sure to be assailed and denounced by the arrogant leaders of the AMA doctors' trust as fakes, frauds and humbugs. Every practitioner of the healing art who does not ally himself with the medical trust is denounced as a 'dangerous quack' and impostor by the predatory trust doctors...at once pounced upon by these medical tyrants and fanatics, bitterly denounced, vilified and persecuted to the fullest extent--J.W Hodge, M.D. (136).

Dr. Gary Null has this to say about using alternative cancer therapies:

> But today in the U.S., and this shows you where fascism really exists, ANY doctor in the United States who cures cancer using alternative methods will be destroyed. You cannot name me a doctor doing well with cancer using alternative therapies that is not under attack. And I KNOW these people; I've interviewed them (136).

All you have to do is read my last book, *Gentle Cures for Tough Cancers,* that details the struggles that people like Dr. Stanislaw Burzynski, Emanuel Revici, Rene Caisse, Joseph Gold, Harry Hoxsey, and many others have undergone during their entire lives in fighting the FDA and other beaurocratic medical agencies (in the U.S. or Canada) while treating their patients with non-toxic cancer therapies, to get a picture of what these physicians are saying.

If you have a child who has recently been diagnosed with autism, Crohn's Disease, type I diabetes, meningitis, Gullain-Barré Syndrome, other rare health disorders, or you've lost a child to SIDS (sudden infant death syndrome), ask yourself this question: when was the last time that they were vaccinated, and what was it for?

Of autism, Dr. David Ayoub, M.D. says:

> I am no longer 'trying to dig up evidence to prove' vaccines cause autism. There is already abundant evidence...This debate is not scientific but is political. There are too many dollars at stake and too many powerful pharmaceutical company lobbyists who stand to lose billions of dollars if the true dangers of vaccines are finally recognized by a public that is weary of being lied to (136).

• SV40 Monkey Virus Contaminates 95 Million Vaccines

Taking a vaccine isn't simply like buying a car that is found to have a defect that you return to the dealer for repairs. Once you are injected, you're stuck for life (or death!) with the contents of that vile vial!

Dianne Jacobs Thompson studies recombinant virology, which is "the combining of unlike viruses into new 'tribes', usually" producing more "dangerous" viruses than the ones you started with, "by men in white coats playing God" (297), as she puts it. One example of such a disaster was the SV40 virus that came from a monkey. Scientists discovered that this virus had the ability to "ride piggyback into the genetic material of a cell where they can take over the 'machinery' and make brand new viruses 'on their own,'" and it was this SV40 virus that opened up the whole science of *recombinant virology*, with its Pandora's box of deadly consequences (297)! This virus contaminated 95 million polio vaccines that were injected into people between 1955 and 1963 (297), and you or I could have received one of them!

Of course the vaccine makers claimed that the virus was insignificant; however, when it was given to guinea pigs they "developed salivary gland tumours and immune deficiency symptoms. The corresponding organ in humans is the pancreas," so is it just a coincidence that since that time "Deadly pancreatic cancer has become epidemic in numbers" (297)? That isn't all; SV40 isn't just linked with pancreatic cancer. It is "now associated with…human mesotheliomas, osteosarcomas, brain tumours, ependymomas, choroid plexus tumours and others," and there is further evidence to support the belief that it was the "same monkey cell cultures…[which] contained other viruses such as SIV (simian immune-deficiency virus)…" that are partly responsible for "…another recombinant virus that we know as HIV" (297). Isn't it time we asked, How much of our current disease (and the death and despair that comes with it) has been caused by these mad-scientist vaccine-makers?

Of vaccines, Dr. W. J. Collins, MD, BS, B.Sc (Lond), M.R.C.S, had this to say:

> I have no faith in vaccination; nay, I look upon it with the greatest possible disgust, and firmly believe that it is often the medium of conveying many filthy and loathsome diseases from one child to another, and no protection whatever against smallpox. Indeed, I consider we are now living in the JENNERIAN epoch for the slaughter of innocents, and the unthinking portion of the adult population (144).

There have recently been reports of a new vaccine for brain cancer (206) that I am sure you will be hearing more about. The vaccine industry has already made it just about impossible for parents to refuse to have their newborns injected with the hepatitis B vaccine, and vaccine makers are feverishly working to try to make it mandatory for all children to take the Gardasil® vaccine. As if your newborn isn't already overloaded with toxic chemicals from multiple vaccine pricks, look for this "new" brain cancer vaccine to be the next one on the list to be foisted on an unwary public. Only time will tell whether this one will be worth its weight in gold, or just another in a long line of Frankenstein vaccine disasters!

The problem with mercury in vaccines isn't the ONLY problem. It has now been revealed that many vaccines contain dangerous levels of aluminum as well, which has also been linked to ADHD, autism, and Alzheimer's (145). Many parents who had autistic kids were told that their children had abnormally high levels of aluminum in their blood and the parents wanted to know why (144)? In one school alone, "90 percent of the children…had developed ADHD during the course of a single year," and testing revealed that they had "massive" levels of aluminum in their "toxicity profiles" (144). "MASSIVE" levels of aluminum?! "90 percent of the children…" in ONE school? This should have made headline news for weeks until the source was thoroughly investigated and uncovered. How do you think those parents feel? Do you think they look favorably upon vaccines?

• The Pigs & the Swine Flu Fiasco

Remember the H1N1 vaccine fiasco? Millions of those vaccines now have to be discarded because no one wanted them, in spite of the media blitz headed up by the vaccine makers who stood to make millions from them. Americans have had just about enough of slick pharmaceutical profiteers trying to make a fast buck at the expense of their lives and the lives of their children. They are wising up and speaking out. (Of course you could end up on a drug company "hit list" for doing so!)

In an article entitled, "The Swines Behind The Flu Pandemic," one of the companies (Baxter International) designated to produce the H1N1 vaccine came under scrutiny because their "Austrian branch sent batches of what was supposed to be human influenza (H3N2) vaccine to 18 different European countries," countries that were supposed to "use these vaccine samples to produce" H1N1 flu vaccine for "their populations" (138). When the Czech Republic ran some tests on the samples they received, they were discovered "to be contaminated with **live Avian influenza virus** (H5N1 – Bird flu)" (138) [emphasis mine]. Had the Czech Republic used the samples to make their vaccine, the results could have been a global disaster (138), starting with the Czechs.

How did the samples end up with bird flu in them? Well, the U.S. government had given Baxter "stocks of Avian influenza virus...so it could" make a "vaccine against any future outbreaks of this disease" (138). [My, my, how generous of them!] Before even getting the virus, Baxter was supposed to agree to "Biosafety Level 3 strict controls," which apparently they did not live up to (138), because either they were "incredibly careless" and the contamination was "accidental," or [and we shudder to think of this possibility] "the contamination was intentional," and the Czechs were smart enough, or just plain lucky enough to catch the problem before it became a disaster (138)! There may have been some very devout Czechs uttering prayers during the flu season that God heard in a bigger way than any of them would ever know!

How many people are aware that the infamous *Weather Underground* group was infiltrated by a man who said that he sat in on a conversation they were having about their plans on reducing the population of the earth? He said that they were sitting around and casually discussing the elimination of millions of people as though talking about the latest pro-football scores. Believe me when I tell you that the same demons that controlled two-legged animals like Hitler, Mao, Idi Amin, and Stalin are still alive and well. They've just found new victims to possess! These people, who have absolutely no moral regard for the lives of others and think nothing of snuffing out the lives of millions, do not deserve to walk the planet that they so worship.

They want the world's population reduced to what they consider "acceptable levels," as long as THEY are in the group left alive! There is a God who sits on high and be assured that HE never sleeps. He is watching them, listening in on their devilment, biding his time, and when their calamity comes, HE will be laughing at them! *(Psalm 2.)*

• Vaccine Effectiveness?

How effective are all those vaccines being given to children? Well, Dr. Kari Simonsen, a pediatrician at the University Of Nebraska Medical Center stated that "one in five children" will get whooping cough even though they receive the vaccine, yet she still condones the use of the vaccine in spite of this failure rate (134). How many people are aware of the fact that just recently the Japanese "changed the start time for vaccinating from 3 months to two years" and immediately "their SIDS rate" dropped (127)? There was "an 85 to 90 percent reduction in severe cases of damage and death" when their infant vaccinations were delayed (127). How revealing is this? If this were done in the U.S., one cannot help but wonder what type of results we would see and how many cases of autism and other vaccination-induced health disasters would be prevented?

Be aware that I am **not** telling you that you should not take vaccines, pneumonia shots, or flu shots. There are even new vaccines in the making for colon cancer and other cancers. How effective they will be is anybody's guess. There are some new individualized vaccines being produced to boost the body's immunity against cancer and some of those are working miraculously. (I am not speaking of Gardasil®.)

As for taking vaccines for childhood diseases and for the flu, that is a decision **you will have to make and live with.** I am telling you to do the research on vaccinations. Be informed about the health decisions that you make, and be sure that your doctor is informed as well. Read and research everything you can before allowing yourself or your child to be the next guinea pig.

For the sake of your health and your kids, if you DO decide to get vaccinated or let your kids get them, at least INSIST (especially with the polio vaccine) that they only be given "an inactivated (dead) virus vaccine that is cultured in human cells, not monkey kidney cells" (246). Get a copy of the VACCINE SAFETY MANUAL by Neil Z. Miller to find out more about the Hepatitis B vaccine, and see the ten minute video presentation about this vaccine at: *http://www.thinktwice.com/hepB_sho.htm.* You may have to go to their main website first at: *http://www.thinktwice.com/hepb.htm,* then to the movie link. If you watch this video (before the government scrubs it), you will understand that the only reason babies are being put at risk with this dangerous vaccine is because it is a money-maker for the vaccine industry!

• FDA & CDC Denials

There was much hype in a recent news report about the FDA and CDC now assuring the public that there is no connection between autism and vaccines in children. Well, not to worry, all you parents out there, right? The good 'ol FDA has quieted all our fears about autism and vaccines by announcing to the world that there is no evidence that all those little vaccine pricks cause autism. So, now we know! We can get all the vaccines we want and be perfectly safe, right? Seems I recall that the FDA also said Vioxx®, Baycol, Avandia and at least 30 or 40 other drugs were safe too. That was before they collectively maimed or killed thousands of Americans! But NOW we can trust what they say about vaccines, right?

Well, what would YOU say if you were the one responsible for approving mercury in vaccines that may have caused thousands of cases of autism in U.S. Children, or if YOU had stock in the pharmaceutical company that made the vaccines? Would you be hasty to acknowledge that this sad travesty has been committed on not only U.S. children, but in other countries solely because of the greed, indifference, and careless disregard for life by many vaccine makers and the FDA? Would you NOW be ready to admit that you were wrong and thousands of children worldwide are afflicted with a permanently disabling disease, or even death, that YOU caused?

Why then, was mercury allowed into the dental profession and approved as safe by the FDA? Mercury not only poisons the heart, it poisons the brain and eventually, the entire body.

At website: *http://www.health-n-energy.com/ARTICLES/mercfill.htm,* we are reminded that dentists often put "retrograde amalgam fillings...directly into bone," and the question is asked "Would any branch of medicine allow the implantation of Mercury into bone" (200)?

They give some of the symptoms of "long term, low level, Mercury poisoning," one reason it is so dangerous: "Fatigue, short term memory loss, poor concentration…phobic, compulsive behavior… suicidal tendencies… shakes and neuro-motor interference…and a 50% reduction in kidney filtration function after just two months in the mouth (Animal studies)" (200), but it "will bind strongly to Selenium," so is it any wonder that Austrian research shows that people with low levels of selenium are at an increased risk for cancer (200)? Mercury is so deadly that only "1 part per ten million [mercury] will actively destroy the membrane of red blood cells" (200). Indeed, microscopic amounts can kill you!

Perhaps it is the heart that suffers the most from mercury damage. According to Dr. Robert Gammel, this toxin causes hypertension, "tachycardia, arrhythmias, damage to the walls of the small blood vessels…reduction of blood supply to the tissues, which will cause cell damage and death", and in the heart "would be called a heart-attack," while "in the extremities it may be called Reynaud's syndrome" (200). Mercury is "stored principally" in the "fatty tissues," which can elevate "levels of cholesterol" (200). If you have your mercury fillings removed, Dr. Gammel believes this could cause your "cholesterol and triglyceride levels" to drop to normal (200), and the one heavy metal that is discovered to be at the highest "concentration in the brains of Alzheimer's patients" is mercury (200). If you are breast feeding, your baby will get mercury in breast milk (200). Don't even think about getting your amalgam fillings removed unless you go to a dentist who is an expert at doing so and knows the dangers involved!

IV. Our Daily Bread & Bromide – Another Poison Approved by the FDA, but Banned in Europe

Much of the bromide in this country is shipped from Israel and comes from the Dead Sea (72). Bread makers used to add iodine to bread, then they got the "bright" (?) idea of adding a worthless toxic filler called "bromide" instead. And we all know that the FDA believes just a little bit of poison won't hurt you (that's why they approved it, of course!) So, for about 40 years now, U.S. consumers have been eating bread laced with bromide instead of iodine. Iodine is good for you, bromide is toxic. According to an article at *www.ehealing.us/article_iodine3.html*, you won't find bromide in the label of ingredients as "bromide." It is hidden under the name *"Azodicarbonamide"* (72). (How's that for stealth?) Check the list of ingredients on the products you purchase. Be a label reader. These people KNOW what they are doing and they know it is wrong. Why else do they intentionally conceal the names of these deadly chemicals from the general public?

The article states that "the Bromilated vegetable oils in bread...are causing obesity... diabetes, brain disorders... but it is the decrease in thyroid hormone from bromilated flour that is killing our youth...and you" (72), and here's the most shocking part of all – bromide or "azodicarbonamide as a food additive is banned in Australia and in Europe," and they are very serious about not using the product there. So serious in fact, that if you are caught using this disgusting additive in Singapore, you can get "up to 15 years imprisonment and a fine of $450,000" (72). Why? Because they don't want their people eating poison! And we have to ask ourselves exactly WHY is it that this **poisonous substance** is allowed to be shipped to bread dough makers in America and baked into our bread supply, when other countries are sending people to prison for using it?! Think about that for awhile...

V. Ractopamine—Another Poison in the Food Chain Approved by the FDA

I discussed the FDA in my last two books, and those who have read my previous writings know that I make no attempts at hiding my utter contempt for this malevolent body that I believe is responsible for the sickness and death of thousands (if not millions) of U.S. citizens over many decades because of their careless disregard for our well-being, their despicable allowance of toxic drugs, deadly hormones, and other chemicals to be placed into our food supply, and their reluctance at removing killer drugs (like Vioxx®) off the market because of their close and cuddly ties with the pharmaceutical industry!

Well, they have managed once again (not surprisingly) to approve the addition of yet another deadly chemical into our food chain. It is known as **ractopamine,** a "beta agonist" (a bronchodilator), which was tested in mice with asthma and it was discovered that the drug increased their muscle mass (242). Voila! A new boon for the cattle industry, much like putting growth hormones in the milk, meat, and dairy supply! Another drug to make the cows and piglets fatter so the farmers could get more money out of them – more GREED at work! Never mind that it might kill off a few thousand Americans!

Here is how the drug is **marked**:

> **Not for use in humans. Individuals with cardiovascular disease should exercise special caution to avoid exposure. Use protective clothing, impervious gloves, protective eye gear, and a NIOSH-approved dust mask** (242).

Yes! This drug with this warning label has been approved by—YOU GUESSED IT—our venerable U.S. FDA for use in "45 percent of U.S. pigs and 30 percent of ration-fed cattle" (242), so that it can be served up on YOUR dinner table! This livestock drug was **BANNED in 160 countries, but not the good 'ol USA,** whose FDA has deemed that it is safe for human consumption, even though it causes "hyperactivity, muscle breakdown" **and KILLS 10% of the pigs that it is used in!** (242). That should GREATLY help all those kids out there taking drugs for their attention deficit disorders, and all those over sixty baby-boomers that can die faster with muscle atrophy so they won't cause such a strain on the failing Social Security/Medicare system, which is already broke! More poison for the American food supply!

We don't need to import deadly drugs from Mexican cartels, not when we already have the good 'ol FDA watching our backs and hovering over our food supply! Oh, and don't worry if you see a teeny-tiny little label on your next pack of chicken or turkey burger that says "may contain small amounts of **Paylean** or **Optaflexx**" **(yes Thanksgiving will never be the same! They're injecting turkeys too!)**, because those are just other names for Ractopamine, and after all, the FDA says it's safe, right? Course, what they won't tell you is that **"1700 people have been 'poisoned' from eating pigs fed the drugs since 1998"** (242). [Emphasis mine.] But what are 1700 people compared to all the MONEY that the massive agricultural lobby can make by increasing the SIZE of their fat little piglets, turkeys, and cows for American consumers? What's the answer? Vote in a totally NEW Senate and Congress—individuals who really ARE concerned about the welfare of their constituents back home, who will revamp the entire FDA, FTC, CDC, Federal Reserve, or get rid of them entirely, and start from scratch, and in the meantime, pray over your food, be a label reader, and **buy organic** whenever possible!

• Organic Versus Conventional

Is it any wonder, folks, that people are lining up to buy ORGANIC meats and vegetables that are guaranteed to be free of pesticides, hormones, herbicides, and poisons like ractopamine? And what do we see on TV? Lovely little news stories (about how there is no difference between eating organic and conventional food) paid for by—you guessed it—the agricultural food growers, etc., ad nauseaum. Expect no help from the FTC (Federal Trade Commission) either. They are currently doing everything they can to try to make it impossible for vitamin and nutritional health food stores to stay in business, and they are trying to put organic farmers out of business. **Congressman Waxman** has just tried to sneak an anti-vitamin amendment into the *Wall Street Reform Bill*, and it isn't the first time this has been tried. Wouldn't the pharmaceutical industry just LOVE to see that passed? It is no secret that big pharma is opposed to natural substances that heal the body. They are making billions off of man-made chemicals that often make people sicker than they already are. They generate the most profit by a society that is sick and stays sick, not one that is well! I know of a nurse practitioner in conventional medicine who actually tells patients to take natural niacin for their high cholesterol. If the drug industry knew she was doing this, I wonder how long before they would be trying to get her fired?

VI. Antibiotic Overkill

• Amalgams & Antibiotics

Amalgam fillings will cause you to be less responsive to antibiotics. When you grind your teeth, chew gum, smoke a cigarette, drink liquids (especially high acid fruit juices or hot liquids), this releases dangerous mercury vapors into your mouth, and make no mistake about it, this toxic metal is continuously released from amalgam fillings. It has been removed from people's mouth and shown to still be releasing mercury FIFTY years later outside the mouth! How's that for peace of mind?

Also, how many people are aware that the more rounds of antibiotics children are given as they grow up, the greater is their risk for developing cancer?

Think of someone you know who may have been on antibiotics for severe infections for weeks, then developed fungal yeast infections, then found out that they had cancer! Well, at least antibiotics are well named! The word literally means AGAINST life, while the word probiotics means PRO-LIFE. Most antibiotics are made from fungi, and when you think about it, they have something in common with chemo drugs. They do not just kill the harmful bacteria, they also kill out the beneficial bacteria needed in the gut to keep us healthy, much like chemo drugs don't know the difference between the cancer cells and the healthy cells, so they kill both. These beneficial bacterial in our intestines actually produce vitamins (like B12) and other nutrients that keep our immune system healthy. That being said, realize that I am not junking all antibiotics because they have been used (and are still being used) to save lives every day. There are times when you may have an infection that will only respond to antibiotics; however, over-prescribed antibiotic usage has opened a Pandora's Box in this country and overseas as well, the implications of which may not be known for decades! Natural pro-life substances like vitamin C (given intravenously) and iodine, would work just as well (if not better than antibiotics) if doctors would simply start giving them in high enough dosages to do the job.

There are many healthy probiotic supplements on the market. Eating organic yogurt, natto, kefir, Lassi (a type of Indian yogurt), sauerkraut and drinking organic green juices will also help build probiotics in the intestines and alkalize the body. Always use the organic, non-pasteurized when available.

As noted by Dr. Vandana Bhide, newborns have none of this beneficial bacterial in their colon, but the colonies begin to grow soon after they are born. It is interesting that breastfed babies grow less harmful bacteria in their gut than babies who are bottle-fed, perhaps one reason that babies on formula have more problems with colic and diarrhea than breastfed babies (172).

Dr. Mark Sircus recommends a probiotic known as *PRESCRIPT-ASSIST®*, which is said to have 29 probiotics. This formula has been helpful for those with IBS (irritable bowel syndrome). You can find this probiotic at the same website that sells transdermal magnesium and

Nascent iodine: *http://www.magneticclay.com/store/prescript-assist-probiotic.aspx*. Garden of Life® also makes a popular probiotic known as Primal Defense® HSO Probiotic Formula, which contains homeostatic soil organisms. You can find their formula at their website: *http://www.gardenoflife.com*, as well as a variety of other nutritional products. Many health food stores carry their products.

Antibiotics wipe out life-sustaining intestinal flora and cause deadly yeast overgrowth to take their place. Iodine does NOT harm this beneficial flora, and it kills yeast, bacteria, fungus, viruses, molds, and even assists in the removal of dangerous heavy metals from the body at the cellular level—the same heavy metals that make us ill.

• Antibiotics, Asthma, Allergies & Crohn's Disease

New studies are showing that physicians might want to reconsider prescribing antibiotics to tots under a year old, because it can double their risks for getting **asthma** by their seventh birthday. The antibiotics destroy the friendly, beneficial bacteria in the baby's gut, making them more susceptible to not only asthma, but allergies and Crohn's Disease as well, and apparently the broad spectrum antibiotics are the worst offenders (121). One of the studies producing this evidence involved **13,000 children** in Mannitoba (49). Not only that, but researchers found that women who take "oral contraceptives" are twice as likely to develop *Crohn's Disease* (121). Other risk factors for developing Crohn's Disease are being left-handed, having your appendix removed during adulthood and using NSAID drugs (e.g. Ibuprofen, Mobic, Advil, Aleve and others) (121). For another source that sells probiotics to help re-establish the normal flora of the intestines, see website *http://www.crohns.net/Miva/education/articles//Risk_Factors.shtml*.

• Antibiotics, Breast Cancer & Diabetes

Research described in the *Journal of the American Medical Association (JAMA)* revealed that using antibiotics may greatly increase your risk for developing breast cancer; the more times you are on antibiotics, the greater your risk (6). The article indicates that they are not claiming antibiotics cause breast cancer, but consider this: antibiotics often destroy large portions of the beneficial flora of your intestines, the biggest part of your immune system! This leaves you with a depressed immunity, overgrowth of yeasts, and ripe for abnormal cellular growth, unchecked because the immune cells that should be there to kill them off, have been wiped out by the antibiotics.

Authors of the *JAMA* report admitted that women who had been given antibiotic prescriptions over a 17-year-period (at least "25 prescriptions"), had greater than "twice the risk of breast cancer" over women not taking the drugs (6). The studies involved thousands of women (6). Human studies, not mice. If you are suffering from cancer, especially BREAST CANCER, think about how many times recently (or in your past) you or your children have taken multiple rounds of antibiotics.

Dr. Lisa Landymore-Lin wrote about this antibiotic peril in her book: *Poisonous Prescriptions.* She believes antibiotics not only cause asthma, but diabetes as well (132). Antibiotic usage is so rampant in Great Britain that researchers believe "70 percent of the British population have a yeast infection" (132). Of course, this could also account for their high cancer statistics.

• Antibiotics & Bacterial Resistance

Many people die every day in hospitals from infections that they get while they are in the hospital—infections caused by deadly drug-resistant bugs like MRSA and C.difficle, and it seems that the more antiseptics a hospital uses, the more resistant these bugs become. Fortunately, bugs do not build up resistance to iodine. While there are many antiseptics you can use to kill pathogens, some of them kill human tissue as well—iodine does not. Bacteria do not ever adapt to iodine's killing power and build up a resistance to it, which is pretty awesome when you consider all the new, virulent strains of bacteria and viruses we now have as a result of the over usage of antibiotics. This resistance does not happen with iodine, perhaps because it works so rapidly.

MRSA attacks the immune system by releasing a toxin called *phenol-soluble modulin or PSM* (109), a substance that creates an inflammatory condition that causes neutrophils to rush to the site, then "blows the neutrophils up" (109), a horrible booby-trap for the immune system!

CHAPTER 15

Detox Steps – Getting the Toxins Out Safely

****

I. The Purpose of Detox

Remember that detoxifying your body will make you feel worse initially. You are ridding your body of poisons that (unless you have detoxed before) have had many years to accumulate. The older you are, the more poisons have built up in your system. You may experience headaches and skin breakouts where poisons are being eliminated from your body right through the skin.

The type detox program or fast that you choose will be up to you, your own strength, and how you feel that the Lord is leading you. Pray and seek the Lord before ever beginning any fast or detox program, and never break a detox or fast of several days immediately. You should gradually begin to introduce more and more solids into the diet, even if you stay with raw foods only. If you begin adding cooked foods, do it slowly, beginning with one meal a day, such as cream of rice with fruit and toasted gluten-free rye bread for breakfast, or a large baked potato for lunch, or items such as organic, poached eggs (unless you are going completely vegan), steamed broccoli, or stewed tomatoes for supper. If you are using cooked foods, you may want to begin eating organic rye breads (great for help in lowering high blood pressure).

Many people who have been on raw food only diets report having a return of their old problems when they begin incorporating cooked meals back into their diet. Do not use gluten cereals if you have allergies to gluten. Be sure to get gluten-free breads. Don't eat organic eggs if you are allergic to eggs. If you have to fight seasonal allergies, consider taking bee pollen capsules, if you are not allergic to bee products. Many people have excellent results with them. I discuss a case in my last book of a physician who cured himself of allergies by taking several capsules of bee pollen daily. Some health food stores even provide bee pollen that is gathered from your local area.

II. Where To Start—Healthy Tips

There are no *quick-fixes* for optimal health, but the very first thing that you need to do is to purchase a good quality **juicer**! By the time you've gotten this far in this book, you should have a pretty good idea which juicer you are going to use (if you don't already have one). Once you've done that, you are ready to begin. You can also begin by taking green powdered drinks before you even get a juicer. See further in this chapter for a sample of various detox programs you may wish to choose. Just be sure to check with your licensed health care provider first, since it does involve fasting. It is not set in stone. You can try the 3 day, 7 day, 21, day or longer program, as you feel led. Always pray first, seeking God's will for you.

III. Nutrient Supplements—Why Do We Need Them?

Most people do not get the amount of vitamins and minerals that they need in their daily diet, especially in this fast-paced society in which we live. You should consider taking a potent multi-vitamin/mineral supplement daily, such as the *OLA LOA®* varieties, found in health food stores, or a mineral drink, such as *Mineral Rich®*, marketed by Maureen Kennedy Salaman. You can find *Mineral Rich®* at her website *www.mksalaman.com*. It is a form of minerals in a good tasting, easily absorbable liquid. Some natural health food stores also carry *Mineral Rich®* and *OLA LOA®*. Do not take grape-seed extracts at the same time that you take Vitamin C. Research suggests that taking them at the same time may raise blood pressure in some individuals.

• Vitamin-Mineral-Herbal Supplement Choices

There are many available choices on the market for vitamin-mineral-herbs and other health ingredients. Many mushroom (and other nutrient) supplements can be found at *www.newchapter.info*. Their supplements are marketed under the brand name Mycomedicinals® or

New Chapter®. Life Extension website (*www.lef.org*) advertises pharmaceutical grade supplements. So does *Usana®* Health at website: *http://www.usana.com,* and Dee Simmons at *www.ultimateliving.com.* (Some of these brands may cost more, but claim to provide you with a pharmaceutical grade product, higher in quality, and often without the unwanted additives found in other brands.) There are also mushroom supplements available at *http://www.advancedbionutritionals.com/immunity* and from *http://www.medicinalmushrooms.net/index.html.* Also, see *http://www.Agaricusfarm.com/index.html* and *http://www.herbalremedies.com,* as well as health supplements at *www.swansonvitamins.com, wwwpuritan.com,* and other websites mentioned in several chapters of this book. (See *Appendix II* at the back of this book.)

Website *http://www.discount-vitamins-herbs.net,* has discount prices, great nutritional information, and a large variety of supplements. You can even buy your own home mushroom growing kits at some websites such as: *http://www.fungi.com/kits/index.html.* There are also places where you can buy vitamins and mineral supplements in bulk, free of additives. Try to avoid supplements which contain undesirable additives like magnesium stearate and titanium dioxide.

IV. Detoxification

Each day you should be drinking (depending on your size) about six to eight (8 ounce) glasses of water per day, unless your physician has you on a special water-restricted diet. There are many ways to detox. You can try drinking only fresh juices for several days, but the key is to remember that you also need plenty of water, whichever detox program you choose. If you have diabetes or other chronic diseases, blood disorders, are pregnant or breast-feeding, or are taking prescription medications, do not attempt to detox (or any type of fasting program) without first consulting with your physician. You should also be praying about it, seeking spiritual guidance.

If you cannot get fruit in season, you can always substitute FROZEN fruit, but do not use canned fruit. Be certain that the water (and ice cubes) you are using does not contain chlorine or fluoride. When drinking the juices, sip them slowly. Always use **organic** produce when possible. It is best to drink most fresh juices within ten minutes of the time that they are juiced. Don't let fresh wheat grass juice sit overnight. Obviously, this won't always be feasible. You can always resort to the powdered green drinks, which I use a lot, along with the little green chlorella pills that you can carry anywhere.

Fresh carrot juice should not be saved longer than two or three days in the refrigerator. Remember, each day that passes, nutrients and enzymes oxidize out of the juice. For those who are already ill, you may need to rely on family members to help with your juicing until you are stronger. Of course, anyone who is severely ill needs to consult with their physician before beginning a new health regimen. Many times, those who are severely ill cannot tolerate fasting and strict detox regimens. They need extra calories, rather than fewer, but fresh juices are excellent for them.

You are flushing out your system, so you will need extra water every day during detox. (You will not be doing strenuous exercise during a detox program. Mild exercise is fine.) I believe that if dietitians would provide organic, fresh-juiced vegetables and fruits to senior citizens at nursing facilities and assisted-living centers, it would greatly improve the health and vitality of our seniors, and what would it do for hospital patients and new moms?

• Getting Started

As always, you will check with your physician before beginning a detox, fasting program, such as the one below. This is just a sample detox that you can follow to cleanse the body. You will also be spending daily time in prayer, seeking God's will and guidance, and presenting your requests before him at this time. Note that the first three days involve water only, except the use of Essiac Tea. Every day of this cleanse, if you already have cancer, you will drink 2 ounces of Essiac upon arising and 2 ounces before retiring for the night. Even if you do not have cancer, feel free to drink the Essiac. (See Chapter 12.)

Do not mix Essiac with anything else. Take it on an empty stomach. Always wait one hour before you ingest Essiac and one hour afterwards before ingesting anything else. Follow the directions on the brand you choose. Day 4 through 7, you are drinking (or eating) fresh grapes or juice. You can choose purple, red, green, or black grapes, or mix them to your taste. Remember to also be drinking water during this detox program. Don't forget to get ten to twenty minutes of fresh air and sunshine in your routine (at least 3 days per week) during this time if you are Caucasian. Darker-skinned individuals need more sunlight. (See earlier precautions if you or a family member has a history of melanoma.) Note that some of this material is also found in Chapters 11 and 12, and a portion of it is also found in my last book, *Gentle Cures for Tough Cancers* in Chapter 35.

• Seven Day Detox Program

Day 1 through Day 3:
Water, at least 7 - 8 glasses per day (8 ounce glasses), if you are not on a water-restricted diet. Do not use water or ice cubes that have chlorine or fluoride. If you already have cancer, drink 2 oz of Essiac tea (as instructed and prepared on the brand you choose) when you first arise in the morning, and 2 oz of the tea on retiring. Be sure to spend time praising God, and in Bible study (e.g., 15-30 min in the am and 15-30 min in the pm) as you are able. Always praise him FIRST, then present your requests before him.

Day 4 through Day 7:
- Essiac tea, 2 oz on arising
- An hour later, drink 6 oz of fresh organic grape juice from your juicer, or you can eat a handful of fresh organic grapes, whichever you prefer (when eating seeded grapes, chew them into tiny bits.) Choose mostly the purple, red, and black grapes. The green grapes are okay, but only occasionally. Try to avoid bitterly sour grapes, and stick to sweeter varieties. (Purple concord grapes and muscadines are great if you can get them organic and in season!) Remember when you juice grapes, you will juice seeds and all. When you eat grapes, eat the seeds and skin.
- Two hours later, you will again drink the grape juice or eat the grapes. You will do this every two hours on day four through day seven, until one hour before bedtime. Drink water as desired.
- At bedtime, again take 2 oz of the Essiac preparation. (Your hours may vary from day to day, depending on when you go to bed at night, and when you rise in the morning.) You may find yourself taking Essiac at 6 or 7 one morning, then at 8 the next. Just be sure that you eat or drink nothing within one hour of taking the Essiac. Remember that ALL your juices should be organic and

fresh-squeezed that you juice yourself, or a family member juices for you. By the end of day 7, you should be well on your way to detox and alkalinity.

• 3 Day Apple Cider Vinegar Detox – Rapid Alkalizer

Mix one teaspoon of apple cider vinegar in 8 ounces of fresh water and drink four to six times each day for three days, adding additional glasses of water during the day as desired. Never under any circumstances should you use water or ice cubes that contains chlorine or fluoride with this program. Doing so will just poison your body! And remember that every time you get a hot shower or bath, or drink a glass of chlorinated water, or clean with chlorine bleach, you lose valuable iodine from your body. If you mop your floors with chlorine water, then walk on them barefoot, some of the chlorine will evaporate, but you will also absorb some through your feet before it all evaporates. So will your kids and pets.

• Lemons & Limes

Though lemons and limes are very acidic, they have an amazing alkaline effect on the body (298). Concerned about yeast infections? Drink plenty of homemade lemonade without sugar. Use a natural herbal sweetener like Stevia instead or a small amount of soda bicarb to remove the tartness. Below is a rapid alkalizer for the body using lemons and/or limes:

(A.) 7 Day Lemonade Detox

Use fresh-squeezed lemon juice (and/or lime juice) diluted in water to concentration of your taste. Use a natural herbal sweetener, such as Stevia®, for sweetening, as desired. Drink as often as you like with extra water as desired for seven days. This is a rapid alkalizer and detox. Use a mineral supplement such as *Ola Loa®* or *Mineral Rich®* once or twice daily on this fast as with any fast you embark on. Remember to discontinue any fast such as this one GRADUALLY.

(B.) 10 Day Lemonade Detox

Lemonade Diet by Stanley Burroughs: Mix 2 tablespoons of fresh-squeezed lemon juice, 2 tablespoons of maple syrup and 1/8 tspn cayenne pepper into 8 oz of water. Drink as often as needed to maintain energy. Follow for a ten day period, but eat and drink nothing else (167). Note that you may wish to try this detox for 3 days and take a break to see how your body responds before doing the full 10 day program.

• Seaweed for Detox & Cancer

Seaweed (sea grass) is consumed in large amounts in Asian countries, but Americans rarely touch it. It is an excellent natural source of iodine. There are many different types of seaweed. If you like eating at sushi bars, you may find your sushi covered with seaweed (254). There is also *brown* alga (or seaweed), including: *kelp, wakame, arame, kombu,* and a red seaweed known as *nori*. Research has shown that there are ingredients in seaweed that may inhibit cancer formation (254). Scientists believe that these substances prevent cancer by boosting the immune system, and that they can help prevent and halt the progression of abnormal cells, lower bad cholesterol levels, and act like magnets, pulling many dangerous heavy metals out of the body (254). Restaurants often put wakame in their salads (254). (Fixing sushi involves raw fish. I never recommend raw fish to anyone.)

Algins like *kelp, dulse (seaweeds), and algaes such as chlorella* are very important in not only removing heavy metals from the body, but taking out dangerous radioactive substances as well. They will also keep your cells from *absorbing radioactive materials*, poisons like *strontium-90* (183). The seriousness of absorbing strontium-90 is that it links up with calcium and will often build up in calcium-rich foods like dairy products and *green leafy vegetables,* where the strontium-90 goes right into "the bones where it damages bone marrow" (183). A seaweed that will keep your body from absorbing strontium-90* is KELP (183). (*Not the same as the mineral, strontium, needed for bone health.)

Researchers conducted a study which revealed that kelp could not only be used as a breast cancer preventative, but it halted the spread of tumors (in animal testing), putting more than half of them into remission (262). It is believed that a chemical in kelp, known as *fucoidan*, contributes to its cancer-preventative effects, but seaweed also has very powerful *antibiotic* effects, which means it may help fight cancerous colon cells as well (262). You can now get fucoidan supplements at health food stores and on the internet.

As described by J. E. O'Brien, author of *The Miracle of Garlic & Vinegar*, research done at the University of Hawaii School of Medicine revealed that "a dried version of...wakame" when *injected* into test animals, helped cure their **lung cancers** (262). Scientists have shown that an ingredient in seaweed has blood pressure lowering effects. It appears to work like an "antidote to excess sodium consumption..." [even though it is high in salt, which is rather strange] and could be important in warding off *strokes* (262). (Check with your doctor before supplementing with seaweed products, especially if you have a chronic condition.)

• Cancer-Fighting Soda-Bicarb Recipe

This is from *Dr. Jim*, the *Country Doctor* who says it will cure just about any cancer:

> Add one part baking soda with three parts maple syrup in a small saucepan. Stir briskly. Heat for five minutes. Take one teaspoon daily, as needed. Be sure you use ALUMINUM FREE baking soda and 100% maple syrup (no synthetics). Use organic syrup (obtain from your health food store) (377a). [Do not use an aluminum pan.]

Note that this formula can be varied. It can be heated just until it foams. You can substitute organic blackstrap molasses or honey for the maple syrup, and if so, you may not necessarily need to heat them. This per Dr. Mark Sircus in his book, *Sodium Bicarbonate Rich Man's Poor Man's Cancer Treatment* (288). *Arm & Hammer®* claims that their soda bicarb is aluminum-free. (Organic honey is useful for those with nausea and vomiting who need extra calories; however, do not give it to children under two without their physician's approval, or to diabetics.)

• Soda-Bicarb Protocol Used to Cure Spreading Prostate Cancer

When Vernon J. ("Vito") was diagnosed with prostate cancer that had gone into his bones, and he was basically sent home to die, he began using a soda bicarb, blackstrap molasses recipe to rapidly alkalize his body (110). Before this patient began using the soda bicarb, he had been treated with *Finasteride*, a drug given for reducing prostate enlargement, and *Casodex*, a drug that treats prostate cancer by reducing levels of testosterone (288).

[The drugs did nothing to stop his cancer.] He cured himself within just **11 days** using oral soda bicarb, which he mixed with blackstrap molasses, as described in detail below:

- **Day 1 through day 4:** he added one teaspoon of soda bicarb and one teaspoon of blackstrap molasses to 8 ounces of water and drank the solution (at room temperature) once a day (288).
- **Day 5**: he began taking 2 teaspoons each of the soda bicarb and the molasses in 8 ounces of water twice a day;
- **Day 6 and 7**: same as day 5 and using pH testing paper to check his urine and saliva.
- **Day 8 and 9**: he drank the same mixture 3 times a day. [This is a lot of salt!]
- **Day 10**: he used the same mixture, but took it only twice a day.
- **Day 11**: he used one-and-a-half teaspoons each of the soda bicarb and the blackstrap molasses in 8 ounces of water twice a day.
- **Day 12**: a bone scan was done. Results were mailed to him and showed that he had no trace of cancer anywhere. He did experience night sweats, some loose stools, and headaches during the process, and said afterwards that he probably should have added some potassium to his diet (110) (288).

I would not recommend this protocol unless you were also taking potassium and magnesium supplements each day, and (as stated earlier) this mixture (especially on days 6 through 10) is very high in sodium. If you are already fighting illness and on a salt-restricted or water-restricted diet, always check with your physician. I am sure individual results would vary depending on your body weight, the rest of your diet, and your overall health to begin with, including the health of your kidneys!

On his website at: *http://www.phkillscancer.com/home,* Vernon also lists some of the vitamins and minerals he was taking during this time. As noted in Chapters 1 and 2, my family member used a modified-version of this formula, but did not take the soda bicarb in such high doses. He was able to reach a high urine pH for several days on a lighter dose and he was taking potassium, though his cancer was unaffected. This was right before he began using the three nutritional formulas that I developed. (See Chapter 2 for exact recipes.)

Eating a lot of cooked foods, meat, or dairy would skew the results of this type of protocol. Vernon's goal was to get his urine and saliva pH at 8.0 or above for 4 or 5 days in a row and, apparently, he accomplished this. Other people could probably get their urine pH up to 8 and keep it there for the same amount of time with a lower amount of the soda bicarb, or by using lemon juice and/or apple cider vinegar (without all that salt). Everyone is different. You would need to adjust accordingly, based on your weight and age and individual tolerance. If you take vitamin C in the form of ascorbic acid in large amounts, it will make your urine acidic and skew the pH readings. You can get the little pH testing strips at most health food stores.

Also, realize that most conventional doctors won't agree to this regimen. You would need the guidance and second opinion of a Naturopathic physician. If you are already fighting illness and on a salt-restricted or water-restricted diet, you should be using great caution and checking with your physician. Vernon did not say what else he was consuming during the day, if anything. I would hope that he was also drinking lots of water to keep his body flushed from all the salt intake.

Remember, if you are fasting, you MUST go off any fast gradually. You cannot immediately begin eating solid and cooked foods in large amounts. It must be gradual, or you can end up in severe distress. You cannot break several days of fasting in ONE day, then immediately go back to eating cooked foods and a regular diet! Your entire digestive system slows down and takes a rest while on a detox program. You don't want to shock your system by immediately going back to a full calorie load. If you already have cancer, you may wish to keep taking the Essiac every day and long after you have healed your immune system. Read the cancer-specific chapter in my last book (*Gentle Cures for Tough Cancers*) for the type cancer you have to see what other supplements you may find helpful.

Also, see Dr. Sircus' book, *Iodine Bringing Back the Universal Medicine,* on the importance of iodine in fighting yeast, bacteria, malaria, flu, and other specific ailments caused by a deficiency in this critical mineral (287), and killing cancer in the process! You can find a food-grade, gentle form of superior iodine called *Magnascent©* at *http://www.magnascent.com.* See Appendix II.

V. Music for the Muted Soul

Music has often been called the universal language. Many people do not realize that music affects not only the body, but the mind, the soul, and the spirit as well. Scientific experiments have been done showing that flowers and animals flourish when they are exposed to long hours of classical music, but shrivel up and die when exposed to long hours of heavy-metal rock music. Why would humans think that they are any different? Why would anyone think that they can subject their body to hours of incessant, deafening cadence and loud rhythmic beats and believe it is good for them? Many teens who thought boom-boxes were *totally rad* twenty years ago, are now having psychological, emotional, and hearing problems! Some cancer treatment centers are using not only music, but comedy, aroma, and color therapy for stress reduction, relaxation, and immune boosting. Just be aware of exactly what you are inhaling when you use aroma therapy.

CHAPTER 16

The Greatest Help of All – Divine Intervention

****

I. Prayer Should Never Be A Last Resort!

Though this chapter regarding prayer is the last chapter in the book, it is the most important chapter, because prayer should be your FIRST response when you are facing any type of illness. Make a covenant with God to spend time every day praising him, not just at the worship service you attend. Search out the many healing verses in the Bible. Memorize them—claim them—and remember that God has also promised that: *"If ye abide in me, and my words abide in you, ye shall ask what ye will, and it shall be done unto you."* (John 15:7.) God operates on faith. Your own words can determine your destiny. If you get up in the morning declaring verbally that everything will go wrong, it probably will! If you start declaring positive outcomes for each day (and for your health), God will honor your faith and move mountains for you. Take healing verses from the Bible, write them down and recite them OUT LOUD every morning when you arise and during your day. Don't wait until you are sick and facing death to develop a prayer life!

One of the best books I have ever read on how to put your faith into action is by Darlene Bishop, *Your Life Follows Your Words.* You can find her book at her website *www.darlenebishop.org.* She was miraculously healed of breast cancer and has a tremendous testimony. Just be aware that I do not advocate avoiding medical care for yourself or your children; however, it is also true that I am not an advocate of chemotherapy and radiation, and those drugs that actually have worse side effects than the treatments that they were originally intended for. On the other hand, there are miracle drugs that many people cannot live without—medications like insulin for example—that save so many lives. I have heard horror stories of so-called "believers," who have children with newly-diagnosed diabetes, refusing to get help for them and letting their children die. This is totally absurd. It is murder!

Realize too that prayer and worship are alkalizing to the body. If you do not know God and have never had a personal relationship with the Lord Jesus Christ, the most important prayer you will ever pray is the one found in **Appendix I** at the end of this chapter.

You may already be struggling against an illness, or perhaps you just want to stay well. Our physical bodies were created by a mighty King—the Creator and King of the Universe. If you are seriously ill, you should be consulting your Creator in prayer for your recovery. If you are going to consult your Creator for your healing, where do you start? Do you know who your Creator is? Do you know God? Do you know what he has said about you and about himself? Not only did he give you life, but he gave you the right kind of food that you need for your body to sustain itself in the very best mode of operation possible! If you want your car to perform at maximum capacity, you feed it quality fuel. Start putting garbage into the gas tank and the car will sputter and die, yet this is what we sometimes do to our bodies without even realizing it. Our bodies are composed not just of flesh and blood, but soul and spirit as well. Many people are struggling to maintain their health, but they have never consulted the Bible to see what God has said about health and healing.

You may be fighting a deadly disease and find an alternative approach in this book that could prolong or save your life, but even if you do, you are not going to live forever in the body you are now in. You will merely prolong the life God himself has been gracious enough to give you! Eventually, somewhere down the road, if Jesus delays his return, you will die just like your ancestors did, just like the rest of humanity. Jesus himself asked, *"For what is a man profited, if he shall gain the whole world, and lose his own soul?" (Matt: 16:26.)* It is your soul that makes you **YOU**. All your dreams, aspirations, desires, loves, dislikes, fears, emotions, and memories make up your soul. It is what makes you unique! There is only ONE of you and there will never be another person to cross this earth again exactly like YOU. You truly are special and unique. However, even if you pray for healing and you are healed, unless you have accepted God's provision for your soul, you would be better off had you never been born! God told us in the Bible that one day our own words will save us or condemn us *(Matt 12:37)*, and that he is a **great King**! *(Mal. 1:14.)* He rules a vast domain far beyond anything you or I could possibly imagine. His throne is encompassed with splendor, honor, majesty, beauty, justice, wisdom, and glory unimaginable by mortal men.

We are told in *THE REVELATION of Jesus Christ to St. John* that a rainbow encircles God's throne, and that out of his throne proceeds thunder, lightning and voices. John, the apostle, was caught up into heaven in *REVELATION* Chapter Four and saw God's great throne. This mighty Sovereign King created everything, including you, and everything that you have. Angelic beings with a splendor brighter than the sun worship and bow before him. He made you, your loved ones, your children, the world you live in and the food that you eat every day, in spite of what you may have been told, or what you believe about coming from a tadpole or a monkey.

Darwin himself knows by now that God exists, but it is too late for him; **don't let it be too late for you!** As long as you still have breath in you, it is not too late. Don't be afraid to talk to someone who is comatose about their soul. It is believed that hearing is the last sense to go. God is totally just and totally holy. When sin entered the world through Adam and Eve's transgression, there was no way that a holy God could justify man and be just himself, unless—and there's the catch. There was a way—only **one way for God to do it**. Man could only be redeemed by someone who had never transgressed the laws of God—someone completely perfect, totally pure, blameless, and willing to take our place. God himself was the only one qualified. He had to pay the price for our transgression, because of the total justice that he demands. He incarnated his only Son into the body of the young virgin Mary, producing Immanuel, God in the flesh, Christ Jesus our Messiah.

Jesus was born with **God's blood in him** because he was and is God. Not Mary's blood, not Joseph's blood, but God's blood. Pure, immortal blood! God arranged it so that the BLOODLINE can only come from the FATHER and that the baby's blood within the womb does not mix with the mother's blood! This is why Mary's blood could never save you! Jesus had his FATHER's blood and his father is GOD! You see, Jesus could never die as long as his blood coursed through his veins and arteries! He had sinless, immortal **LIFE** in his blood! He was and is **God in the flesh**. When he was crucified by the Romans, they had no idea that the only way Jesus could die was for all of his blood to be drained from his body. As long as his eternal, sinless blood kept coursing through that beating heart, and that last beat ended, he could not die. Only after his precious blood had been drained from his body through the crucifixion, did he expire. You can see the awful representation of that in the movie, *The Passion,* released a few years ago. That same blood is physical, spiritual, immortal, and pure! When you turn from your sins (repent) and accept Jesus' sacrifice on your behalf, a spiritual *circumcision* takes place between your body and your soul. Your sins are forever cut loose from your soul. The blood of the Lamb of God is applied to your body, soul, and spirit. When you die, you are free to join God in heaven, your soul forever free from the sins that Jesus himself paid for. You are justified by the blood of the Lamb. If you never repent and turn from sin, and do not accept God's free gift of pardon, when you die your sins are still attached to your soul. God is holy, perfect and just. He cannot allow sin into his presence. Your soul is forever consigned to hell—a place of the **lost**—a place where your sins are a permanent part of your eternal soul. A place you will NEVER escape from, a never-ending prison of unimaginable horror and permanent separation from God. You will never hear the sound of beautiful music again, the rich nature sounds of a waterfall, birds singing, or the laughter of a baby.

Your soul never dies, neither do you! You may look different at sixty than you did at fifteen, but inside you don't feel any different. (Apart from a few aches and pains, maybe!) Ever wonder why? It is because your soul never ages. Go ahead—pay for it yourself, if you like. Don't you know—that's what all those other "religions" are doing out there? They are trying to pay their own way without JESUS. The Buddhists think Buddha will save them, but Buddha did not have immortal blood and he wasn't resurrected! Neither were any of the other prophets of the world's major religions. Their bones are still in the grave awaiting the great resurrection, some to eternal life and some to eternal damnation. Jesus' bones were never found! That's because all those other "gods" out there are still in the GRAVE! Jesus is alive today because he is the only one that was resurrected. He had immortal blood. Your blood is stained with Adam's sin. You have the wrong blood. When a sick person is in the hospital, that's exactly what they do every single day – check out the BLOOD. It's because there is something wrong with the blood! You need a blood transfusion and you get it by faith. Not faith in something, but faith in SOMEONE! You need a Savior with **pure, immortal** blood! Nothing else can ever save you! Forget about praying to statues, dead saints, exalted humans, and false prophets. Only the Lord Jesus Christ can save you. He had the right kind of blood! No one else does! Of all the billions of people that have crossed this planet down through the ages, only Jesus himself had the RIGHT kind of blood to save humanity! Are you trying to get into heaven without going through Jesus? If you are, then God says you are a thief and a robber. And if this sounds narrow-minded to you, I didn't say it, Jesus did, so take it up with him when you see him! John 10:1-4: *Verily, verily, I say unto you, He that entereth not by the door into the sheepfold, but* **climbeth up some other way, the same is a thief and a robber.** *But he that entereth in by the door is the shepherd of the sheep. To him the porter openeth; and the sheep hear his voice: and he calleth his own sheep by name, and leadeth them out. And when he putteth forth his own sheep, he goeth before them, and the sheep follow him: for they know his voice...* So, WHAT *door* are you going through to get to heaven? Are you trusting in your religion, your prayers, statues, some other prophet, your priest, a dead saint, an icon, your church, an angelic vision, a sacrament, your own good works to get you through that door? According to God himself, there is only one way and one door, and it is through the Lord Jesus Christ, no exceptions! See Appendix I.

II. Health & Healing From God

God sometimes heals instantly—other times—he heals gradually, but either way, he expects you to cooperate with him in your healing. If you are praying to him to heal you of some disease, such as cancer, you need to be doing your part. If God has healed you and you go back to eating fast-food burgers and fries every day and living a very unhealthy lifestyle, don't expect to maintain your good health. You have to do your part in staying healthy. Praise God that he has more compassion on us than we sometimes have on each other. He is very forgiving, but he requires accountability and responsibility on our part. If you want healthy kids, feed them a healthy diet. Reach them with good nutrition while they are small, so it will stick when they are adults. I made the mistake of researching alternative health and nutrition when my child was already a teenager. Try to convince a teen to eat a nutritious diet! They already know everything, right? So you are wasting your time.

God has already provided for us exactly the type food that we need in the most natural, nutritious forms possible. There is an old expression which states that we spend the first half of our lives acquiring wealth and the second half using our wealth to regain our health! How many of us have spent twenty or more years living on "dead foods," only to wind up complaining that we are beset with arthritis, gout, diabetes, high blood pressure, fatigue, coronary artery disease, poor circulation and migraine headaches, yet we continue to live this way and wonder why we cannot get well.

Only **live** food has the **enzymes** already within it that enables you to digest it. If you take a raw vegetable, like an onion, with the roots still attached and put it in the ground, it will sprout and live. Cook it, then put it in the ground and it will rot. Why? Because, once cooked, you have destroyed all the life in the vegetable and it is dead. It no longer has within it the living enzymes needed for the body to digest it. Thus, your body will have to produce the enzymes to digest it—a taxing process on your entire digestive system. Not only that, cooked food moves through the bowels sluggishly, fermenting on the way. Raw food moves through the bowels much quicker, its roughage acting as a broom to sweep out the colon along the way. If you are eating cooked foods, always combine your meals with raw, fresh vegetables, but eat fresh fruits on an empty stomach only. Do not combine them with other foods.

III. Being Prepared

If you have a young child or other family member or friend who is fighting a terminal illness, obtain some CD and/or DVD praise songs and play them at your relative's bedside 24 hours a day. During sleep time, turn the volume down if the music keeps them awake. The WORD of God is so powerful. You may wish to get a CD of the Bible that is being read aloud and play it at your sick relative's bedside. Immerse them in the Word of God. Remember to proclaim these same verses over your loved one throughout the day. You can also claim *Psalm 118:17* for them. Get several family members and friends together. Go to your child's (or friend's) hospital room. Form a circle around the bed, join hands, and pray for them. Lay hands on them. Anoint them with oil (use olive oil or some other type of edible oil that is fresh and not rancid). Then raise both arms and begin to praise God over the one who is ill. Praise music will clear evil spirits out of an area in a hurry! Evil spirits do NOT like worship music, especially songs elevating the Blood of Jesus. Sing to God and praise him at your child's bedside, and most importantly—if they are old enough to learn and well enough that they can participate—teach your children to praise the Lord!

IV. Final Steps

You can follow every guideline in this book and help your body stay well and recover from serious illness, but it won't do a bit of good if your soul is still stained with sin. If you have terminal cancer, and you are not healed, you will be meeting God face-to-face in the very near future. Think about that. Are you ready? None of us are promised tomorrow, even if we are strong and healthy. This chapter will prepare you to meet God tomorrow or twenty years from now. Simply bow your head where you are—tell God that you are sorry for your sins and that you repent (forsake your sins and determine to leave them behind you)—change of heart, change of attitude—tell him that you are turning your life over to him and turning against sin. We are told in his word: *"That if thou shalt confess with thy mouth the Lord Jesus, and shalt believe in thine heart that God hath raised him from the dead, thou shalt be saved."* (Romans 10:9-10.) For a sample of a prayer that you can pray, see **Appendix I** at the end of this chapter.

You should be willing to tell others that you are a new Christian, confessing it with your mouth as God requires. Find a spirit-filled local Bible-believing church to join, be willing to follow the Lord's example in baptism, and begin growing in faith by reading your Bible every single day. It is your lifeline to the future! As a Christian, you can claim the Blood of Jesus over your mind, spirit, soul, and body for divine protection, instruction, and wisdom, and you need to be under the guidance of a shepherd (or pastor) of a local Bible-believing Church.

Are you bitter with God because you have lost someone that you deeply love? Consider this. When Jesus came to earth as a tiny infant, totally dependent on the care of Mary and Joseph, imagine the overwhelming love that God felt for his Son as that tiny baby, then watching him grow day-by-day, just as you do your own children. Right up until that fateful day when heaven stormed over as Jesus hung on the cross for the sins of the world. Imagine the heartbreak of God the Father when he watched everything that Jesus went through in order to become the world's sin offering. His heavenly Father went through the same sorrow and heartache that you have faced in losing a loved one, only magnified a trillion+ times! You haven't suffered any tears or pain that he himself has not already endured.

It amazes me how many people who claim to be *Christians* never darken the door of their local church; never give a dime to help the needy; balk at the thought of tithing their income; would rather die than fast for one meal; watch T.V. for two or more hours a day (then claim that they haven't time for prayer or for church); cringe at the thought of any sort of open expression of praise and worship to God; then come and ask **you** to pray for them because they need healing, all the while expecting God to give them a miracle and heal them when they haven't obeyed a single thing that Jesus commanded of them! Remember, God knows that we are far from perfect. He knows the framework of our bodies—that we are just clay—but he also knows what we are capable of. As his creation, we are to worship God with all of our hearts and with our lives. His Word tells us that *"Whoso offereth praise glorifieth me"* (Ps. 50:23). I am not telling you that you need to be interrupting people around you where you work at and singing out worship songs during an inappropriate time where your employer is paying you to do a certain job. There is a time and place for everything, but we are also to worship God with our thoughts. What's on your mind during your free time? Do you want peace of mind? Try worshipping God with your thoughts. Exalt him, think about him, memorize his words and think on them, for he promises: *"Thou wilt keep him in perfect peace, whose mind is stayed on Thee: because he trusteth in thee"* (Isa 26:3). Try renting nature movies, just so you can admire God's great creation. **Keep your mind on God and you won't lose it!** Did you know that if you are depressed, Isaiah 61:3, says that you can actually lift DEPRESSION by putting on the "garment of praise!" Been depressed lately? Start PRAISING GOD! Are your children depressed? Teach them to PRAISE and worship God! You may argue that you have no idea HOW to worship God. Well, here is a good way to get started—take Bible verses exalting God and memorize them by SINGING them. Verses like: *O give thanks unto the Lord; for he is good; because his mercy endureth forever.* (Ps 118:1.) Or, if you would rather, just pick a psalm, such as Psalm 149, and memorize it. It is only nine verses—or Psalm 150—which is only six verses. There is even a promise from God you can claim when you are worshipping him. It is Psalm 37:4: *"Delight thyself also in the Lord; and he shall give thee the desires of thine heart."*

Worship is so powerful that God actually used praise and worship to win a battle for him in the Old Testament: II Chronicles 20:17-22. It reveals the story of Jehoshaphat who was concerned about being surrounded by powerful enemies that he felt were going to overwhelm him and his small army. God revealed through one of his prophets that he himself would fight the battle. Jehoshaphat **"appointed singers unto the LORD, that they should praise the beauty of holiness, as they went before the army, and to say, Praise the LORD; for his mercy endureth forever."** When these praisers began singing and praising, their enemies were soundly defeated, yet Jehoshaphat and his army never lifted one finger against them—just their voices and musical instruments were all that was needed, and God did the fighting. Notice that they used SCRIPTURE to praise God. What do you think would happen if our modern army had enough faith to try this approach? Pure hatred for the name of Jesus is rapidly growing in a godless world, just as he predicted for the last days before his return. Just try walking down any public street in Saudi Arabia or Iran with a Bible under your arm and see where it gets you.

What you choose to do with the information in this book you have just read is up to you. If you are fighting a terminal illness, pray Psalm 119:17 every day: *"Deal bountifully with thy servant, that I may live, and keep thy word,"* and declare Psalm 118:17 BOLDLY every day: *"I shall not die, but live, and declare the works of the Lord."* Take these verses, type and print them off on your PC, and tape them on your mirror so that you can memorize them and repeat them when you get up in the morning. Declare them or sing them throughout the day all day long! Verbally declare Jesus as your HEALER!

APPENDIX I

Below is a sample prayer that you can pray asking Jesus to come into your life. As you pray this prayer, God knows your heart and he can tell how sincere you are. As you say the words—mean them. When you finish, sign your name at the bottom and put the date. (You will always REMEMBER this date as the most important of your life—because it is the day that you were BORN AGAIN!)

Prayer:

Dear Jesus: I am a sinner. I realize that I can do nothing to save myself and that you have done everything necessary for me to be saved. I am willing to put my trust for eternal life in you alone. I have broken your holy commandments. I am guilty and deserving of your wrath, but I am trusting your holy WORD where you have said in Romans 10:9 *"That if thou shalt confess with thy mouth the Lord Jesus, and shalt believe in thine heart that God hath raised him from the dead, thou shalt be saved."* I am confessing you now as my Savior and willing to tell others that I have done so. I forsake my own righteousness and take yours. I repent and turn from my sinful life. Right now, I ask you to let your Holy blood cleanse me of all my sins. Come into my life and change me and be the Lord of my life. Show me your will for my life. Guide me and direct me. Fill me with your Holy Spirit right now and make me a new creature forever. Amen.

_____   _____
            Your Name   Today's Date

Be willing to follow Jesus in the commandment of being baptized and most importantly, find a Bible-believing church where you can fellowship with other Christians and GROW as a Christian! It is God's will that you fellowship with other believers, and always keep your EYES on Jesus, not on the performance or failures of others. Remember, other Christians, even family and friends will always come up short and disappoint you because no Christian is perfect. Only Jesus was and IS perfect. Keep your eyes on other Christians, and if they fail, you will become discouraged and disheartened. Keep your eyes on

JESUS, and he will NEVER forsake you, fail you, or disappoint you! *Fear thou not; for I am with thee: be not dismayed; for I am thy God: I will strengthen thee; yea, I will help thee; yea, I will uphold thee with the right hand of my righteousness. (Isa 46:10.)* The right hand of God's righteousness is none other than JESUS!

APPENDIX II

Valuable Links: Note that these links are given for informational purposes only. What you do with this information is up to you.

- **Aloe vera** website: *aloeverahealthbenefits.info.*

- **Alternative health doctor list** is at this link: *http://heartspring.net/naturopathic_directory.html* and here: *http://www.altmedangel.com.* Also check out this site: *http://www.naturopathic.org.* For the American Holistic Medical Association's link to finding a physician in your area, see website: *http://www.holisticmedicine.org/displaycom mon.cfm?an=1&subarticlenbr=49.*

- **Alternative health websites**: for more information about Johanna Budwig, and many other alternative health websites, see this link: *http://www.healingcancernaturally.com/budwig_protocol.html,* and for a link which has dozens of testimonials of people who cured their cancers using natural non-toxic therapies, some of which are discussed in this book, see: *http://www.healingcancernaturally.com/naturalcancer-cure testimonials.ht ml#herbal%20healing%20of%20cancer.*

- **Budwig Formula** – for more on this protocol, see this website: *http://www.west.net/~cure/budwig_diet.htm*

- **Burzynski Patient Group**: *http://www.burzynskipatientgroup.org/stori es.htm* and also see link: *http://www.burzynskipatientgroup.org.* At these two links you can read the amazing true case histories of many of Dr. Burzynski's patients who were cured of all forms of cancer using his non-toxic antineoplastons and PBs (oral form). See trailers on his new movie at: *http://www.burzynskipatientgroup.org.*

- **Burzynski's website**: *http://www.burzynskiclinic.com/ph/index.html* - here you can get all the details about his amazing non-toxic cancer cure known as antineoplastons and PBs (oral form). Also see website: *http://www.cancure.org/burzynski_institute.htm.*

- **Cancell testimonial** - here is a link for a testimonial on a person who used Cancell for curing a bone tumor and a brain tumor: *http://cancerfighter.wordpress.com/2008/06/19/cancell-testimony.*

- **Cansema-like skin formula**, see website: *http://www.mnwelldir.org/docs/cancer1/altthrpy.htm#formula.*

- **Dental Revisions** – information can be obtained by calling: Scientific Health Solutions, Inc. at 800-331-2303 or 719-548-1600 or email at: *dentists@bestdentalmaterials.com.* Also, see Dr. Thomas E. Levy's book on STOP AMERICA'S #1 KILLER for more details.

- **Encyclopedia** for health: *http://www.polymvahealthclub.com/hd.* This website by Poly-MVA has an encyclopedia of more than 75,000 health-related items that you can search.

- **eXcella™ sweetener** – for a sweetener that does not affect blood sugar, see website: *livonlabs.com.* This sweetener is a natural sucrose substitute.

- **Gentle cures** website: *gentlecures.org*

- **Herbs in bulk** can be purchased here: *http://www.sunbreezeherbshop.com,* *http://www.herbalhealer.com/bulk-herbs.html,* and *http://esutras.com/index.Php?cPath=1.*

- **Hodgkin's Lymphoma cure testimonial** - To read the interview with Sue Best whose son, Billy, was healed of Hodgkin's lymphoma several years ago, and also a resource for dozens of other links, see this site: *http://curezone.com/forums/fm.asp?i=67143.*

- **I.P.T.** (insulin potentiation therapy) - see the LifeWorks Wellness Center at 301 Turner Street in Clearwater, Florida; their link is here: *http://www.lifeworkswellnesscenter.com/succan.asp.* You can also email them here: *lifeworksinfo@bodyhealth.com.*, and another link to some of their success stories at: *http://www.lifeworkswellnesscenter.com/success.asp.*

- **IMVA Website**: *http://publications.imva.info/index.php.*

- **Dr. T. Simoncini's** website: *http://www.cancerisafungus.com/*

- **Liposome-encapsulated vitamin C (Lypo-Spheric™)** - see website: *livonlabs.com*. Also, see Dr. Thomas Levy's website for info on this product as well: *peakenergy.com* and *http://tomlevy.com*.

- **Lugol's Solution.** For a website with a link that will give you directions on making your own Lugol's Solution, see website: *http://www.veggieterryann.com/?q=node/39*.

- **Magnascent© Iodine** can be obtained from: *http://www.magnascent.com/index.php*.

- **Transdermal Magnesium** Sources: *http://magnesiumforlife.com/transdermal-magnesium* and *http://www.ancient-minerals.com/* and *http://www.swansonvitamins.com/SWU481/ItemDetail?n=0*.

- **Mercury-free dentists** close to your area: see this link: *http://library.altmedangel.com/2a.htm*. and website: *http://www.dentalwellness4u.com/freeservices/find_dentists.html*, as well as this one: *http://mercuryfreedentists.com*.

- **Morgellon's Disease cure**: see website: *http://www.loveforlife.com.au/node/4578*.

- **Non-Hodgkin's lymphoma testimonial** - to read the amazing testimonial from Maryjo Siegel who was healed of non-Hodgkin's lymphoma using non-toxic antineoplastons, see this link: *http://burzynskipatiengroup.org/maryjo.htm*. You can also email Maryjo if you have questions about her experience at: *maryjo@siegel.net*.

- **Poly-MVA** info and amazing case histories of cancer survivors who used Poly-MVA to completely heal their cancers, see this link: *http://www.polymvasurvivors.com*.

- **Probiotic specialists** – NATREN® - see their website at *www.natren.com*.

- Testimonials of people who used natural methods to cure deadly cancers - see this link: *http://www.cancure.org/cancer_victors.htm*.

- Tour alternative health facilities in Mexico - see this website: *http://cancercontrolsociety.com/forms/trip/bus_tours.html*.

- **USANA** pharmaceutical-grade products: *http://www.usana.com,* and also see Dee Simmons website: *www.ultimateliving.com.*

- Vitamin site with nutrient information: *http://www.mcvitamins.com/default.htm.*

- **Whey protein** – the best I have found that is cold-processed and contains no aspartame is called *Miracle Whey*™ and can be found at Dr. Joseph Mercola's website: *http://proteinpowder.mercola. com/Miracle-Whey-Protein.html,* and for those who may have a hard time digesting protein, try his *Whey Protein Powder with Aminogen®,* located at: *http://proteinpowder.mercola.com/Whey-Protein-With-Aminogen.html.*

- **Whitaker Wellness Center** is in Newport Beach (4321 Birch Street), California, see this link: *http://whitakerwellness.com/about_us/medical_team.* Dr. Julian Whitaker runs this health care center, and has written many books on alternative healing. He has an excellent website with a great deal of helpful information. They use many of the alternative health treatments that I have mentioned in my books, including chelation, hyperbaric oxygen, and IV therapies. (Also, for those suffering from depression, obsessive-compulsive disorders, and anxiety, Dr. Whitaker says that he has had excellent results treating his patients with low-dose **Dilantin** for these problems. Contact them for more info.) He also has a great newsletter.

- **Zeolites** websites: *http://liquidzeolite.zoxic.com,* or *http://www.ghchealth.com/zeotrex.php?gclid=CKnb0c25iZcCFQFqxwodh1p6dA* and *http://www.zeoliteshealth.com.* There are many others that either carry the product or discuss it in detail.

REFERENCES

1. "Agaricus Blazei Murill." Newsletter August 2001, from the Wellness Directory of Minnesota™'. Updated 05/05/07. Online posting. Accessed 8 Nov. 2007. <http://www.mnwelldir.org/docs/Cancer1/altthrpy.htm#Agaricus.htm>. Copyright © 1995-2004 International Wellness Directory.

2. "Agaricus." Wellness Directory of Minnesota™, Alternative Cancer Therapies, updated 05/05/07. Online posting. Accessed 8 Nov 8, 2007. <http://www.mnwelldir.org/docs/Cancer1/altthrpyhtm>. Copyright © 1995-2004 International Wellness Directory.

3. "Alternative Cancer Treatment with Liquid Cesium Chloride." Article – the Puna Wai Ora Mind-Body Center. "Liquid Cesium Chloride / DMSO – Directly Targets and Kills Cancer Cells and Stops Pain." Online posting from www.alternative-cancer-care.com website. Accessed 23 Mar 2010. <http://www.alternative-cancer-care.com/Liquid_Cesium_Chloride.html>.

4. American Association for Cancer Research (2007, April 17). "Marijuana Cuts Lung Cancer Tumor Growth in Half, Study Shows." Online posting. Accessed 25 Mar 2010. <http://www.sciencedaily.com/releases/2007/04/070417193338.htm>. © 1995-2009 Science Daily LLC.

5. "An overview of medicinal mushrooms, mushroom preparations and their medicinal properties." From Mushroom Harvest website online posting "Medicinal Mushrooms." Accessed 31 Dec. 2007. <http://www.mushroomharvest.com/extra_pages/med_mush rooms.htm>.

6. "Antibiotic Use and Increased Risk of Breast Cancer," from the National Cancer Institute. Online posting. "Study Shows Link Between Antibiotic Use and Increased Risk of Breast Cancer." Accessed 23 Mar 2010. <http://www.cancer.gov/newscenter/pressreleases/antibiotics>.

7. "Antineoplastons." Online posting. Alternatives in Cancer Therapy, from their excerpt of the book *Alternatives in Cancer Therapy*, by Ross, R., Ph., Pelton, Lee Overholser. Accessed 8 Nov. 2007. <http://www.curezone.com/diseases/cancer/anti-neoplastons.asp>.

8. "Anti-Tumor Effect of Cranberry." Online posting. "Health News Archive 105 - Cancer." Accessed 4 Nov 2007. <http://www.discount-vitamins-herbs.net/n-105-cancer-cranberry.htm. © 2001-2007, Discount Herbs & Vitamins, Inc.

9. "Apple Juice May Help Keep Colon Cancer At Bay." By ANI. From OneIndia™ website, online posting. Accessed 29 Jun. 2008. <http://living.oneindia.in/health/wellbeing/2008/apple-juice-colon-cancer-treatment-280308.html>. © Greynium Information Technologies Pvt. Ltd.

10. "Are your dental fillings poisoning you?" Online posting at Encognitive.com website. Accessed 20 Mar. 2010. <http://www.encognitive.com/node/4750>.

10a. "Asparagus cancer recoveries and remissions," from the article "Asparagus for cancer," from the *Cancer News Journal*, Dec. 1979. Online posting at healingcancernaturally.com. Accessed 15 Jun. 2010. <http://www.healingcancernaturally.com/cancer-diet-and-nutrition.html>. © 2004, 2005, 2006, 2007, 2008, 2009 & 2010 www.healingcancer naturally.com.

11. "Autism Therapy: Vitamin B6 and Magnesium." From Healing Thresholds website online posting. Accessed 20 Mar. 2010. <http://autism.healingthresholds.com/therapy/vitamin-b6-and-magnesium>. © 2010 Healing Thresholds.

12. "Autism Treatment Options." Online posting. Accessed 25 Mar 2010. <http://www.child-autism-parent-café.com/autism-treatment.html>. © 2005-2010 ASD Concepts, LLC.

13. "Beating Ovarian Cancer at 80 with RM-10." Interview with Rose Menlowe. "Jordan Rubin's Grandmother from Garden of Life." "Rose Menlowe cured of ovarian cancer with Jordan Rubin RM 10." Online posting. Accessed 23 Jun. 2008. <http://www.crohns.net/Miva/education /testimonial_rosemenlowe.shtml>.

14. "Blueberries Contain Chemical That May Help Prevent Colon Cancer." From American Chemical Society (2007, March 26). *ScienceDaily*. Retrieved July 8, 2008, from <http://www.sciencedaily.com/releases/2007/03/070325111552.htm>. Online posting from Science Daily website. Also related article: "Blueberry Compound Shows Promise of Lowering Cholesterol as Effective as Drug" (from Aug. 31, 2004) © 1995-2008 ScienceDaily LLC.

15. "Bone Cancer - Another Flax Cure." Online posting. Accessed 8 Nov. 2007. <http:// www.curezone.com/diseases/cancer/testimonials/Bone-cancer_another_flax_cure.asp>. Copyright © 1996 - 2005 Curezone.com.

16. "Bone Cancer." Online posting. Accessed 8 Nov 2007. <http://www.herbs2000.com/disorders/cancer_bone.htm>. © 2002-2007 herbs2000.com.

17. "Breast Cancer Choices Supplement Strategy – Iodine." From Breastcancerchoices.org online posting. Accessed 29 Mar 2010. <http://www.breastcancerchoices.org/iodine>. © 2004-2010 Breast Cancer Choices, Inc.

18. "Broccoli sprouts cut bladder cancer risk by half. From CHINESE MEDICINE NEWS online posting. A "CM NEWS, American Association for Cancer Research release," 02/28/2008. Accessed 24 Jul. 2008. <http://chinesemedicinenews.com/2008/02/28/broccoli-sprouts-cut-bladder-cancer-risk-by-half>. © 2007-2008 CHINESE MEDICINE NEWS.

19. "Burzynski Patient Group." "Crystin S." Online posting. Accessed 8 Nov 2007. <http://burzynskipatientgroup.org/crystins.htm>.

20. "Burzynski Patient Group." "Dustin K." Online posting. Accessed 8 Nov. 2007. <http://www.burzynskipatientgroup.org/dustink.htm>.

21. "Burzynski Patient Group." "Jodi G." Online posting. Accessed 8 Nov. 2007. <http://www.burzynskipatientgroup.org/jodig.htm>.

22. "Burzynski Patient Group." "Roy H." Online posting. Accessed 8 Nov. 2007. <http://www.burzynskipatientgroup.org/roy_hash.htm>.

23. "Burzynski Patient Group." "Sophia G." Online posting. Accessed 8 Nov. 2007. <http://burzynskipatientgroup.org/sophiag.htm>.

23a. "Burzynski The Movie." Online posting. Accessed 15 May 2010. <http://www.burzynskimovie.com>. © 2010 Burzynski Movie.

24. "Cancer-fighting Foods and Spices." The Cancer Cure Foundation. Online posting. Accessed 27 Dec. 2007. <http://cancure.org/cancer_fighting_foods.htm>.

25. "Cancer vaccine programme suspended after 4 girls die." Online posting from truthaboutgardasil.org website. Accessed 19 Apr 2010. <http://truthaboutgardasil.org/breaking news-india-halts-hpv-vaccine-program/cancer-vaccine-programme-suspended-after-4-girlsdie>

26. "Candida, Yeast and Fungus a Cancer – Baking Soda to Cure." From an online posting at http://aromatherapy4u.wordpress.com website. Accessed 25 Mar 2010. Information from Dr. T. Simoncini. <http://aromatherapy4u.wordpress.com/2008/08/05/974>.

27. "Cervical Cancer." Online posting. Accessed 10 Nov. 2007. <http://www.herbs2000.com/disorders/cancer_cervical.htm>. © 2002-2007 herbs2000.

28. "Cesium Chloride Alternative Cancer Treatment Comparison." Online posting. Accessed 13 Jan. 2008. <http://www.alternativecancer.us/cesiumchloride.htm>.

29. "Cesium Plus with Rubidium and CESIUM & DMSO PROTOCOLS." From the WOLFE CLINIC website online posting. Accessed 25 Mar 2010. <http://thewolfeclinic.com/supplements/ionic_cesium_plus_with_rubidium.html>.

30. "Chlorophyll and Cancer Prevention." From an online posting 06/28/2008 at cancersolutions.org website. Accessed 29 Jun. 2008. <http://www.cancersolutions.org/2008/06/chlorophyll-and-cancer-prevention.html>.

31. "Chlorine, Cancer, and Heart Disease." From the article: "The Effects of Chlorine in Your Water: Chlorine, Cancer and Heart Disease." Online posting at healthynewage.com website. Accessed 23 Mar 2010. <http://www.healthnewage.com/chlorine-cancer.htm>. © Heart Core Corp. 2001-2010.

32. "Chlorine in the bathwater is linked to cancer." Last updated 26 Jan 2007. From Mail Online, www.dailymail.co.uk website. Online posting. Accessed 23 Mar 2010. <http://www.dailymail.co.uk/news/article-431777/Chlorine-bathwater-linked-cancer.html>. © Associated Newspapers Ltd.

33. "Chronic Fatigue An Answer?" From the Magnesium Website Magnesium Online Library, Nov. 22, 2002. Online posting. Accessed 07 Mar. 2010. <http://www.mgwater.com/chronic lz.shtml>.

34. "Cilantro: A Common Spice/Herb That Can Save Your Life." Online posting. Wellness Directory of Minnesota™. Accessed 10 Nov. 2007. <http://www.mnwell.dirorg/docs/detox/cilantro.htm> © 2004, 2005 International Wellness Directory.

35. "Cilantro Helps Eliminate Mercury, Lead, and Aluminum." From an article at shirleys-wellness-café.com "Dental Amalgam a source of mercury poisoning," online posting. Accessed

26 Mar 2010. <http://www.shirleys-wellness-café.com/amalgam.htm> © 1996-2010 Shirley's Wellness Café.

36. "Comparison of Glutathione in Fresh vs. Cooked Foods in milligrams per 3 ½ oz. (100 gm serving)." Online posting. Accessed 10 Nov. 2007. <http://www.nutritionadvisor.com/glutathione_foods.php>. © Nutritionadvisor, Inc.

37. "Compound Identified In Grapes May Fight Cancer And Diabetes." American Chemical Society (2002, May 22). *ScienceDaily*. Retrieved July 8, 2008 from http://www.sciencedaily.com/releases/2002/05/020522073916.htm. © 1995-2008 ScienceDaily LLC.

38. "Conditions Linked to Deficiencies of Magnesium." Online posting from www.ctds.info website. Accessed 27 Mar 2010. <http://www.ctds.info/5+13_magnesium.html>. © 1999-2009 Pine Canyon Media, LLD.

39. "Country Doctor Cures Cancer With Baking Soda & Maple Syrup." "Cancer, Cure, Cure for, Alternative Method." Online posting Ashville, N.C. Website "Clayton's Canine Closet." "Country Doctor" is actually a truck driver with no medical degree, but 185 of the patients he has used his simple remedy on (out of 200) with "terminal cancer," lived "at least 15 more years." Accessed 31 Aug 2008. <http://www.claytonscaninecloset.com/cureforcancer>. © Ann Clayton Photographic Imaging Fernley, NV.

40. "Cup of Black Tea Could Defend Against Anthrax Threat, Research Suggests." From an article at *ScienceDaily* 16 March 2008. Their information from Cardiff University. Online posting. Accessed 25 Dec. 2008. <http://www.sciencedaily.com/releases/2008/03/080312100045.ht m>. © 1995-2008 *ScienceDaily LLC*.

41. Daily Mail Reporter. "Red Grapes 'are wonder cure for high blood pressure and cholesterol'" Mail Online health. Last updated 20th Aug 2008. Online posting. Accessed 21 Aug 2008 <http://www.dailymail.co.uk/health/article-1047217/Red-grapes-wonder-cure-high-blood-pressure-cholesterol.html#>. © 2008 Associated Newspapers Ltd.

42. "Deficiency" [of magnesium]. From the Linus Pauling Institute at Oregon State University Micronutrient Information Center. Online posting. Accessed 27 Mar 2010. <http://lpi.oregonstate.edu/infocenter/minerals/magnesium>. © 2001-2010 Linus Pauling Institute.

43. "DHEA, magnesium and CWR An Interview with C. Norman Shealy, M.D., Ph.D. Normalizing DHEA through topical magnesium supplementation." Online posting. Accessed 20 Mar. 2010. <http://www.yourlifesource.com/cwr-dhea.htm>. YourLifeSource.com. © 2002 Loren & Kathy Schiele.

44. "Dietary Supplement Fact Sheet: Selenium". Online posting from the NIH (National Institutes of Health) Office of Dietary Supplements. USA.gov. Accessed 27 Mar 2010. <http://dietary-supplements.info.nih.gov/factsheets/selenium.asp>.

45. "Docs Show Eli Lilly Knew Mercury In Vaccines Was Known Dangerous in 30's" 3-17-2. From an online posting of www.rense.com. Accessed 27 Mar. 2010. <http://www.rense.com/general21/vacc.htm>.

46. "Doctors Say, Reader's Digest is Wrong Physicians and Researchers Set the Record Straight about Vitamins." From Orthomolecular Medicine News Service, April 3, 2010. The Reader's Digest article can be found here: <http://www.rd.com/living-healthy/5-vitamin-truths-

and-lies/article175625. html>. Orthomolecular Medicine News Service (OMNS) has a free subscription link at: http://orthomolecular.org/subscribe.html and an archive link at: http://orthomolecular.org/resources/omns/index.shtml. The Editor and contact person at OMNS is Andrew S. Saul, Ph.D. (USA). I received this information sent to me in an email 04/03/2010 from omns@cihfimedia services.org

47. "Dr. Budwig's Diet & Cancer Healing Protocol," at website *Healing Cancer Naturally*. "Dr. Budwig's Protocol." The quote is from Dr. Johanna Budwig in *Flax Oil as a True Aid*. Online posting. Accessed 7 Nov. 2007. <http://www.healingcancernaturally.com/budwig_protocol. html>. © 2004, 2005, 2006 & 2007 www.healingcancernaturally.com.

48. "Dr. Budwig's Diet & Cancer Healing Protocol." at website Healing Cancer Naturally. Online posting 17 Jan. 2005. <http://www.healingcancernaturally.com/budwig_protocol.html> from Dr. Budwig in "Der Toddes Tumors, Band II." (The Death of the Tumor, Vol. II) transcribing an interview broadcast by the Siddeutscher Rundfunk Stuttgart (South German Radio Station) on 11 Sept. 1967. © 2004, 2005, 2006 & 2007 www.healingcancernaturally.com.

49. "Early antibiotic use can cause asthma, study finds." By The Vancouver Sun June 11, 2007. Online posting. Accessed 23 Mar 2010. <http://www.canada.com/vancouversun/news/arts/story.html?id=0497dbe6-a3f8-4ce6-b797-f4206a810ddd>. © 2008-2010 Canwest Publishing, Inc.

50. "Eli Lilly (Satan's Chemist)." Online posting. From the article "Is Eli Lilly Milking Cancer by Promoting *and* Treating It? Oct 2009 by Jeffrey Smith. Accessed 27 Mar 2010. <http://www.whale.to/a/eli_lilly.html>.

51. "Epsom Salts." Online posting from Enzyme Stuff the Wonderful World of Digestive Enzymes website. Accessed 27 Mar 2010. <http://www.enzymestuff.com/epsomsalts.htm>. © Kd2002.

52. "Extracts From Reishi Mushroom And Green Tea Shows Synergestic Effect To Slow Sarcoma." Federation of American Societies for Experimental Biology. Online posting from *ScienceDaily,* 14 April 2008, who adapted their article from the information provided by Federation of America Societies for Experimental Biology, via *EurekaAlert,* a service of AAS. Accessed 25 Dec. 2008. <http://www.sciencedaily.com/releases/2008/04/08040 8175308.htm>. © 1995-2008 *ScienceDaily LLC*

52a. "FDA: Pfizer Concealed Serious Harm from Drugs. Oft-Cited Drug Giant Did Not Report Patient Complaints That Caused Serious Injuries." From the Associated Press and CBS News June 9, 2010. Online posting. Accessed 9 Jun 2010. Also see the article: "FDA Warns Pfizer For Unreported Drug Complaints. Pfizer Gets FDA Warning Letter For Failing to Submit Drug Side-effect Reports." Also from the Associated Press and CBS News June 9, 2010 online posting. Accessed 9 June 2010. See websites: <http://www.cbsnews.com/stories/2010/06/09/business/main6566003.shtml?tag=channelMore,latestRight> and http://www.cbsnews.com/stories/2010/06/09/ap/health/main6565877.shtml?tag=channelMore,latestRight>. © Copyright 2010 The Associated Press.

53. "Fluoride and Osteosarcoma." From the article: "Dog Food Comparison Shows High Flouride (sic) Levels: Fluoride and Osteosarcoma." From Environmental Working Group website online posting. Accessed 23 Mar 2010. <http://www.ewg.org/pethealth/report/fluoride-in-dog-food/FlourideandOsteosarcoma>. © 2007-2009 Environmental Working Group.

54. "Food as Medicine: Protective Foods Other Phytochemicals. How Other Phytochemicals Help Protect Against Cancer." Online posting. The Cancer Project. 12 Nov. 2007. <http://www.cancerproject.org/protective_foods/phytochemicals.php>.

55. *FOODNEWS from ENVIRONMENTAL WORKING GROUP* - foodnews.org. Online posting - shows ranking of 43 fruits and vegetables in order of those having highest pesticide load (non-organic foods). Accessed 16 Aug 2008. <http://www.food news.org>.

56. "Fungi Can Change Quickly, Pass Along Infectious Ability." From the ScienceDaily.com website online posting Mar 22, 2010. Accessed 25 Mar 2010. <http://www.sciencedaily.com/releases/2010/03/100317144634.htm>. © 1995-2009 ScienceDaily LLC.

57. "Glutathione for people & animals. Protects against disease, toxins." From Shirley's Wellness Café online posting. Accessed 26 Mar 2010. See the book by Alan H. Pressman, D.C., PhD., CCN: *Glutathione The Ultimate Antioxidant.* <http://www.shirleys-wellness-café.com/glutathione.htm>. © 1996-2010 Shirley's Wellness Café.

58. "Grape Juice Inhibits Breast Cancer Cell Growth in Animal Study." From Health News Archive 21 – Breast Cancer. Online posting. Accessed 2 Nov 2007. <http://www.discount-vitamins-herbs.net/health-news21.htm#127>. © 2001–2007 Discount Herbs & Vitamins, Inc.

59. "Green Tea Compound Blocks Bladder Tumors in Rats." Online posting. Accessed 2 Nov. 2007. <http://www.discount-vitamins-herbs.net/health-news5.htm>. © 2001 – 2007 Discount Herbs & Vitamins, Inc.

60. "Green Tea Fights Killer Disease." Online posting. FoodNavigator.com, News Headlines—Science & Nutrition, 2/4/2004. Accessed 12 Nov. 2007. <http://www.foodnavigator.com/news/news-NG.asp?id=51104>. © 2000/2007 - Decision News Media SAS.

61. "Green tea may cut the risk of gastric cancer in women." Research Update article #2 online posting at *swansonvitamins.com* website. From Cancer Epidemiology, Biomarkers & Prevention 17(2):343-351, 2008. Accessed 29 Mar. 2008. <http://video.swansonvitamins.com/c_files/ResearchUpdate/080327_Rua2.html>.

62. "Harvard Researchers Link Vitamin D Levels to Colon Cancer Survival." GEN News Highlights online posting Jun 19, 2008. Accessed 21 Jun. 2008. <http://www.genengnews.com/news/bnitem.aspx?name=37488385>. © 2008 Genetic Engineering & Biotechnology News.

63. *Healing With Vitamins,* by the Editors of Prevention Health Books (City, State, not given), Rodale, Inc. 1996.

64. "Health Alert: Cancer treatment with Vitamin C." Posted & Updated Aug 29, 2008. Online posting. Accessed 04 Sep 2008. Wistv.com. <http://www.wistv.com/Global/story.asp?S=8922907&nav=menu36_8>. Copyright © 2000-2008 WorldNow and WISTV, a Raycom Media Station.

65. "Hepatitis B Vaccines: Adverse Reactions. Think Twice!" From Think Twice Global Vaccine Institute. Online posting. Also, see the Vaccine Safety Manual by Neil Z. Miller, and see "Testimony of Michael Belkin Before the Advisory Committee on Immunization Practices – Centers For Disease Control and Prevention (Feb 17, 1999) – Atlanta, Georgia." Website www.thinktwice.com. Accessed 27 Mar 2010. <http://www.thinktwice.com/hepb.htm>. © 1996-2010.

66. "Herbs & Supplements." "Milk Thistle." See under "Dosage and Administration." Online posting from Express Scrips website (updated 16 Oct. 2007). Accessed 03 Jul. 2008. <http://www.drugdigest.org/DD/DVH/HerbsTake/0,3927,551935%7CMilk%2BThistle,00.html>. Copyright © 2008 Express Scripts, Inc.

68. "Hoelen." Online posting. Accessed 12 Nov. 2007. <http://www.herbs2000.com/herbs/herbs_hoelen.htm>. © 2002-2007 herbs2000.com.

68a. "Homemade Liposomal C." Online posting. Updated July 2010. Accessed 25 Jul 2010. <http://www.pdazzler.com/archives/62>. © 2010 pdazzler.

69. "How to Get More Magnesium in Your Diet." Online posting from www.ctds.info. Accessed 27 Mar 2010. <http://www.ctds.info/magdiet.html>. © 2002-2009 Pine Canyon Media, LLC.

70. "Inate Response Selenium." From Crusador Enterprise, Inc. website. Online posting. Accessed 20, Mar 2010. <http://www.healthtruthrevealed.com/item-IRS.html> © 2010 Crusador Enterprise, Inc.

71. "Intravenous Therapy" "ORTHO-IMMUNE." Online posting, accessed 20 Jan. 2008. <http:www.alternative-doctor.com/cancer/ca_advanced.htm>. © 2003 Keith Scott-Mumby.

72. "Iodine And The Halogen Revolution." From e-Healing.us. "Avoid Bromilated Vegetable Oils in Breads & Baking Products." Online posting. Accessed 23 Mar 2010. <http://www.ehealing.us/article_iodine3.html>.

73. "Iodine and the Heart." From New Frontiers in Cardiology. Online posting. Accessed 25 Mar 2010. <http://naturalallopathiccardiology.com/cms/index.php?option=com_content&view+article&id=121>.

74. "Iodine - Candida, Chelation, more." Online posting. Accessed 23 Mar 2010. <http://veggieterryann.com/?q=node/39>.

75. "Iodine Deficiency." Online posting from The Vitamin C Foundation. Accessed 06 Apr 2010. <http://www.vitamincfoundation.org/iodine.htm>. Article © 2005 by Robert Sarver.

76. "Iodine (I) General Discussion." Online posting. "Final Thoughts on Iodine:" W.W. Greene, D.C. Accessed 07 Apr 2010.<http://www.dcnutrition.com/Minerals/Detail.CFM?RecordNumber=73>. © 2000-2006 DCNutriton.com.

77. "Iodine Therapy Guidelines." From Breastcancerchoices.org "Iodine Protocol." Online posting. Accessed 29 Mar 2010. <http://www.breastcancerchoices.org/iprotocol.html>. © 2004-2010 Breast Cancer Choices, Inc.

78. "Is There a Diabetes Iodine Link?" Online posting from Healthy Eating Politics Alternative Views on Food and Health. Accessed 27 Mar 2010. <http://www.health-eating-politics.com/diabetes-iodine.html>. © 2008 Healthy-Eating-Politics.com.

79. "Israeli Science – Green Tea Is Good For the Brain?" Oct 16, 2007. From an online posting accessed 13 Nov. 2007. "Kosher News About Israeli Jews." <http://www.isragood.com/2007/110/israeli-science-geen-tea-is-good-for.html>. IsraGood © 2006-2007.

80. "Is the Budwig Protocol 'just flax seed oil and cottage cheese'"? Online posting. Accessed 13 Nov. 2007. <http://www.healingcancernaturally.com/budwig_protocol.html>. © 2004, 2005, 2006 & 2007 www.healingcancernaturally.com.

81. "Johanna Budwig Revisited," "or How to Heal Cancer." Online posting. Wellness Directory of Minnesota™. Accessed 13 Nov. 2007. <http://www.mnwelldir.org/docs/cancer1budwig.htm>. Copyright © 2001 International Wellness Directory.

82. "Kiwifruit." The World's Healthiest Foods: Eating-Healthy Cooking-Healthy Feeling-Great, George Mateljan Foundation. "Protection Against Asthma. Online posting. Accessed 13 Nov. <http://www.whfoods.com/genpagephp?tname=foodspice&dbid=41>. Copyright © 2001-2007 The George Mateljan Foundation.

83. "Lead contamination in Washington, D.C. drinking water." From Wikipedia, the free encyclopedia online posting. Accessed 23 Mar 2010. <http://en.wikipedia.org/wiki/Lead_contamination_in_Washington,_D.C._drinking_water>.

84. "Liver Cancer." Online posting. Liver Cancer – Healing with Herbs, Vitamins and Minerals. Accessed 13 Nov. 2007. <http://www.herbs2000.com/disorders//cancer_liver.htm>. © 2002-2007 herbs 2000.com.

85. "Lorraines Healing Therapies." Ancient Minerals Magnesium Gel Plus. Online posting. Accessed 20 Mar 2010. <http://www.health.freemotion.com.au/magnesium_gel.htm>.

86. "Lung Cancer." Online posting. Accessed 13 Nov. 2007. <http://www.herbs2000.com/disorders/cancer_lung.htm>. ©2002-2007 herbs2000.com.

87. "Lyprinol." Online posting. Accessed 13 Nov. 2007. <http://www.primohealth.com/PILyprinol.a.html>.

88. "Magnesium." Magnesium Uptake. Online posting from www.krispin.com. Accessed 25 Mar 2010. <http://www.krispin.com/magnes.html. © Krispin Sullivan, CN 1997.

89. "Magnesium." Online posting at website: http://www.ithyroid.com/magnesium.htm. Accessed 20 Mar. 2010. <http://www.ithyroid.com/magnesium.htm>.

90. "Magnesium and Calcium Fight Heart Disease, Alzheimers and More." Online Posting from greatestherbsonearth.com website. Accessed 27 Mar 2010. <http://www.greatestherbs.onearth.com/articles/heart_disease.htm>. © 2000-2010 from Greatest Herbs On Earth© Nature's Sunshine Products.

91. "Magnesium and inflammation," from the Blog of Michael R. Eades, M.D. 29, July 2005. Online posting. Accessed 07 Mar. 2010. <http://www.proteinpower.com/drmike/uncategorized/magnesium-and-inflammation>.

93. "Magnesium Articles & Citations." 03-25-2010. Online posting from Dr. Gary Erkfritz, D.C. Online posting. Accessed 25 Mar 2010. <http://www.drgarye.com/DesktopDefault.aspx?tabid=879>. © 2004 © 2002-2010 by DotNetLuke.

94. "Magnesium Deficiency: A Growing Health Crisis." Online posting. Accessed 27 Mar 2010. <http://www.charlespoliquin.com/Articles/Multimedia/Articles/Article.aspx?ID=208>. © 2010 Poliquin, Inc.

95. "Magnesium, Drinking Water, & Health. Are you getting enough magnesium to keep yourself healthy?" From The Magnesium Web Site Magnesium Online Library. Online posting. Accessed 27 Mar 2010. <http://www.mgwater.com.

96. "Magnesium, The Nutrient That Could Change Your Life: Chapter 16. Kidney Stones." From Magnesium Online Library. This is from the book: *Magnesium The Nutrient That Could Change Your Life* by J. I. Rodale with Harald J. Taub. The book is from Pyramid Books, New York, N.Y. © 1968 by J. I. Rodale. Online posting. Accessed 26 Mar 2010. <http://www.mgwater.com/rod16.shtml>.

97. "Maitake." Herbs 2000.com. Online posting. Accessed 13 Nov. 2007. <http://www.herbs 2000.com/herbs/herbs_maitake.htm>. ©2002–2007 herbs2000.com.

98. "Managing Your Child's Asthma with Natural Medicine." Online posting from mercola.com website article: "New Study Suggests Asthma Could Have A Natural Fix." Posted by Dr. Mercola 04/06/2010. Accessed 06 Apr. 2010. <http://articles.mercola.com/sites/articles/archive/2010/04/06/managing-your-childs-asthma-with-natural-medicine.as px>. © 2010 Dr. Joseph Mercola.

99. "Medical Conditions." "Botanicals." Online posting. Accessed 13 Nov. 2007. <http://www.naturalopinion.com/nmp/Sample.html>. Natural Medical Protocols. A reference program for doctors on natural medicine.

100. "Melanoma, Cancer, Metastasis." Online posting. Accessed 4 Nov. 2007. Vitasearch website. <http://search.vitasearch.com/get-clp-summary35010>. Also, see reference: "Low plasma coenzyme Q10 levels as an independent prognostic factor for melanoma progression," Rusciani L, Proietti I., et al, Jam Acad Dermatol, 2006;54(2):234-41. From *Vitasearch Clinical Pearls* website.

101. "Mercury." Online posting at www.ithyroid.com website. Accessed 26 Mar 2010. <http://www.ithyroid.com/mercury.htm>.

102. "Mercury – A Dangerous Toxin." Online posting from The Free Library website by Farlex at www.thefreelibrary.com. Accessed 27 Mar 2010. <http://www.thefreelibrary.com/Alter native+Medicines+-+Mercury+and+Human+Health-a01073742805>. © 2010 Farlex, Inc.

103. "Mercury, Candida and the Die-Off Reaction." Online posting. Accessed 23 Mar 2010. <http://www.mercurypoisoning.me/Candida_and_mercury_poisoning.html>.

104. "Mercury." See "Mercury – Mercury Detoxification." Online posting from tuberose.com website. Accessed 26 Mar 2010. <http://tuberose.com/Mercury.html>.

105. "Mercury Exposure of Dentists and Assistants." Updated 09-2007. Online posting. Accessed 26 Mar 2010. <http://www.mercurypoisoned.com/dental_personnel.html>.

106. "Mercury fillings pose health risks, FDA warns." From CBC News article online posting (updated Thurs. June 5, 2008.) Accessed 03 July 2008. <http://www.cbc.ca/consumer/story/2008/06/05/dental-amalgam.html>. © CBC 2008.

107. "Metal Toxicity And Candida Yeast Infection Shown To Be Linked." See under "Research Proves Link between Metal Toxicity and Candida Yeast Infections." Online posting from MicoNutra Health™ Journal. Accessed 25 Mar 2010. <http://www.micronutra.com/

journal/yeast-infection/metal-toxicity-and-Candida-yeast-infection-shown-to-be-linked>. Copyright © 2009 Micro Nutra Health™ Journal.

108. Moore, Charles W. "Mercury Fillings: A Time Bomb In Your Head." Online posting from Natural Life Magazine, green family living – Jan/Feb 1997. Accessed 27 Mar 2010. <http://www.naturallifemagazine.com/9702/mercury.htm>. © 1976-2010 Life Media.

109. "MRSA germ undermines body's defences" (sic) CTV News. Online posting. Accessed 23 Mar 2010. <http://www.ctv.ca/servlet/ArticleNews/story/CTVNews/20071112/staph_defences_071112/20071112?hub=TopStories>.

110. "My Dance With Cancer." Website of Vernon J ("Vito"). Online posting. Accessed 07 Apr 2010. <http://www.phkillscancer.com/home>. © 2009 My Dance With Cancer.

111. "New breakthrough boosts immune cell activity 45.2% more than ordinary mushrooms." "MycoPhyto® Complex." Online posting. Accessed 28 Dec. 2007. <http://www.advancedbionutritionals.com/immunity>.

112. "New Research on Cancer-fighting Foods, Supplements." (Also see: "Drinking cloudy apple juice daily may help prevent colon cancer.") American Chemical Society (2007, March 26). *ScienceDaily*. Retrieved July 8, 2008, from http://www.sciencedaily.com/releases/2007/03/0703 25111619.htm. © 1995-2008 ScienceDaily LLC.

113. "NK-Immunomodulation by AHCC in 17 Cancer Patients." From Health News Archive 62 – Cancer and AHCC Research at the www.discount-vitamins-herbs.net website online posting. Accessed 8 Dec. 2007. <http://www.discount-vitamins-herbs.net/health-news62.htm>. © 2001-2007, Discount Herbs & Vitamins, Inc.

114. "No Harmful Synthetic Chemicals." From innvista website online posting. Accessed 27 Mar. 2010. <http://www.innvista.com/health/foods/organics/synchem.htm>.

115. "Poly-MVA New hope for cancer patients. New hope for brain cancer patients." Online posting. Accessed 14 Nov. 2007. <http://www.mnwelldir.org/docs/cancer1/poly.htm>. Wellness Directory of Minnesota™. Copyright © 2001, 2002 International Wellness Directory.

116. "Preterm birth: Magnesium sulphate (sic) cuts cerebral palsy risk." Jan 20, 2009. Online posting. Source: Wiley-Blackwell. From Esciencenews.com website. Accessed 27 Mar 2010. © 2010 Eureka Science News.

117. "Range Guide Products – Chelorex – Heavy Metal Detox." Online posting from ranguide.net website. Accessed 23 Mar 2010. <http://www.rangeguide.net/chelorex.htm>.

118. "Red Wine Antioxidant May Help Destroy Pancreatic Cancer." From living.Oneindia.in/health/wellbeing website – by ANI from the March edition of *Advances in Experimental Medicine and Biology* journal. Online posting article accessed 29 Jun. 2008. © Greynium Information Technologies Pvt. Ltd.

119. "Researchers Discover That A Protein In Grape Skins Can Kill Cancer Cells." University of Virginia Health System (2004, May 28). *ScienceDaily*. Retrieved July 8, 2008, from <http://www. sciencedaily.com-/releases/2004/05/040526065457.htm>. © 1995–2008 Science Daily LLC.

120. "Resveratrol—Another Look Some call it the Fountain of Youth," Newsletter Update from Minnesota Wellness Publications, Inc. Online posting, accessed 26 Aug 2008. <http://www.mnwelldir.org/nw_current.htm>. Copyright © 2008 Minnesota Wellness Publications, Inc. Also see their reference: Gunnlaugsdoitter, E., et al., "Prevalance and causes of visual impairment and blindness in Icelanders aged 50 years and older: the Reykjavik Eye Study," Acta Opthamol, 2008 May 3, in regards to the info on resveratrol and cataracts.

121. "Risk factors for crohn's disease include smoking and NSAIDs and antibiotics for crohns." Online posting at www.crohns.net website. "Risk Factors For Crohn's Disease." Accessed 23 Mar 2010. <http://www.crohns.net/Miva/education/articles/Risk_Factors.shtml>.

122. "Selenium May Protect Against Viruses, Heart Disease, Arthritis, Hepatitis, and Cancer." New Research Centreforce MSM online posting. Accessed 03 Apr 2010. <http://health.centreforce.com/health/selenium.html>. From Centreforce Australia, P O Box 227, Gin Gin Qld 4671 Australia. Note from website: Andrew Holtz and the Associated Press contributed to this CNN article which can be found at http://www.cnn.com/HEALTH/9612/24/nfm/index.html, and the Journal of the American Medical Association can be found in the archives at http://jama.ama-assn.org/.

123. "Selenium Reduces Cancer Risk." From the British Journal of Urology 81(5):730-4, 1998 May. Online posting at website alkalizeforhealth.net. Title: "Decreased incidence of prostate cancer with selenium supplementation: results of a double-blind cancer prevention trial." Accessed 25 June 2008. <http://www.alkalizeforhealth.net/Lselenium.htm>. © 2000–2008 AlkalizeForHealth.

124. "Sodium Bicarbonate – The Natural Wonder Drug." An online posting by THE COFAH NETWORK BLOG 04/11/2009. From The Healing of a Nation – The Hebrew People. Accessed 25 Mar 2010. <http://naturalhealing.cofah.com/2009/04/11/sodium-bicarbonatethe-natural-wonder-drug.aspx>.

125. "Stroke and Magnesium Deficiency The Two Often Come Together." Online posting at Magnesium™ Direct website. Accessed 07 Mar. 2010. <http://www.magnesiumdirect.com/stroke.aspx>. © 2010 Magnesium Direct.

126. "Studying Great Salt Lake's High Mercury Levels," by The Associated Press 08-09-2008. Great Salt Lake, Utah (AP). Online posting. Accessed 27 Mar 2010. <http://www.nytimes.com/2008/08/10/science/earth/10saltlake.htm?_r=1>. From The New York Times. © 2008 The New York Times Company.

127. "Sudden Infant Death Syndrome: is there a vaccine connection?" Online posting. Accessed 26 Mar 2010. <http://www.shirleys-wellness-café.com/vaccine_sids.htm>. © 1996-2010 ShirleysWellnessCafe.com. aka: MyWellnessHouse.com.

128. "Supplement Sampler." "Magnesium." From the University of Wisconsin Integrative Medicine Department of Family Medicine. U of W School of Medicine and Public Health website online posting. Accessed 20 Mar. 2010. <http://www.fammed.wisc.edu/files/webfm-uploads/documents/outreach/im/ss_magnesium.pdf>.

129. "Susan Hale." Article from Burzynski Patient Group. Online posting. Accessed 28 Aug 2008. <http://www.burzynskipatientgroup.org/susanhale.htm> on Glioblastoma multiforme.

130. "Test Magnesium Levels." From Diagnose-Me Treatment online posting at www.diagnose-me-com/treat/T347488.html. Accessed 10 Apr 2010. <http://www.diagnose-me.com/treat/T347488.html>.

131. "The Deadly Dangers Of Mercury Contamination." From an interview with John Moore Nov 2003 Vol 23, No. 11 12-20-2003, from www.rense.com website. Accessed 27 Mar 2010. <http://www.rense.com/general46/merc.htm>.

132. "The End of Antibiotics – Yeast infection natural cures – Zimbio. Online posting. From kandylini.wordpress.com and http://www.naturalnews.com/z022892.html. Accessed 23 Mar 2010. <http://www.zimbio.com/Yeast+infection+natural+cures/articles/240/The+End+of+Antibiotics>.

133. "The Healing Power of Vitamins, Minerals, and Herbs." *Reader's Digest*, Pleasantville, N.Y. Reader's Digest Assoc., Inc. 1009, 1999, 2000.

134. "The Herd Immunity Theory – Treating Our Children Like Cattle." Online posting. Accessed 27 Mar 2010. <http://text.vaccineriskawareness.com/The-Herd-Immunity-Theory-Treating-Our-Children-Like-Cattle>.

135. "The Issels Treatment: Comprehensive Immunotherapy for Cancer." Online posting. "Co-Enzyme Co-Q10." Accessed 30 Nov. 2007. <http://www.issels.com/TreatmentSummary.aspx>. © 2005–2007 Issels Treatment.

136. "The Medical Mafia" and "Medical Fascism". Online posting from website: http://www.whale.to/a/medical_mafia.html. Accessed 21 Mar 2010.

137. "The Role of Caffeine in Diabetes." From Diabetes website, the www.diability-resource.com site online posting. Accessed 27 Mar 2010. <http://www.disability-resource.com/diabetes/the_role_of_caffeine_in_diabetes.htm>. © 1996-2010 Disability Resource Directory.

138. "The Swines Behind The Flu Pandemic." Online posting. Accessed 27 Mar 2010. <http://vaccineriskawareness.com/The-Swines-Behind-The-Flu-Pandemic>. Also see website from article: <http://www.bild.de/BILD/news/bild-english/world-news/2009/04/28/swine-flu-scare-in-switzerland/container-with-virus-explodes-in-train.html>.

139. "The Water Flouridation Hoax". From the article "Adverse Health Effects on Water Fluoridation." Online posting. Accessed 23 Mar 2010. <http://www.blatantpropaganda.org/propaganda/articles/water_fluoridation.html>.

140. "Thyroid Health - Interactions Between Selenium and Iodine." Online posting from The Green Willow Tree website April 27, 1999. Accessed 27 Mar 2010. <http://www.greenwillowtree.com/Page.bok?file=selenium.iodine.html>.

141. "Thyroid Nascent Iodine For Less." Online posting. Accessed 23 Mar 2010. <http://www.thyroidnascentiodine.com/cancer.htm>. © 2007 Thyroidnascentiodine.com.

142. "Toxins – Heavy Metals, Toxins Removed Safely, Effective & Naturally." Also see: "AUTISM The figure of one autistic infant for every 150 is now widely documented." Online Posting. Accessed 23 Mar 2010. <http://www.i-amperfectlyhealthy.com/Toxins.html>.

142a. "UK Recommends Against Buying Breast Cancer Drug. UK Health Watchdog Recommends Against Breast Cancer Drug For Patients With Advanced Disease." From the Associated Press article. Online posting at CBS News Jun 9, 2010. Accessed 9 Jun 2010. <http://www.cbsnews.com/stories/2010/06/09/ap/health/main6566088.shtml>. Copyright 2010 The Associated Press.

143. "Uncovering Mushroom's Magic." "BREAST CANCER." From "Shiitake–Enoki–Lenti nan," Online posting. Accessed 31 Dec. 2007. <http://www.a-zbreastcancer.com/articles/amus hroom.htm>. © a-zbreastcancer.com © 1999-2008.

144. "Vaccination Quote by Medical Doctors." From whale-to-whale.com. From website: www.oasisadvancedwellness.com. Online posting. Accessed 23 Mar 2010. <http://www.oasisadvancedwellness.com/learning/vaccination-quotes-medical-doctors.html>. © 2010 Oasis Advanced Wellness, Inc.

145. "Vaccine Ingredients Aluminum." Online posting from www.novaccine.com. See article: "New Warning About Everyday Poison Linked to Alzheimer's, ADHD, and Autism," from Dr. Mercola, Food Consumer – 03/20/2010. Accessed 27 Mar 2010. <http:www.novaccine.com/vaccine-ingredients/results.asp?sc=91>. © 2008 WAVE, Inc. – World Association for Vaccine Education.

146. "Vitamin A may prevent prostate cancer." Yourhealthbase.com. Online posting. Accessed 16 Nov. 2007. <http://www.yourhealthbase.com/cancer_prostate.htm>. © 2002–2007 by Hans R.Larsen. *International Health News* website.

147. "Vitamin B6 (and Magnesium) in the Treatment of Autism." From the Autism Research Institute website, *Autism Research Review International*, 1987, Vol. 1, No. 4, page 3. Online posting. Accessed 07 Mar. 2010. <http://www.autism.com/ari/editorials/ed_vitb6.htm>.

148. "Vitamin C Injections Slow Tumor Growth in Mice," from the U.S. Department of Health and Human Services - NIH - National Institutes of Health. From an article "Embargoed for Release Monday Aug 4, 2008 5:00 pm EDT. Contact given is J. Chamberlain, NIDDK. Online posting. Accessed 29 Aug 2008. <http://www.nih.gov/news/health/aug2008/niddk-04.htm>. For more information about NIH and its programs, visit www.nih.gov.

149. "Vitamin D Cuts Pancreatic Cancer Risk by 43%." Online posting. Accessed 2 Nov. 2007. <http://www.discount-vitamins-herbs.net/n-417-pancreatic-cancer_vitamin-D.htm>. © 2001 - 2007 Discount Herbs & Vitamins, Inc.

150. "Vitamin D Deficiency Found in Patients with Lupus." From article: "Vitamin D deficiency in patients with active systemic lupus erythematosus," Borba VZ, Vieira JG, et al, Osteoporosis Int, 2008 July 4; [Epub ahead of print]. (Address: Division of Endocrinology, Universidade Federal de São Paulo, São Paulo, Brazil. E-mail: familiabborba@terra.com.br). Online posting. Accessed 10 Jul. 2008. <http://www.vitasearch.com/get/PC/summaries/get.php?id=37506>. Copyright © Vitasearch.

151. "Vitamin D deficiency rickets in black US children." From Nutrition Research Newsletter, Sept. 1994 © 1994 Frost & Sullivan, © 2008 Gale, Gengage Learning, Online posting. Accessed 07 Mar. 2010. <http://findarticles.com/p/articles/mi_m0887/is_n9_v13/ai_15855205>.

152. "Vitamin D: How Much is Enough?" "Many Americans are deficient, studies show." Online posting from Harvard Public Health Review website, Harvard School of Public Health. Spring/Summer 2007. Nutrition. Accessed 09 Feb. 2008. <http://www.hsph.harvard.edu/review/spring07/spr07vitaminD.html>. Copyright © 2007, President and Fellows of Harvard College.

153. "What's in Garden of Life's RM 10 Formulated by Jordan Rubin?" Online posting. Accessed 23 Jun. 2008 <http://www.crohns.net/Miva/productinfo/whatsinR10.shtml>. For the story of Jordan's grandmother, who was cured of advanced ovarian cancer using RM 10, see website: <http://www.crohns.net/Miva/education/testimonial_rosemenlowe.shtml>.

154. "Wheat Grass Treatment For Cancer." Cancer Tutor website. Online posting. Alternative Cancer Treatments Information Center™. Accessed 19 Nov. 2007. <http://www.cancertutor.com/Cancer/Wheat grass.html>.

155. "Wiki: Sodium Bicarbonate." Online posting from http://wapedia.mobi website. Accessed 27 Mar 2010. <http://wapedia.mobi/en/Bakng_soda>.

156. Adams, Mike. "Cancer profiteering? New chemo drug costs $30,000 a month." Online posting from NaturalNews.com Dec 10, 2009 by Mike Adams, the Health Ranger, Editor of NaturalNews.com. Accessed 09 Apr 2010 <http://www.naturalnews.com/027705_chemotherapy_fraud.html>. Natural News Network © 2009.

157. Adams, Mike. "Cordyceps mushroom is an effective cancer treatment, says new research." By Mike Adams, the Health Ranger, NaturalNews Editor. Online posting. Accessed 20 Mar. 2010. <http://www.naturalnews.com/z028409_cordyceps_cancer.html>.

157a. Adams, Mike. "Grapeseed Extract Kills 76% of Leukemia Cancer Cells in 24 Hours." From an online posting at Natural News website Jan 6, 2009 by Mike Adams, Natural News Editor. Accessed 08, Jan. 2009. <http://www.naturalnews.com/025249.html>. Natural News Network © 2008.

157b. Adams, Mike, The Health Ranger. "Pharmacists give themselves cancer from dispensing toxic chemotherapy chemicals." Online posting from Natural News website Tues July 13, 2010. See the section under "Why pharmacists are dying from cancer," and "Secondhand chemo," and "The great contradiction in cancer treatments." Accessed 13 Jul 2010. <http://www.naturalnews.com/029191_secondhand_chemotherapy_cancer.html>. Natural News Network © 2009.

157c. Adams, Mike. "Pig virus contaminates rotavirus vaccines, but FDA says no problem." Online posting from Natural News website. Accessed 20 Jun 2010. <http://www.naturalnews.com/028832_rotavirus_vaccines_contamination.html>. Natural News Network © 2009.

158. Adams, Mike. "Why Moxxor makes fish oil, krill oil and many painkiller medications obsolete." From an article at Natural News website. "The safe, natural way to ease inflammation." Online posting. Accessed 8 Jan. 2009. <http://www.naturalnews.com/moxxor_health_benefits.asp>. Natural News Network © 2008. Moxxor can be purchased at website http://www.mymoxxor.com/productListPage.aspx?ID=consumerwellness.

159. Adler, Tina. "Diet causes viral mutation in mice – selenium deficiency." Article initially from Science News, May 6, 1995. Online posting. Accessed at website http://findarticles.com

on 23 Mar 2010. <http://findarticles.com/p/articles/mi_m1200/is_n18_vf147/ai_16858569>. © 1995 Science Service, Inc. and © 2004 Gale Group.

160. Aldhous, Peter. "Vitamin C jabs may combat cancer." From an online posting at newscientist.com 08/04/08. Accessed 04 Aug. 2008. <http://www.newscientist.com/article/dn14460-vitamin-c-jabs-may-combat-cancer.html>. © Reed Business Information, Ltd.

161. Altman, Lawrence K. "A Study Finds Magnesium Cut Deaths by Heart Attack." From an online posting of *The New York Times* June 28, 1992. Accessed 07, Mar 2010. <http://www.nytimes.com/1992/06/28/world/a-study-finds-magnesium-cut-deaths-by-heart-attack.html?pagewanted=1>. © 2010 The New York Times Company.

162. Antol, Marie N. *Healing Teas: How to Prepare and Use Teas to Maximize Your Health*, (City, State, n.g.) Avery Publishing, Penguin Group (USA), Inc., 1996.

163. Arthur, John R., Geoffrey J. Beckett and Julie H. Mitchell "The interactions between selenium and iodine deficiencies in man and animals." Division of Micronutrient and Lipid Metabolism, Rowett Research Institute, Bucksburn, Aberdeen and University Department of Clinical Biochemistry, The Royal Infirmary, Edinburgh EH3 9YW, UK. Online posting. Nutrition Research Reviews (1999), 12, 55-73 doi:10.1079/095442299108728910. Accessed 23 Mar 2010. <http://journals.cambridge.org/action/displayFulltext?type=1&fid=2511804&jid=NRR&volumeId=12&issueID=01&aid=547592>. Also, see link: http://journals.Cambridge.org/action/displayAbstract?aid=547592.

164. Attiyeh E, London W, Mosse Y, et al. "Chromosome 1p and 11q Deletions and Outcomes in Neuroblastoma." *New England Journal of Medicine*. 2005; 353:2243-2253. Taken from website CancerConsultants.com article: "Chromosome Abnormalities Affect Outcomes of Neuroblastoma." Online posting 11-29-2005. Accessed 26 Aug 2008. <http://patient.cancerconsultants.com/CancerNews_Neuroblastoma.aspx?DocumentId=35491. Copyright © 1998-2008 CancerConsultants.Com.

165. Balch, James F., M.D. *The Super Antioxidants–Why They Will Change the Face of Healthcare in the 21st Century*. New York: M. Evans and Co., Inc., 1998.

166. Balch, Phyllis A., C.N.C and J.F. Balch, M.D. *Prescription for Nutritional Healing*. New York: Avery Publishing, 2000.

167. Baroody, Theodore A., N.D., D.C., Ph.D. Nutrition, C.N.C. *Alkalize or Die – Superior Health Through Proper Alkaline-Acid Balance*. Waynesville, N.C: Holographic Health Press, 1991.

168. Bergener, Kenneth E. From Burzyski Patient Group website online posting, Updated 24 May, 2005. Accessed 6 Nov 2009. <http://burzynskipatientgroup.org/kenb.html>. Also, see testimonies of other prostate cancer survivors using antineoplastons at: http://burzynskipatientgroup.org/john.htm; http://burzynskipatientgroup.org/ronaldm.htm; http://burzynskipatientgroup.org/robertm.htm; http://burzynskipatientgroup.org/ronaldg.htm; http://burzynskipatientgroup.org/carle.htm, and http://burzynskipatientgroup.org/isaiahc.htm.

169. Berkson, B.M. "A conservative triple antioxidant approach to the treatment of hepatitis C. Combination of alpha lipoic acid (thioctic acid), silymarin, and selenium: three case histories." Online posting from the National Library of Medicine. Accessed 15 May, 2009. <http://www.ncbi.nlb.gov/pubmed/10554539?dopt-abstract.> PubMed ID is 10554539.

170. Berkson, Bert, M.D., Ph.D. *The Alpha Lipoic Acid Breakthrough.* New York: Prima Publishing, Division of Random House, Inc., 1998.

171. Bharat B, Aggarwal, Anjana Bhardwaj, et al. "Role of Resveratrol in Prevention and Therapy of Cancer: Preclinical and Clinical Studies." Anti-cancer Research 2004 online posting. Accessed 25 Jan. 2008. <http://www.agrawal.org/PDF/ACR-Resveratrol1.pdf>. Study from M.D. Anderson Cancer Center and the UCLA Center for Human Nutrition.

172. Bhide, Dr. Vandana. "Probiotics, Prebiotics and Symbiotics: Lactobacillus, Saccharomyces, Bifidobacteria." "The Gut – Where Probiotics work." Online posting from naturalmedicine.suite101.com. Accessed 23 Mar 2010. <http://naturalmedicine.suite101.com/article.cfm/probiotics_ prebiotics_and_symbiotics>.

173. Black, John F. "Increase Health With Vitamin D Supplements." From an online posting Ezine articles, accessed 25 Mar 2010. <http://ezinearticles.com/?Increase-Health-With-Vitamin-D-Supplements&id=3970829>. © 2010 EzineArticles.com.

174. Blauer, Stephen. *The Juicing Book: A Complete Guide to the Juicing of Fruits and Vegetables for Maximum Health.* (City, State, n.g.) Avery Publishing, 1989.

175. Blaylock, Russell. L., M.D. *Natural Strategies For Cancer Patients.* New York: Twin Streams, Kensington Publishing Corp. © 2003.

176. Block, Betsy. "Barley Green: On the Medicinal Benefits of Barley Grass Powder." From an article at healingcancernaturally.com, "Barley Green as Medicine in Cancer And Other Diseases." Online posting. Accessed 16 Jan. 2008. <http://www.healingcancernaturally.com/barley-green-powder-medicine.html>. © 2004, 2005 & 2006 www.healingcancernaturally.com.

177. Bragg, Paul C., N.D., Ph.D. and Patricia Bragg, N.D., Ph.D. *Apple Cider Vinegar Miracle Health System.* Santa Barbara, Ca. HEALTH SCIENCE. Their website is at www.bragg.com.

178. Brandt, Johanna. *The Grape Cure.* Yonkers, New York: Ehret Literature Publishing Co., Inc., P.O. Box 24, Dobbs Ferry, N.Y., 10522, 1971. Their website is at www.arnoldehret.org.

179. Brewer, AK. "The high pH therapy for cancer tests on mice and humans." Pharmacol Biochem Behav. 1984;21 Suppl 1:1-5. Online posting from PubMed National Institutes of Health and U.S. National Library of Medicine. PMID: 6522424. NCBI. Accessed 23 Mar 2010. <http://www.ncbi.nlm.nih.gov/pubmed/6522424?dopt=Abstract>.

180. Brownstein, D. "Clinical Experience with Inorganic Non-radioactive Iodine/Iodide." From The Original Internist, 12(3):105-108, 2005. Online posting at iodine4health.com. Accessed 23 Mar 2010. <http://iodine4health.com/ortho/brownstein_ortho.htm>. © Zoe, 2006.

181. Cameron, Ewan, M.B., Ch.B., F.R.C.S., and Linus Pauling, Ph.D. *CANCER AND VITAMIN C. A Discussion of the nature, causes, prevention, and treatment of cancer with special reference to the value of vitamin C.* Philadelphia, PA., Linus Pauling Institute of Science and Medicine, Camino Books, 1979, 1993.

182. Carper, Jean. *The Food Pharmacy – Dramatic New Evidence That Food Is our Best Medicine.* New York: Bantam Books, 1988.

183. Cassel, Ingri. "A practical guide to removing toxins from the body." From the Feb 2008 Idaho Observer. Online posting. Accessed 23 Mar 2010. <http://proliberty.com/observer//20080201.htm>.

184. Cathcart, Robert F., M.D. "Vitamin C – Orthomed.com," "Polio (Klenner's Cure 1949)." Online posting. Accessed 26 Nov. 2007. <http://www.orthomed.com>. © 2005 & prior years, Robert F. Cathcart, M.D.

185. Chen, Q, Espy MG, Krishna MC, Mitchell JB, Corpe CP, Buettner GR, Shacter E, Levine M. "Pharacologic ascorbic acid concentrations selectively kill cancer cells: action as a pro-drug to deliver hydrogen peroxide to tissues." From Molecular and Clinical Nutrition Section, National Institute of Diabetes and Digestive and Kidney Diseases, National Institutes of Health, Bethesda, MD 20892, USA. PMID 16157892, PubMed website. Proc Natl. Acad Sci USA 2005 Sep 20; 102(38):13604-9. Epub 2005 Sep 12. Online posting. Accessed 20 Mar 2010. NCBI. <http://www.ncbi.nlm.nih.gov/pubmed/16157892>.

186. Clark, Hulda Regehr, Ph.D., N.D. *The Cure For All Cancers: Including Over 100 Case Histories Of Persons Cured*, Chula Vista, CA: New Century Press, 1993.

187. Claudino, Marcela, Danielle Santi Ceolin, Sandra Alberti, Tania Mary Cestari, Cesar Tadeu Spadella, Izabel Regina Fischer Rubira-Bullen, Gustavo Pompermaier Gariet, Gerson Francisco de Assis. "Alloxan-Induced Diabetes Triggers the Development of Periodontal Disease in Rats." From the Dept of Biological Sciences, School of Dentistry of Bauru, Sao Paulo University, Bauru, Sao Paulo, Brazil. Dept of Stomatology, School of Dentisty of Bauru, Sao Paulo University, Bauru, Sao Paulo, Brazil, Dept of Surgery and Orthopedics, School of Medicine of Botucatu, Sao Paulo State University, Botucatu, Sao Paulo, Brazil. Online posting of their research article. Accessed 27 Mar 2010. <http://www.plosone.org/article/info:doi%2F10.1371%2Fjournal.pone.0001320>. (cc) is licensed under a Creative Commons Attribution License.

188. Colbert, Don, M.D. *Toxic Relief.* Lake Mary, FL: Siloam, A Strang Co., 2001, 2003.

189. Condor, Bob. "Oregano Stops Inflammation of Lupus, Rheumatoid Arthritis." Insider's Health. Blog for *Altrnative Health Journal.* 21 May, 2009. Online posting. Accessed 07 Mar. 2010. <http://www.insidershealth.com/blog/1/oregano_stops_inflammation_of_lupus_rheumatoid_arthritis/226>. © 2010 InsidersHealth.com.

190. Condor, Bob. "Researcher: Flax meal beats flax oil to prevent colon cancer." June 4, 2008. Online posting from bartonpublishing.com. Accessed 22 Jun. 2008. <http://www.bartonpublishing.com/blog/2008/06/04/flax-meal-beats-flax-oil-to-prevent-coloncancer>. © 2008.

191. Connor, John G. "Cancer Prevention and Diet." Online posting. Accessed 26 Nov. 2007. <http://www.compassionateacupuncture.com/cancer.htm>. Copyright © 2005 John G. Connor. Updated Oct. 2004.

192. Dean, Carolyn, M.D., N.D. *The Magnesium Miracle.* © 2003, 2007, Ballantine Books, N.Y.

193. Derry, Dr. David. "Iodine is by far the best antibiotic, antiviral and antiseptic of all time." Online posting. Accessed 23 Mar 2010. <http://curezone.com/blogs/fmp.asp?i=1413057>.

194. Diwan, Piyush. "Consumption Of Magnesium Rich Foods Can Cut Colon Cancer Risk In Men." Online posting 03-17-2010 from TopNews.in website. Accessed 18 Mar 2010. <http://www.topnews.in/consumption-magnesium-rich-foods-can-cut-colon-cancer-risk-men-2256487>.

195. Doheny, Kathleen, HealthDay Reporter. "Magnesium Sulfate Reduces Threat of Cerebral Palsy." 08/27/2008. Online posting. HealthDay News. Accessed 01 Sept. 2008. <http://www.washingtonpost.com/wp-dyn/content/article/2008/08/27/AR2008082702634.html>. © 1996 - 2008 The Washington Post Company. Their sources for this article: Dwight J. Rouse, M.D., professor of obstetrics and gynecology, University of Alabama at Birmingham; William Zinser, M.D., pediatric neurologist, Children's Medical Center, Dallas, and associate professor of pediatric neonatology, University of Texas Southwestern Medical Center at Dallas; Aug 28, 2008, *New England Journal of Medicine.*

196. Dubin, Reese. From *Miracle Food Cures From The Bible* by Reese Dubin. © 1999 by Prentice-Hall.

197. Edelson, Stephen M., Ph.D. "Vitamin B6 and Magnesium." Online posting. Autism Research Institute. Accessed 27 Mar 2010. <http://www.autism.com/treatable/supplement/vitamin b6.htm>. © 2007-2008 Autism Research Institute.

198. Fallon, Sally and Mary G. Enig, PhD. "Dangers of Statin Drugs: What You Haven't Been Told About Popular Cholesterol-Lowering Medicines." Online posting from the Weston A. Price Foundation®. Accessed 26 Mar. 2010. <http://www.westonaprice.org/Dangers-of-Statin-Drugs-What-You-Havent-Been-Told-About-Popular-Cholesterol-Lowering-Medicines.html>. © The Weston A. Price Foundation for Wise Traditions in Food, Farming, and the Healing Arts.

199. Forgionne, Guisseppi. A., Ph.D. "Nutritional Therapy for Primary Peritoneal Cancer: A Case Study." From the CancerLynx website. Jul. 8, 2002. Online posting. Accessed 26 Nov. 2007. <http ://www.cancerlynx.com/peritonealcase.html>.

200. Gammel, Dr. Robert. This is from his 1995 article "Mercury Amalgam Fillings." This is from Health-n-Energy websites article: "Mercury Amalgam Fillings – potential health dangers." Online posting. Accessed 18 Mar. 2010. <http://www.health-n-energy.com/ARTICLES/ mercfill.htm>.

201. Gendel, Wayne. from "Tips for Great Health in the Sun - Avoid Chemicals." From the website: Sunshine is Good!- living raw foods – Naturally Savvy Get Savvy about Healthy Living. Online posting. Accessed 23 Mar 2010. <http://www.naturallysavvy.com/living-raw-foods/ sunshine-is-good>. © 2010 Healthy Shopper.

202. Goh Yl, Bollano E, Einarson TR, et al. "Prenatal multivitamin supplementation and rates of pediatric cancers: A meta-analysis." *Clinical Pharmacology and Therapeutics,* online posting, Feb 21, 2007. DOI: 10:1038/sj.clpt.6100100. From "Neuroblastoma News" CancerConsultants.com website 02/23/07. Accessed 26 Aug 2008. <http://patient.cancerconsultants.com/CancerNews_Neuroblastoma.aspx?DocumentId=39373>. Copyright © Brain Cancer Information Center on CancerConsultants.com. © Leukemia Information Center on CancerConsultants.com. © 1998 -2008 CancerConsultants.Com.

203. Gopinathan, U., Reddy MK, Nadkami MS, Desari S, Rao GN. "Antimicrobial effect of ciprofloxacin, povidone-iodine, and gentamicin in the decontamination of human donor globes." Devchand Nagardas Jhaveri Microbiology Centre, Hyderabad, India. From PubMed

website, US National Library of Medicine and the National Institutes of Health. PMID 9436880. Online posting. Accessed 23 Mar 2010. <http://www.ncbi.nlm.nih.gov/pubmed/9436880>.

204. Gottlieb, Bill. *Alternative Cures – The Most Effective Natural Home Remedies for 160 Health Problems.* (City, State, n.g.) Rodale, Inc., 2000.

205. Griffith, H. Winter, M.D. *Vitamins, Herbs, Minerals & Supplements, The Complete Guide.* Rev. Edition. (City, State, n.g.) Fisher Books, Member of Perseus Books Group, 1988, 1998.

206. Gupta, Sanjay, MD. "Smart Bomb: Vaccine for Brain Cancer; Interview with Dr. Peter" (Dr. Peter Pronovost). By the Associated Press. Online posting. Posted in Life Sciences. Accessed 18 Mar 2010. <http://www.rdmag.com/News/FeedsAP/2010/03/life-sciences-smart-bomb-vaccine-for-brain-cancer-interview-wi>.

207. Gursche, Siegfried. *Fantastic Flax, A Powerful Defense Against Cancer, Heart Disease and Digestive Disorders.* Burnaby BC V5J 5B9: Vancouver, Canada: Alive Books, 2003.

208. Gursche, Siegfried. *Good Fats and Oils, Why We Need Them and How to Use Them in the Kitchen.* Vancouver, Canada: Alive Books, 2000.

209. Hawken, C.M. *Green Foods, "Phyto Foods" for Super Health.* Pleasant Grove, UT: Woodland Publishing, 1998.

210. Hayes, Norvel. *Worship Your Foundation For The Victorious Life.* Tulsa, OK: Harrison House, 1997.

211. Heinerman, John. *Heinerman's New Encyclopedia of Fruits & Vegetables,* Reward Books 1995, p. 75 by Penguin Putnam, Inc., New York, 1995.

212. Hoffer, Abram, M.D., Ph.D., "Clinical Procedures in Treating Terminally Ill Cancer Patients with Vitamin C." Supportive Vitamin C Therapy for Cancer Patients. Online posting. Accessed 27 Nov. 2007. <http://www.doctoryourself.com/hoffer_cancer_2.html>.

213. Hoffer, Abram, M.D., Ph.D., with Linus Pauling, Ph.D. *Healing Cancer—Complementary Vitamin & Drug Treatments,* Toronto, Ontario Canada: CCNM Press, Inc. 2004.

214. Hollingsworth, Elaine. "Selenium: Prevent and Cure Cancer." From Ms. Hollingsworth book: *Take Control Of Your Health And Escape The Sickness Industry.* From Articles – Selenium at website: Doctors Are Dangerous Take Control Of Your Health And Escape The Sickness Industry. Online posting. Accessed 27 Mar 2010. <http://www.doctorsaredangerous.com/articles/selenium.htm>. © www.doctorsaredangerous.com.

215. Horne, Steven H. Co-authored by Kimberly Balas. "Iodine Robbers." April 3, 2008, Natural Healing. From heal it yourself article database. Accessed 23 Mar 2010. <http://www.healityourself.com/articlelive/articles/18/1/Iodine-Robbers/Page1.html>.

216. Howard, J.M.H. "Magnesium deficiency in peripheral vascular disease." From the *Journal of Nutritional Medicine.* From CABI Abstract www.cabi.org. Online posting. Accessed 07 Mar. 2010. <http://www.cababstractsplus.org/abstracts/Abstract.aspx?AcNo=19901450777>.

217. Howenstine, James, M.D. "How Can Iodine Deficiency Be Detected?" "Iodine is Vital For Good Health." Online posting from www.newswithviews.com website. Accessed 25 Mar 2010. <http://www.newswithviews.com/Howenstine/james37.htm>. © 2005 Dr. James Howenstine.

218. Howenstine, James, M.D. 11/05/2005. "IODINE IS VITAL FOR GOOD HEALTH." NewsWithViews.com website online posting. Accessed 23 Mar 2010. <http://www.newswithviews.com/Howenstine/James37.htm>. © 2005 Dr. James Howenstine.

219. Howenstine, James, M.D. 12/23/2003. "USE OF CoQ10 TO TREAT MALIGNANCIES." NewsWithViews.com website online posting. Accessed 20 Mar. 2008. <http://www.newswithviews.com/Howenstine/james2.htm>. Copyright © 2003 Dr. James Howenstine.

220. Hyman, Mark, M.D. "How to Rid Your Body of Mercury and Other Heavy Metals. A 3-Step Plan to Recover Your Health." from The Huffington Post 03-13-2010. Accessed 23 Mar 2010. <http://www.huffingtonpost.com/dr-mark-hyman/autism-mercury-toxicity_b_497047.html>. © 2010 HuffingtonPost.com, Inc.

221. Keegan, Lynn, Ph.D., R.N. *Healing Nutrition.* Albany, N.Y: Delmar – A Division of Thomas Learning, www.thomsonrights.com. Fax 800-730-2215. From *Healing Nutrition* 2nd Edition by KEEGAN. © 2002.

222. Kennedy, Robert F, Jr. From his article "Deadly Immunity – Autism." June 16, 2005. From the article "Deadly Immunity" at website: I-am Perfectly Healthy.com. Online posting. Accessed 23 Mar 2010. <http://www.i-amperfectlyhealthy.com/DeadlyImmunity.html>.

223. Kerfoot, Jessica. From the Burzynski Patient Group website online posting at: <http://burzynskipatientgroup.org/jessicak.htm>. Accessed 12 Dec. 2008.

224. Kimura Y. Kido T, Takaku T, Sumiyoshi M, Baba K. "Isolation of an anti-angiogenic substance from Agaricus blazei Murrill: its antitumor and antimetastatic actions." Online posting. Cancer Sci 2004 Sep;95(9):758-64, from U.S. National Library of Medicine and the National Institutes of Health PubMed NCBI website. Accessed 20 Jan 2008 PMID 15471563. <http://www.ncbi.nlm.nih.gov/pubmed/15471563?ordinalpos=1&itool=EntrezSystem2.Pentrez.Pubmed.Pubmed_ResultsPanel_RVAbstractPlus>.

225. Kloosterman, Karin. "Seaweed Biogel Heals Broken Hearts." August 18, 2008. Online posting from www.canadaisrael.ca website. Accessed 25 Mar 2010. <http://www.canadaisrael.ca/2008/8/seaweed-biogel-heals-broken-hearts>. © 2008 Canada's Israel.

226. Kowalska, Elzbieta, Steven A. Narod, Tomaz Huzarski, Stanislaw Zajaczek, Jowita Huzarska, Bohdan Gorski and Jan Lubinski. "Increased Rates of Chromosome Breakage in BRCA1 Carriers Are Normalized by Oral Selenium Supplementation." Online posting at Cancer Epidemiology, Biomarkers & Prevention website Vol. 14, 1302-1306, May 2005. © American Association for Cancer Research. Accessed 25 June 2008. <http://cebp.aacrjournals.org/cgi/content/full/14/5 /1302>.

227. Lam, Michael, M.D. "Medicinal Mushrooms." "Cancer and Immunity." Online posting. "An Insider's Guide to Natural Medicine." Accessed 27 Nov. 2007. <http://www.drlam.com/A3R_brief_in_doc_format/cancer_and_immunity.cfm>. © 2001–2004 by Dr. Michael Lam, M.D.

228. Last, Walter. "MAGNESIUM CHLORIDE for Health & Rejuvenation." Online posting. Accessed 27 Mar 2010. <http://www.health-science-spirit.com/magnesiumchloride.html>.

229. Laurance, Jeremy, Health Editor. The INDEPENDENT. "Research backs theory that vitamin C shrinks tumours." Online posting from Independent News and Media Limited. March 28, 2006. Accessed 06 Apr 2010. <http://www.independent.co.uk/life-style/health-and-families/health-news/research-backs-theory-that-vitamin-c-shrinks-tumours-471757.html>. © 2006 Independent News and Media.

230. Levy, Thomas, M.D. *Curing the Incurable Vitamin C, Infectious Diseases, and Toxins.* Henderson, NV: LivOn Books, 2002. Third Edition: 2009.

231. Levy, Thomas, M.D., J.D. GSH MASTER DEFENDER Against Disease, Toxins, and Aging. Henderson, NV: LivOn Books, 2008.

232. Levy, Thomas E., M.D., J.D. *Stop America's #1 Killer! Reversible Vitamin Deficiency Found to be Origin of ALL Coronary Heart Disease.* Henderson, NV: LivOn Books, 2006.

233. Levy, Thomas, M.D. "Vitamin C For Heart, Cancer & Infectious Diseases." From a speech given by Dr. Levy at the 35th Annual Cancer Convention – Sept. 1-4, 2007, the Cancer Control Society.

233a. Li, Dr.William. "Dramatically Effective New Natural Way to Starve Cancer and Obesity." Online posting Jun 8, 2010 from Dr. Joseph Mercola's website. Accessed 8 Jun 2010. <http://articles.mercola.com/sites/articles/archive/2010/06/08/dramatically-effective-new-natural-way-to-starve-cancer-and-obesity.aspx>. © 2010 Copyright Dr. Joseph Mercola.

234. Lloyd, Emma. "What is Medical Cannabis?" Online posting. Accessed 25 Mar 2010. <http://www.wisegeek.com/what-is-medical-cannabis.htm>. Copyright © 2003—2010 Conjecture Corporation.

235. Lockwood, K, S. Moesgaard and K. Folkers. "Partial and complete regression of breast cancer in patients in relation to dosage of coenzyme Q10." PubMed, NCBI, Biochem Biophys Res Commun. 1994 Mar 30;199(3):1504-8, p 1. Online posting. Accessed 27 Nov. 2007. <http://www.ncbi.nlm.nih.gov/sites/entrez>. PMID: 7908519.

236. Lockwood, K., S. Moesgaard, T. Yamamoto and K. Folkers. "Progress on therapy of breast cancer with vitamin Q10 and the regression of metastases." PubMed, NCBI Online posting. Entrez PubMed, Biochem Biophys Res Commun 1995 Jul. 6;212(1)72-7. Accessed 27 Nov. 2007. <http://www.ncbi.nlm.nih.gov/entrez/query.fcgi?cmd=Retrieve&db=pubmed&dopt=Abstract&list_uids=7612003>.

237. Martin, Daniel. "Aspirin a day may HARM your health and 'does not cut heart attack risk in worried well'." Online posting at www.dailymail.co.uk MAIL ONLINE website, last updated 03 March 2010. Accessed 26 Mar 2010. <http://www.dailymail.co.uk/health/article-1255005/Aspirin-day-HARM-health-does-cut-heart-attack-risk-worried-well.html>. © Associated News papers Ltd.

238. McClure, Bob. "Local doctor discovers panacea for diabetes." From the Largo Leader – Tampa Bay Newspapers. 09-03-2008. Online posting. Accessed 25 Mar 2010. <http://www.tbnweekly.com/pubs/largo_leader/content_articles/090308_lle-01.txt>. © 2003-2010 Tampa Bay Newspapers.

239. Ma E, Sasazuki S, Inoue M, Iwasaki M, Sawada N, Takachi R, Tsugane S. "High Dietary Intake of Magnesium May Decrease Risk of Colorectal Cancer in Japanese Men." From the journal Nutrition 2010 Feb. 17. For the Japan Public Health Center-based Prospective Study Group. Epidemiology and Prevention Division, Research Center for Cancer Prevention and Screening, National Cancer Center, Tokyo 104-0045, Japan. U.S. National Library of Medicine and National Intitutes of Health PubMed website, NCBI. Online posting. Accessed 07 Mar. 2010. <http://www.ncbi.nlm.nih.gov/pubmed/20164369. PMID 20164369.

240. Mauskop A, Altura BT, Cracco RQ, Altura BM. "Intravenous magnesium sulfate rapidly alleviates headaches of various types." Department of Neurology, State University of New York, Health Science Center of Brooklyn 11203, USA. From PubMed's website U.S. National Library of Medicine National Institutes of Health. Headache 1996 Mar;36(3):154-60. PMID 8984087. <http://www.ncbi.nlm.nih.gov/pubmed/8984087?dopt=Abstract>.

241. Melli, G, M Taiana, F.Camozzi, D. Triolo, P. Podini, A. Quattrini F. Taroni, G. Launa. "Alpha-lipoic acid prevents mitochondrial damage and neurotoxicity in experimental chemotherapy neuropathy." From PubMed website online posting. Accessed 26 Mar. 2010. <http://www.mitochondrial.net/showabstract.php?pmid=18809400>.

242. Mercola, Dr. Joseph. "Banned in 160 Nations…Yet U.S. FDA Regards it as Safe?" Online posting 03/06/2010. Accessed 07 Mar. 2010. <http://articles.mercola.com/sites/articles/archive/2010/03/06/why-does-fda-allow-banned-drugs-to-be-fed-to-livestock.aspx>. © 2010 Dr. Joseph Mercola.

243. Mercola, Dr. Joseph. "Drug Company Had Hit List for Doctors Who Criticized them." Online posting 04-23-2009. Accessed 13 June, 2009 <http://articles.mercola.com/sites/articles/archive/2009/04/23/Drug-Company-Had-Hit-List-for-Doctors-Who-Criticized-Them.aspx>. Copyright © by Joseph Mercola.

244. Mercola, Dr. Joseph. "Is This the New Silver Bullet for Cancer?" From an online posting Mar 11, 2010 at his website. Accessed 18 Mar 2010. <http://articles.mercola.com/sites/articles/archive/2010/03/11/is-vitamin-d-the-silver-bullet-for-cancer.aspx>. © 2010 Dr. Joseph Mercola.

245. Mercola, Dr. Joseph. "Sunlight Actually Prevents Cancer." 04-03-02. Online Posting. Accessed 27 Nov. 2007. <http://www.mercola.com/2002/apr/3/sun_prevents_cancer.htm>. Cancer March 2002;94:1867-75.

246. Mercola, Dr. Joseph. "The FDA Shuts Down Common Infant Vaccine After Startling Discovery." Online posting by Dr. Mercola April 17, 2010, from CNN March 22, 2010. Accessed 17 Apr 2010. <http://articles.mercola.com/sites/articles/archive/2010/04/17/major-vaccine-suspended-due-to-contamination-with-pig-virus.aspx>. © 2010 Dr. Joseph Mercola.

247. Meresmaa, Randolph. "Magnesium and Cancer - How Magnesium Cures Cancer." Online posting. Accessed 04 Mar. 2010. From e-zine articles® website: <http://ezinearticles.com/?Magnesium-and-Cancer---How-Magnesium-Cures-Cancer&id=2238016>. Copyright © 2010 EzineArticles.com.

248. Merkle, Jason, Jay and Patty Merkle. "Jason Merkle," from Burzynski Patient Group stories website. Online posting. Accessed Nov. 2005, Mar, Apr. 2008 and Jun. 2008. <http://www.Burzynskipatientgroup.org/jasonm.html>.

249. Miller, Donald W., Jr., MD. "Iodine for Health." Online posting from www.lewrockwell.com. Accessed 23 Mar 2010. <http://www.lewrockwell.com/miller/miller20 html>. © 2006 LewRockwell.com.

250. Miller, Donald W, Jr., MD. "Iodine in Health and Civil Defense." Presented at the 24th Annual Meeting of Doctors of Disaster Preparedness at Portland State University Aug 6, 2006. Online posting. Accessed 30 Mar, 2006. <http://www.donaldmiller.com/Iodine%20Talk.doc>.

251. Miller, Donald W., MD. "Iodine Metabolism." Online posting. Accessed 23 Mar 2010. <http://iodine4health.com/overviews/clinicians/miller_clinician.htm>. © Zoe, 2006.

252. Mindell, Earl L., R.Ph., Ph.D. with V.L. Hopkins. *Dr. Earl Mindell's What You Should Know About The Super Antioxidant Miracle.* New Canaan, CT: Keats Publishing, Inc., 1996.

253. Mindell, Earl, R.Ph., Ph.D. *Earl Mindell's Food As Medicine: What You Can Eat To Help Prevent Everything From Colds To Heart Disease To Cancer,* New York: Simon & Schuster Adult Publishing Group, 1994. © by Earl Mindell, R.Ph., Ph.D., and Carol Colman.

254. Mindell, Earl, R.Ph., Ph.D. *Earl Mindell's Soy Miracle.* New York: A fireside book, Simon & Schuster Adult Publishing Group. © 1995 by Earl Mindell, R.Ph., Ph.D.

255. Moss, Ralph W., Ph.D. *Antioxidants Against Cancer.* State College PA: Equinox Press, Inc., 2000.

256. Moss, Ralph W., Ph.D. *Cancer Therapy: The Independent Consumer's Guide to Non-Toxic Treatment & Prevention.* New York: Equinox Press, 1992.

257. Moss, Ralph W., Ph.D. *The Cancer Industry.* Brooklyn: Equinox Press, 2002.

258. Mrozikiewicz, A., D. Kielczewska-Mrozikiewicz, Z. Lowicki, E. Chmara, K. Korzeniowska, and P.M. Mrozikiewicz. "Blood levels of alloxan in children with insulin-dependent diabetes mellitus." From the Department of Clinical Pharmacology, Karol Marchinkowski University of Medical Sciences Dluga ½, 61-848, Poznad, Poland. Third Clinic of Children's Diseases, Karol Marcinkowski University of Medical Sciences, Poznad, Poland. Online posting. Accessed 27 Mar 2010. From SpringerLink – Journal Article. <http://www.springerlink.com/content/r001211h96j18266>. © Springer. Part of Springer Science+Business Media.

259. Mulwane, Marilla. "Risks of fluoride poisoning from Iceland's volcanic eruptions." Online posting from helium.com website. Accessed 14 May 2010. <http://www.helium.com/items/1829970-affects-of-fluoride-toxic-ash-on-animals-in-iceland>. ©2002-2010 Helium, Inc.

260. Nadler, Jerry L., M.D. "Diabetes and Magnesium: The Emerging Role of Oral Magnesium Supplementation." *The Magnesium Report* – Clinical Research, and Laboratory News for Cardiologists Third Quarter 2000. Paul Mason, Editor of The Magnesium Website Online Library. From the Magnesium Online Library. Online posting. Accessed 07 Mar. 2010. <http://www.mgwater.com/diabetes.shtml>.

261. Null, Gary and Martin Feldman. "Mercury dental amalgams: the controversy continues." Journal of Orthomolecular Medicine, Vol. 17. No 2, 2nd Quarter 2002, pp. 85-110. From "Amalgam dental fillings are a health hazard." Online posting at www.yourhealthbase.com.

Accessed 26 Mar 2010. From International Health News www.yourhealthbase.com "Amalgam (Silver) Fillings" and "Summaries of the latest research concerning amalgam fillings" by Hans R. Larsen MScChE. <http://www.yourhealthbase.com/amalgams.html>. © 1998-2009 by Hans R. Larsen.

262. O'Brien, James E. *The Miracle of Garlic & Vinegar and other Exciting Natural Wonders.* Globe Mini Mags®. Boca Raton, FL: Globe Communications Corp., 1991.

263. Olsen, Cynthia with contributions by Jim Chan and Christopher Gussa. *Essiac A Native Herbal Cancer Remedy* by Cynthia Olsen, Lotus Press, P. O. Box 325, Twin Lakes, WI. 53181. © 1996.

264. Passwater, Richard A, Ph.D. "New Discoveries Expand Our Knowledge About Selenium's Importance." Online posting. Accessed 27 Mar 2010. <http://www.healthy.net/scr/article.aspx?ID=477>.

265. Patrick, Kirk, citizen journalist, Aug 20, 2009. "Top Ten Natural Ways to Remove Heavy Metals." From www.naturalnews.com website. Accessed 23 Mar 2010. <http://www.naturalnews.com/026885_zeolite_heavy_metals_cilantro.html>. © 2009 Natural News Network.

266. Patton, D. "Vitamin E has protective role in bladder cancer." Online posting. News & Analysis Science and Nutrition 30/03/2004. Accessed 3 Nov. 2007. <http://<http://www.foodnavigator.com/news/news-NG.asp?id=51009>. DECISIONNEWSMEDIA SAS © 2000-2007.

267. Paul, Regina. "Holistic Use of Lugol's Iodine." Online posting at www.ehow.com. Accessed 23 Mar 2010. <http://www.ehow.com/way_5720715_holistic-use-Lugol's-iodine.html>.

268. Peterson, Dr. Dan. "Periodontal Disease Linked with Pancreatic Cancer." From "Periodontal Disease Rick (sic) Factors." Online posting at www.dentalgentlecare.com. Accessed 27 Mar 2010. <http://www.dentalgentlecre.com/periodontal_disease_rick_factors.htm>. © 1998-2008 Family Gentle Dental Care.

269. Phillips, Gavin. "The Cancer Racket." "The Hoxsey Remedies." Online posting. Accessed 28 Nov. 2007. <http://www.getipm.com/personal/cancer-racket.htm>.

269a. Proksch E., Nissen, HP, Bremgartner M, Urquhart C. "Bathing in a magnesium-rich Dead Sea salt solution improves skin barrier function, enhances skin hydration, and reduces inflammation in atopic dry skin." Online posting from Int J Dermatol. 2005 Feb;44(2):151-7. Department of Dermatology, University of Kiel, Kiel Germany from PubMed website: the U.S. National Library of Medicine and National Institutes of Health, online posting. PMID: 15689218. Accessed 30 May 2010. <http://www.ncbi.nlm.nih.gov/pubmed/15689218>.

270. Raloff, Janet. "Selenium's Value to Prostate Health." Online posting. Accessed 3 November 2007. <http://www.sciencenews.org/articles/20030510/food.asp>. © 2003 Science Service from Science News Online website.

271. Rath, Matthias: "It is the multinational pharmaceutical companies that control the world." Online posting. Accessed 4 Mar. 2010 from <http://www4.dr-rath-foundation.org/publication_library/interviews/dsalud_interview.html>. © 2010 by Dr. Rath Health Foundation.

272. Reid, Melanie. "MS link to Vitamin D deficiency hailed by politicians as giant leap forward." Online posting from The Times Online website. Accessed 8 Jun 2009. <http://www.timesonline.co.uk/tol/news/uk/scotland/article5672308.ece>. © 2009 Times Newspapers Ltd.

273. Rossi, Carey, Natural Health Expert, from an online article: "Magnesium Can Keep Your Cells Young. Getting enough of this mineral is essential for slowing aging at the cellular level." 22 May, 2008 at website STOP-AGING-NOW, America's Best Anti-Aging Vitamins & Supplements. Online posting. Accessed 07 Mar. 2010. <http://www.stopagingnow.com/news/news_flashes/4193/Magnesium-Can-Keep-Your-Cells-Young>. © 2001-2010 Stop Aging Now, LLC.

274. Rowen, Robert, MD. "Chronic iodine deficiencies and the use of Iodoral—an iodine/iodate supplement." Online posting from iodine4health.com. Accessed 23 Mar 2010. <http://iodine4health.com/overviews/clinicians/rowen_clinician.htm>.

275. Ryan, Caroline. BBC News. "Sunshine 'Prevents Cancer.'" Feb. 15, 2002. From website The Greatest Herbs on Earth™. Online posting. Accessed 28 Nov. 2007. <http://www.greatestherbsonearth.com/articles/sunshine_prevents_cancer.htm>. Copyright © 2000-2007 Greatest Herbs on Earth.

276. Sahelian, Ray, M.D. "Atrial fibrillation treatment with natural supplements, diet and food." Online posting. Accessed 07 Mar. 2010. <http://www.raysahelian.com/atrialfibrillation.html>.

277. Salaman, Maureen Kennedy. *All Your Health Questions Answered Naturally*. MKS, Inc., 1998.

278. Salaman, Maureen Kennedy. *Nutrition: The Cancer Answer II*. Menlo Park, Ca: Statford Publishing, 1995, 2002.

278a. Sampalis, Tina, M.D., Ph.D. *The Healing Power of Neptune Krill Oil*, New York, N.Y. Rebus LLC, 2005.

279. Saunders, Terri L. "Are Your Dental Fillings Making You Sick?" Online posting at www.sunherb.com. Accessed 26 Mar 2010. <http://www.sunherb.com/dental.htm>. See their herb shoppe at: http://www.sunherb.com. © 2000-2009 Sunrise Herb Shoppe.

279a. Schauzer, Gerhard, PhD., CND, FACN. "Nutritional Selenium Supplements: Product Types, Quality, and Safety." From the *Journal of the American College of Nutrition JACN*, Vol. 20 No. 1, 1-4 (2001). Online posting. Accessed 30 May 2010. <http://www.jacn.org/cgi/content/full/20/1/1>.

280. Scott, C., and Lust, John, Naturopath. *Crude Black Molasses, The Natural "Wonder Food."* (City, State, n.g.) Benedict Lust Publications, 1980, 1992.

281. Siegel, Maryjo. See website Burzynski Patient Group at http://burzynskipatientgroup.org/maryjo.htm. Accessed 05-18-2008. Site updated 02-19-2008 <http://burzynskipatientgroup.org/maryjo.htm>.

281a. Simoncini, Tullio, M.D. *Cancer Is A Fungus*. From the online posting article at cancerisafungus.com, accessed 06 Mar. 2008 <http://www.cancerisafungus.com/cancer-fungus-content.html>. Also see article "Cancer therapy with sodiumbicarbonate by Dr. Simoncini," at http://www.curenaturalicancro.com/2-treatment-sodiumbicarbonate.html Accessed 12 Jan. 2009. Also see website: <http://www.cancerfungus.com> and website: <http://www.curenaturalicancro.com, as well as <http://www.curenaturalicancro.com/treatment-simoncini-protocol.html> and website: <http://www.curenaturalicancro.com/2-side-effects-sodiumbicarbonate.html> and website: <http://www.curenaturalicancro.com/2-treatment-sodiumbicarbonate.html>.

282. Sinatra, Stephen.T., M.D., F.A.C.C. *Coenzyme Q10 and the Heart*, New York: The McGraw-Hill Companies, 1999.

283. Sinatra, Stephen, M.D., F.A.C.C. *The Coenzyme Q10 Phenomenon: The breakthrough nutrient that helps combat heart disease, cancer, aging and more*, New York: the McGraw-Hill Companies, 1998.

284. Sircus, Mark Ac., OMD. "A Magnesium Deficiency Increases Cancer Risk Significantly." Online posting from naturalnews.com. Accessed 18 April 2008, and 04 Mar. 2010, <http://www.naturalnews.com/023279_magnesium_cancer_calcium.html>. See Natural News Network © 2008, 2009.

285. Sircus, Mark Ac, OMD. *Iodine: Bring Back the Universal Nutrient Medicine* e-book. Available at website: http://publications.imva.info/index.php.

286. Sircus, Mark, Ac., OMD. *Iodine: Bring Back the Universal Nutrient Medicine.* From IMVA – International Medical Veritas Association, May 18, 2007. Online posting at website: <http://www.thenhf.com/articles/articles_502/articles_502.htm>. Accessed 08 April, 2010.

287. Sircus, Mark, Ac., O.M.D. *Magnesium Medicine. Magnesium The Lamp of Life* e-book. Also, see e-book: *Magnesium The Ultimate Heart Medicine,* also by Mark Sircus, Ac., O.M.D., and see website: http://magnesiumforlife.com/medical-application/magnesium-the-ultimate-heart-medicine, as well as website: http://publications.imva.info/index.php, and the main IMVA International Medical Veritas Association website at: http://imva.info.

288. Sircus, Mark Allan, Ac., OMD. *Sodium Bicarbonate Rich Man's Poor Man's Cancer Treatment.* From IMVA Books Dec 28, 2008. Available at online bookstores and website: <http://publications.imva.info/index.php/sodium-bicarbonate-rich-man-s-poor-man-s-cancer-treatment-e-book.html>.

289. Slahin, Guurses, Ulya Ertem, Feride Duru, Dilek Birgen, Nazmiye Yuuksek. "High Prevalence of Chronic Magnesium Deficiency in T Cell Lymphoblastic Leukemia and Chronic Zinc Deficiency in Children with Acute Lymphoblastic Leukemia and Malignant Lymphoma." From informahealthcar.com website. Online posting. *Leukemia & Lymphoma* 2000 Vol. 39, No 5-6, pp 555-562. Accessed 20 Mar. 2010.

290. Stengler, Mark, N.D. *The Natural Physician's Healing Therapies – Proven Remedies that Medical Doctors Don't Know About.* Stamford, CT: Bottom Line Books – Prentice-Hall Press, 2001. Avery Publishing, Penguin Group USA, Inc.

291. Stone, Irwin. "The Genetics of Scurvy and the Cancer Problem." "I 1331 Charmwood Square, San Jose, California 95117. This is a Transcript of a talk presented at the meeting of The California Orthomolecular Medical Society, San Francisco, 14 Feb., 1976." Online posting. Accessed 14 Aug 2008. <http://www.seanet.com/~alexs/ascorbate/197x/stone-i-ortho

mol_ psych-1976-v5-n3-p183.html>. From Orthomolecular Psychiatry, 1976, Vol 5, Number 3, PP. 183-190. HTML Revised 22 Feb, 2003. Formatting © 2001-2003 Ascorbate Web.

292. Strand, Ray., M.D. *What Your Doctor Doesn't Know About Nutritional Medicine May Be Killing You.* Nashville: Thomas Nelson Publishers®, 2002.

293. Tanner, Lindsey. "Lack of Vitamin D Raises Risk of Death." Online posting accessed 23 Jun. 2008. <http://news.aol.com/story/_a/lack-of-vitamin-d-raises-risk-of-death/20080624101309990001>. © 2007 AOL, LLC.

294. Teas J., Baldeon ME, Chiriboga DE, Davis JR, Sarries AJ, Braverman LE. "Could dietary seaweed reverse the metabolic syndrome?" Asia Pac J Clin Nutr. 2009; 18(2):145-54. University of South Carolina Cancer Center, Dept of Epidemiology and Biostatistics, 15 Greene Street 2nd Fl, Columbia SC 29208, USA. Online posting at National Library of Medicine NCBI PubMed site. US National Library of Medicine. National Institutes of Health. Accessed 07 Mar. 2010. <http://www.ncbi.nlm.nih.gov/pubmed/19713172>. PMID 19713172.

295. Tenney, D. *Medicinal Mushrooms: Cancer-fighters and Immunity Enhancers.* Pleasant Grove, UT: Woodland Publishing, 1997.

296. Thomas, Richard. *The Essiac Report Canada's Remarkable Unknown Cancer Remedy.* Los Angeles, CA. The Alternative Treatment Information Network, 1993.

297. Thompson, Dianne Jacobs. "Seawater – A Safe Blood Substitute?" Online posting. Accessed 25 Mar. 2010. <http://www.whale.to/v/Thompson.html>. Extracted from Nexus Magazine, Vol 13, Number 6 (Oct - Nov 2006), which is from their website <www.nexusmagazine.com>. © 2006 by Dianne Jacobs Thompson. From the web page: <http://www.truthquest2.com/oceanplasma.htm>.

298. Tietze, Harald W. *Papaya The Healing Fruit.* Vancouver, Canada: Alive Books, Alive Natural Health Guides, 2000 (from Andrea Ehring, author of Das Krebsheilmittel Der Aborigines: Papaya: The Cancer Healing Remedy of the Aborigines.) <http://www.alive.com>. Alive Group, Inc., Canada.

299. Tsikas, Mick. "Study finds why vitamin D is crucial – Immune system cells rely on 'sunshine' nutrient to fight infection." From a Reuters article updated March 8, 2010. An online posting at msnbc.com. Accessed 18 Mar 2010. <http://www.msnbc.msn.com/id/35762978/ns/health-diet_and_nutrition>. © 2010 Reuters.

300. Udall, K. Gilbert. *Immune and Stamina Booster Cordyceps Sinensis.* Pleasant Grove, UT: Woodland Publishing, 2000.

301. Ullyett, Joan, B.A., R.H.N. "Mercury Fillings: The Enemy Within." Online posting from MyYogaOnline.com website. Accessed 19 Mar 2010. <http://www.myyogaonline.com/healthy_living_203_MERCURY_FILLINGS:_THE_ENEMY_WITHIN.html>. © 2005-2009 Fresh Eye Productions, Inc. MyYogaOnline.com.

302. Veracity, Dani, citizen journalist. From online posting at NaturalNews.com. Jun 02, 2005. Accessed 27 Mar 2010. "White flour contains diabetes-causing contaminant alloxan." <http://www.naturalnews.com/008191.html>.

303. Weatherby, Craig and Hartnell, Randy. "Extra Virgin Olive Oil Seen Superior for Reducing Cardiac and Cancer Risks: Antioxidants Get Credit. FDA OK's heart-health claim for 'mono' fats; Antioxidants abundant only in EVOO offer added health benefits." "Antioxidants in Extra Virgin Olive Oil Add Extra Cardiac Benefits. Phenols in extra virgin grade add cardiac benefits to those imparted by its 'mono' fats." Also see section 3 on "Olive Oil's 'Mono' Fats Seen Cutting Risk of Breast Cancer. New results support and explain hypothesized anti-cancer effect of the 'Mediterranean Diet.'" From Vital Choices website online posting. Jan 2, 2006. Accessed 01 January 2008. Vol. 3, Issue 55. <http://newsletter.vitalchoice.com/e_article000507623.cfm?x=b6qDMGw,blkJpvRw>. See section 4 - "Antioxidants in Extra Virgin Olive Oil May Curb Colon Cancer" - "Findings apply only to unrefined oils; standard 'pure' oils fall short in protective polyphenols." From Vital Choices website online posting. Jan 2, 2006 Accessed 01 Jan. 2008. Vol. 3, Issue 55. <http://newsletter.vitalchoice.com/e_article000507623.cfm?x=b6qDMGw.blkJpvRw>. Source given as: Gill CI, Boyd A, et al. "Potential anti-cancer effects of virgin olive oil phenols on colorectal carcinogenesis models in vitro. Int. J. Cancer. 2005 Oct 20;117 (1):1-7.

304. Weintraub, N.D. Skye. *Selenium Heart Disease and Free-Radical Fighter.* Pleasant Grove, UT: Woodland Publishing, 1997.

305. West, Dr. Bruce. "Iodine Fulfillment Therapy." From the "Health Alert" Newsletter by Dr. BruceWest, Dec 2005, Volume 22, Issue 12. Online posting from oasisadvancedwellness.com website. Accessed 23 Mar 2010. <http://www.oasisadvancedwellness.com/learning/iodine-fulfillment-therapy.html>. © 2010 Oasis Advanced Wellness, Inc.

306. West, Larry. "Can Vaccines Cause Autism in Children?" Online posting. Accessed 27 Mar 2010. <http://environment.about.com/od/earthtalkcolumns/a/autismhtm>. From About.com: Environmental Issues. © 2010 About.com a part of the New York Times Company.

307. Wigmore, Ann. *The Hippocrates Diet and Health Program.* (City, State, n.g.) Avery Publishing, 1984.

308. Wigmore, Ann. *The Sprouting Book: How to Grow and Use Sprouts to Maximize Your Health and Vitality.* Wayne, N.J: Avery Publishing Group, Inc., 1986.

309. Wigmore, Ann. *The Wheat grass Book: How to Grow and Use Wheat Grass To Maximize Your Health and Vitality* Nov. 1984 (City, State, n.g.) Avery Publishing, member of Penguin Putnam, Inc., and The Hippocrates Health Institute, Inc., 1985.

310. Wilder, Bee. "How to Overcome Candida (Pt3)." From the Dec 2008 Nourished Magazine. Online posting. Accessed 23 Mar 2010. <http://nourishedmagazine.com.au/blog/articles/how-to-overcome-Candida-pt3>.

311. Williams, Sandra. "Dental Amalgam and Mercury Bans - Norway and Sweden Ban Mercury and Reduce Pollution." Online posting. Jan 02, 2008. Online posting. Accessed 20 Mar. 2010. <http://pollution-control.suite101.com/article.cfm/dental_amalgam_and_mercury_bans>. Sources: Health Canada, The Safety of Dental Amalgam, 2002, Stason.org, Amalgam and Mercury Free Dentistry, 2002.

312. Willner, Robert, M.D., Ph.D. "Dr. Johanna Budwig Diet Cancer, Arthritis, Multiple Sclerosis, Psoriasis, Eczema, Acne...Flax seed oil and cottage cheese." Accessed 1 Dec. 2007. <http://www.alternativehealth.co/nz/cancer/budwig.htm>.

313. Winters, Jason. "Sir Jason Winters Story – About Sir Jason Winters." Online posting. Accessed 1 Dec. 2007. <http://www.sirjasonwinters.com/story.htm>. © 1997-2007 Tri-Sun International.

314. Yeager, Selene, et al. *The Doctors Book of Food Remedies: The Newest Discoveries in the Power of Food to Cure and Prevent Health Problems - From Aging and Diabetes to Ulcers and Yeast Infections.* (City, State, n.g.): Rodale, Inc., 1998.

315. Young, Robert O., Ph.D., and Shelley Redford Young. *The pH MIRACLE Balance Your Diet, Reclaim Your Health.* New York: Warner Books, Inc. 2002. From *The pH Miracle* © 2002 by Robert Young, Ph.D.

316. Zamani M., Sharifi Tehrani A, Ali Abadi AA. "Evaluation of antifungal activity of carbonate and bicarbonate salts alone or in combination with biocontrol agents in control of citrus green mold." Dept of Plant Protection, Collage (sic) of Horticultural Science & Plant Protection, University of Tehran, Karaj, Iran. From online posting of PubMed, U.S. National Library of Medicine and National Institutes of Health. PMID 18396809. Accessed 25 Mar 2010. <http://www.ncbi.nlm.nih.gov/pubmed/18396809>.

317. Zeltner, Brie. The Plain Dealer 00-08-09. "Risk from mercury in 'silver' fillings still prompts dental debate." From Health and Fitness Northeast OH Healthy Living and Medical Consumer News. Online posting. Accessed 27 Mar 2010. <http://www.cleveland.com/health fit/index.ssf/2009/09/risks_from_mercury_fillings_st.html> © 2010 Cleveland Live, Inc.

318. Zidan, Jamal, Shetver, Likta, et al. "Prevention of chemotherapy-induced neutropenia by special honey intake." Online posting from SpringerLink Journal Article. Accessed 13 Jan. 2008. © Springer, Part of Springer Science+Business Media.

319. Ziff, S., Ziff, M.F., D.D.S. *Dentistry Without Mercury.* Orlando, FL: Bio=Probe, Inc., 1985.

INDEX

1p36LPH (chromosome), 259
24-hour Iodine Loading Test, 173
2aG4, 230
95 million vaccines contaminated, 314

A

abdominal cancer
 & grapes, 229-230
 & zinc, 138-139
ABM mushroom:
 & breast cancer, 280
 & colon cancer, 280
 & liver cancer, 280
 & lung cancer, 280
 & ovarian cancer, 280
 & sodium pyroglutamate, 280
 & solid cancers, 280
abscisic acid in wheat grass, 243-244
acai berries, 233
acetaminophen & ascorbyl palmitate, 52
acidity & cancer, 204
acidophilus milk, 54
acne :
 & kombucha, 278
 & magnesium, 121, 127
 & selenium, 148-149, 152
ADA & mercury, 287, 294
 endorses use of mercury, 297
ADD: 23,
 & magnesium, 120
additives in supplements, 329
ADHD, 23
 & aluminum, 315
 & iodine, 174
 & magnesium, 121
Adriamycin, 192-193
aflatoxin & chlorophyll, 206-207
agaricus blazeil murrill, 280
aging & magnesium, 133-134
AHCC, 212
 & immunity, 281
 & multiple myeloma, 281
akashiba (red reishi), 284
ALA & chemo, 149
 & hepatitis C, 149
 & liver transplants, 149
 & neuropathy, 149
alcohol & atrial fib, 119
alcohol use & cancer, 237
alcohol use & magnesium, 119

alfalfa, 221
 & lupus, 221
 sprouts, 221
alkalinity:
 & *Alka-Seltzer Gold®,*167, 212
 & apple cider vinegar, 208-209
 & asparagus, 207-208
 & flax, 49-50
 & grapes, 232-234
 & juice-fasting, 245
 & lemons, 245-246
 & oxygen levels, 246
 & raw foods, 216
 & raw vegetables, 232
 & wheat grass, 226-229
alkalinity, maintaining, 246
Alka-Seltzer® Gold, 167, 212
ALL (acute lymphocytic leukemia) & flax, 52
 leukemia & thymulin, 285
 leukemia & zinc, 285
allergies & dairy, 46
 & mag chloride, 127
 & magnesium, 119
 & Pycnogenol®, 237
allergies cured with bee pollen, 328
allergies-antibiotic link, 324
alloxan toxin in white flour, 155-156:
 & caffeine, 156
 & gum disease, 155-156
 causes diabetes, 155-156
almond oil, 59
aloe vera, 284, 351
 & colon problems, 49
alternative docs, 351
aluminum & ADHD, 315
 in vaccines, 303-304, 315
Alzheimer's Disease, 23
 & aluminum, 127
 & Epsom Salt, 209-210
 & magnesium, 120, 127
 & mercury, 309
 risk with flu shots, 309
amalgam fillings, danger of, 287-294
AminoSweet® (has aspartame), 34-35, 210
amla fruit & cholesterol, 224
anaplastic astrocytoma cure, 253-254
Ancient Minerals, 116, 117
anemia & fluoride, 213
 & green drinks, 227
 & spirulina, 225

INDEX

angina & magnesium, 120
Ann Wigmore, 130, 222, 226-229, 242
anorexia & leukemia, 119
anthrax & black tea, 271
anti-American groups, 316-317
anti-angiogenesis foods & tumors, 230
   sources of, 230
antibiotics:
   & allergies link, 324
   & asthma link, 324
   & autistic kids, 304
   & bacterial resistance, 325
   & breast cancer link, 324-325
   & cancer risk, 323
   & Crohn's link, 324
   & diabetes link, 324-325
   & fungal infections, 323, 325
   & mercury retention, 304
   & MRSA, 325
   & mercury vapors, 322-323
   & overkill with, 322-325
   & yeast infections, 325
   resistance & C.difficle, 325
antihistamine, reishi mushroom, 284
   & cholesterol, 85
antineoplastons:
   & anaplastic astrocytoma, 253-254
   & astrocytoma cure, 248, 249
   & bladder cancer, 260
   & brain cancers, 248-249, 258
   & brain stem tumor, 251-254
   & breast cancer, 257
   & cancer, 247-270
   & colon cancer cure, 268
   & esophageal cancer, 257-258
   & FDA fight, 255-258
   & fibrous histiocytoma, 258
   & glioblastoma cure, 254
   & glioblastoma multiforme, 260
   & Hodgkin's lymphoma cure, 261-268
   & leukemia, 258
   & lupus, 258
   & lymphomas, 257
   & mantle zone lymphoma, 258
   & Medulloblastoma, 250
   & melanoma cure (stage IV), 267-268
   & mesothelioma, 258, 268
   & multiple myeloma, 257
   & myxopapillary ependymoma, 254
   & neuroblastomas, 259

   & neuro-endocrine tumors, 258
   & optic pathway gliomas, 259
   & ovarian cancer, 257
   & pancreatic cancer, 269
   & pilocytic astrocytoma, 249
   & pinoblastoma cure, 255
   & prostate cancer, 257, 269-270
   & rhabdoid brain tumor, 251
   & stage IV melanoma cure, 267-268
   & terminal cancers, 248
   & Wilm's tumor, 258
antineoplastons vs. antineoplastics, 247-248
anti-tumor B, Chinese remedy, 286
anxiety & magnesium, 121
aosiba (blue reishi), 284
APL leukemia & vitamin A, 285
APM (aspartame), 210
apple cider vinegar & rapid alkalinity, 208-209
   & colon health, 49
   & detox, 209
   3 day alkalizer formula, 332
apple skin & cholesterol, 224
apples & colon cancer 42
arame sea vegetable, 244, 333
Arm & Hammer®, 166-167
aroma therapy for healing, 337
arrhythmias & fish oil, 119
   & magnesium, 119
arsenic & vitamin C, 62
arterial plaque & green tea, 276
arthritic pain, 23
   & krill, 57
   & kombucha, 278
   & *Pycnogenol®*, 237
   & soda bicarb, 203-204
artichoke & cancer, 230
AS2-1 & A10 antineoplastons, 249
asbestos exposure, 295
ascorbate flush, 96
ascorbyl palmitate & the liver, 62
asparagus:
   & alkalinity, 207-208
   & bladder cancer, 208
   & cancer (overall), 207-208
   & Hodgkin's, 208
   & kidney disease, 208
   & lung cancer, 208
   & skin cancer, 208
aspartame (*Equal®*), 34, 35, 210
aspartic acid, 210
aspartyl-L-phenylalanine, 210

INDEX

aspirin therapy, 188
asthma:
   & antibiotic link, 324
   & cordyceps sinesis, 281
   & glutathione, 177
   & *Lyprinol®*, 58
   & magnesium, 118-119, 121, 127
   & selenium, 147
   & vitamin C, 87
   & vitamin D, 106
asthma cure & cordyceps, 281
astrocytoma cured with antineoplastons, 248, 249
astrocytoma III, 257
astrocytomas & antineoplastons, 249
atherosclerosis & magnesium, 121
ATP Cofactor, 173
atrial fib:
   & alcohol, 119
   & *Fosamax*, 119
   & magnesium, 119
   & *Novartis AG*, 119
attacks against alternative medicine, 312-313
atypical teratoid/rhabdoid tumors, 250
autism:
   & B6, 123-124
   & Epsom Salt, 209-210
   & magnesium, 118-119, 123-124
   & measles virus, 304
   & statistics for, 302-304
   & *Super Nuthera*, 210
   & thimerosal, 302, 304
   & turmeric, 281
   & vaccines, 301, 313
   & vaccine gamble, 306
autism rates & Hep B vaccine, 303-304
autistic children & Epsom Salt, 117
autistic children:
   & antibiotics, 304
   & sulfur, 117
   & treatment for, 121
   & vaccines, 301
autoimmune disorders & vitamin D, 106
autoimmunity & wild oil of oregano, 126
Avandia & heart disease, 308, 318
avian bird flu found in measles vaccine, 311-312
avocados, 55, 182
azodicarbonamide (bromide), 320

B

B vitamins & stones, 231
B12, 189:
   & chlorella, 223
   & raw food diet, 231-232
   in spirulina, 225
   injections 225
   mist spray, 225
   nasal form, 225
   patches, 232
   sublingual, 225, 231-232
B6:
   & autism, 121, 123-124
   & cancer, 188
   & zinc & magnesium, 128
babies & honey, precautions, 244
baby's death & Hep B vaccine, 304-306
bacteria & raw foods, 217-218
bacteria & resveratrol, 236
bacteria & wine, 217-218
bacterial resistance & antibiotics, 325
Bakuryokuso barley juice, 222
baldness & fluoride, 213
banning mercury fillings, 289
barberry & cancer, 278
barley & cholesterol, 224
barley grass & carcinoma, 221-222
Barley Green™, 242
Bartter's Syndrome, 120
basal body temperature, 175
bathing & vitamin D, 96
Baycol, 318
bed sores & bentonite clay, 296
bee pollen, 213
   for allergies, 328
bee propolis & ulcers, 49
being prepared, 344-345
Bell's palsy & magnesium, 120
beneficial bacteria, 323
bentonite clay, 116:
   & bed sores, 296
   & chicken pox, 296
   & dermatitis, 296
   & itchy skin, 296
   & measles, 296
   & mercury, 296
   & MRSA, 296
   & poison ivy, 296
   & poison oak, 296
   & radiation, 296

INDEX

    & resources for, 298
benzene & vitamin C, 62
benzene, dangers of, 295
berries fight cancer, 230
best blood transfusion, 343
best food choices, 344
beta carotene & cholesterol, 224
beta carotene & esophageal cancer, 139
beta-glucan & cancer, 283
beta-sitosterol & colon problems, 50
beta-sitosterol & ulcers, 50
bicarb & kidney health, 246
Big Pharma hypocrisy, 307-308
billberry:
    & cholesterol, 224
    & colon problems, 49
    & ulcers, 49
bindweed & cancer, 230
Biogel for heart disease, 124-125
bi-polar disorders, 23:
    & GSH, 180
    & magnesium, 120
    & vaccines, 303
bird flu in the H1N1 vaccine, 316
birth defects & selenium, 148-149
black currants, 56
black seed oil, 59
black tea & anthrax, 271
bladder cancer:
    (also, see *Orange Wunder Formula*, ch. 2)
    & antineoplaston cure, 260
    & asparagus, 208
    & broccoli sprouts, 246
    & chlorine, 215
    & cure for, 20, 260
    & green tea, 277
    & *Orange Wunder Formula* (chap. 2)
    & pH, 245-246
    & polyporus umbellatus, 283-284
    & sunlight, 104
    & vitamin C, 75
    & vitamin D, 101
    & vitamin E, 153
bladder health & cranberries, 229
bladder tumors & vitamin C, 64-65
bladderwrack, 162
    heavy metal remover, 298
blindness & spirulina, 225
blood & ocean water, 138
blood acidity & cancer, 232
blood cleanser, chlorophyll, 227

blood clots (also see under blood-thinners):
    & chondroitin sulfate, 87
    & magnesium, 120
    & vitamin C, 86
blood disorders & spirulina, 225
blood pressure (also see under HTN & under high blood pressure):
    & flax, 56
    & kombucha, 278
    & magnesium, 134
    & seaweed, 334
blood sugar & hoelen, 282
    & pterostilbene, 237
blood that saves, 341-343
blood thinners & chlorophyll, 221-222
    & grapes, 233
    & maitake, 283
    & reishi, 284
Blue Ice™ cod liver oil, 95
blueberries & pterostilbene, 237
blueberries for children's cancer, 237
blurred vision & mercury, 310
Bob's Red Mill, 166-167
boils & magnesium chloride, 127
bone cancer, vitamin A & selenium, 144
bone density & vitamin C, 113
bone spurs, 232
bone tumor & *Cancell*, 352
borage oil, 43, 55, 56
    & leukemia, 52
    & retina problems, 55
botulism & vitamin C, 79
bovine cartilage, 195:
    & peritoneal cancer, 229
bowel growth & molasses, 205-206
bowel problems, 23
bowel tolerance level, 62, 98, 148
brain cancers & antineoplastons, 248-249
brain stem tumor cure, 251-254
brain tumors, 258:
    & Budwig diet, 47
    & *Cancell*, 352
    & folic acid, 99
    & prevention of, 259-260
    & vaccines, 301
    & vitamin C, 75
BRCA-1 gene & selenium, 144
breast cancer, 212-213, 257:
    & ABM, 280
    & antibiotic link, 324-325
    & chaparral tea, 271

INDEX

& chemo, 169
& chlorine, 213-214
& concord grapes, 235
& CoQ10, 143, 188, 189-190
& dairy, 109
& divine healing, 339-340
& goiter, 168-169
& iodine, 145, 163-166
& iodine protocol, 172-173
& kelp, 333-334
& lignans, 50
& *Lugol's*, 161
& magnesium, 129
& molasses, 205-206
& pterostilbene, 237-238
& resveratrol, 234-235, 237
& selenium, 137, 143, 144, 145
& sunlight, 104
& vitamin A, 95, 137
& vitamin C, 72, 74, 95, 137
& vitamin D, 95, 102, 110
& vitamin E, 95
& wheat grass juice, 228
breast cancer iodine protocol, 172-173
breast cancer rates in Japan, 163-164
breathlessness, 152
brewer's yeast, 142:
   & selenium, 151
broccoli (raw), & colon problems, 50
   & ulcers, 50
broccoli sprouts & bladder cancer, 246
bromide & iodine, 137, 159-160, 168
   & poison in white bread, 319-320
bromide banned in Europe, 320
bromide replaces iodine by bread makers, 319-320
bromide sedation, 174
bromide users fined in Singapore, 320
bromism, symptoms of, 169
bronchitis & mag chloride, 127
brown alga, 333
brucellosis & vitamin C, 79
Bubonic plague, 217-218
Budwig Formula, 23-24, 38, 45-49
   & Hodgkin's, 53
Budwig, Johanna, 44-45
buffered C, 97-98
burdock root, 272
burdock, 278:
   heavy metal remover, 298
Burzynski links, 268, 351

Burzynski, Dr. Stanislaw, 247-270
Burzynski, The Movie, 256-257
butter, 51-52

C

C.difficle & antibiotic resistance, 325
cachexia & cancer, 183
CAD (coronary artery disease) 23:
   (also, look under vitamin C)
   & GADF from grapes, 230
   & magnesium, 121
   & *Pycnogenol®*, 237
   & resveratrol, 236
caffeic acid in grapes, 229
caffeine creates alloxan, 156
Caisse, Rene, 272-276
calciferol D3, 108
calcium:
   & chick peas, 226
   & colon cancer, 145
   & magnesium, 134-135
   & oxalates, 231
   & sesame sprouts, 226
   & sunflower seeds, 226
calcium bentonite clay & mercury, 296
Calcium D-glucarate, 187:
   & cholesterol, 224
calcium lactate gluconate, 110
calcium oxalate stones, 88
calcium, excess of, 109
calcium, natural sources of, 111
calcum & prostate cancer, 135
calendula & colon problems, 49
calendula & ulcers, 49
Cancell & bone tumor, 352
Cancell & brain tumor, 352
cancer:
   & ABM mushroom, 280
   & acidity, 204
   & alcohol use, 237
   & antibiotic risk, 323
   & antineoplastons, 247-270
   & artichoke, 230
   & asparagus, 207-208
   & B6, 188
   & barberry, 278
   & berries, 230
   & beta-glucan, 282
   & bindweed, 230
   & blood acidity, 232

INDEX

& cachexia, 183
& cesium, 202-203
& chaga mushroom 280
& cherries, 230
& chlorine, 215-216
& enoki mushroom, 282
& Essiac tea, 272-276
& fish oil, 56
& flax, 50
& fucoidan, 333-334
& fungus, 197-198, 204, 212
& glutamine, 183
& green tea, 230
& iodine, 160-161, 167
& kale, 230
& lentinan (shiitake), 285
& lignans, 50
& *Lodamin*, 230
& magnesium, 118-119, 167
& *Maitake D-fraction*, 283
& maitake mushroom, 230, 282-284
& mesima mushroom, 280
& molasses, 205
& mushrooms, 280-285
& niacinamide, 70
& nutmeg, 230
& oral soda bicarb, 200
& oxygen, 48
& parsley, 230, 278-279
& pawpaw, 230
& *PRIMA-1*, 230
& *PSK* (from coriolus), 281-282
& pterostilbene, 237-238
& *Pycnogenol®*, 237
& red grapes, 230
& reishi mushroom, 284
& resveratrol, 230, 233-238
& root canals, 85
& seaweed, 333
& selenium, 150, 151
& shark cartilage, 230
& *Sir Jason Winter's* tea, 279
& soda bicarb, 334
& spirulina, 225
& split-gill mushrooms, 280
& strawberries, 230
& tea, 270-279
& THC, 183
& tinder polypore mushroom, 280
& tomatoes, 230
& turmeric, 230

& *Ukrain*, 230
& umbelliferae, 230
& vitamin C, 94
& vitamin D, 101-103
& wakame, 334
& yeast infections, 325
Cancer Control Society tours, 353
cancer diet & raw foods, 227
cancer in kids & blueberries, 237
cancer prevention & folic acid, 259-260
cancer profit cycle, 91-92
cancer rates & iodine, 170
cancer risk & selenium levels, 318
Canderel™, 210
Candida yeast, 95-96:
   & chlorophyll, 200
   & iodine, 161
   & mercury, 290, 291
   & protocol for, 96
   & *THREELAC™*, 199
Candida killers, 161
Cansema, 352
carbonated sodas, 89:
   & kidney damage, 231
   & stones, 231
carcinoma:
   & barley grass, 221-222
   & vitamin C, 75
carcinoma of stomach & vitamin C, 76
cardiomyopathy:
   & mercury, 155
   & vitamin C for, 86
carotenoids, 233
carrot juice & ulcers, 49
Casodex, 335
cat's claw, 284
cataracts, 113, 151, 180, 236:
   & selenium, 148-149
cayenne & cholesterol, 224
CDC denials, 318
Celebrex vs. *Lyprinol®*, 58
celery, 187, 189
   & cholesterol, 224
Celtic Salts, 117, 206
cerebral palsy:
   & magnesium sulfate, 120
   & magnesium, 121
cernitin & cholesterol, 187, 224
cervical cancer:
   & glutathione, 180-181
   & vitamin E, 180-181

INDEX

cesium & cancer, 202-203
CFS (chronic fatigue syndrome), 23
  & *Lyprinol®*, 58
  & mag chloride, 127
  & mag malate, 135-136
  & magnesium, 119, 120
  & malic acid, 120
chaga mushroom & cancer, 280
chaparral tea:
  & breast cancer, 271
  & colon growths, 271
  & leukemia, 271
  & melanoma, 271
Chediak-Higashi Disease & vitamin C, 83-84
Chelorex™ for selenium, 142, 151
chemical poisons, 156-157
chemotherapy:
  & ALA, 149
  & breast cancer, 169
  exposure to, 299-301
  toxicity of, 299-300, 301
cherries & cancer, 230
CHF, congestive heart failure, 23:
  & CoQ10, 191-192
  & magnesium, 118-119
chia seeds, 55
  & ulcers, 49
chick peas & calcium, 226
chicken pox & bentonite clay, 296
  & vitamin C, 63
children & mercury fillings, 296
  & root canal fillings, 296
Chinese herbs:
  & esophageal cancer, 286
  & mouth cancer, 286
Chinese parsley (cilantro), 299
Chinese red yeast rice, 187:
  & cholesterol, 224
  & guggol, 224
Chinese remedy, anti-tumor B, 286
chlorella:
  & B12, 223
  & colon health, 223
  & heavy metal detox, 222
  & interferon, 222
  & T cells, 222
  & tumors, 223
chlorella, 182, 222, 333:
  & mercury removal, 222, 291, 297
  growth factor, 222
chlorinated pools, 215

chlorine:
  & bladder cancer, 215
  & breast cancer, 213-214
  & cancer (overall), 215-216
  & chronic illness, 310
  & heart disease, 215
  & iodine, 209
chlorine bath, 215
chlorine destroys iodine, 215
chlorine in cleaning, 332
chlorine showers, 215
chlorophyll, 221-228:
  & aflatoxin, 206-207
  & Candida yeast, 200
  & colon cancer, 206-207
  & endocarditis, 221
  & hemoglobin, 227
  & liver cancer, 206-207
  & pancreatic health, 221
  & PCN, 221
  & ulcers, 221
  & wound healing, 221
  blood cleanser, 227
  blood thinner, 221-222
  in mouth washes, 227
  vs sulfa, 221
chlorophyllin, 206-207
cholesterol:
  & amla fruit, 224
  & antihistamines, 85
  & apple skin, 224
  & barley, 224
  & beta carotene, 224
  & bilberry, 224
  & *Calcium D-glucarate*, 224
  & cayenne, 224
  & celery, 224
  & cernitin, 224
  & Chinese red yeast rice, 224
  & cinnamon, 224
  & citrus pectin, 224
  & *Ecklonia Cava*, 224
  & exercise, 224
  & fenugreek, 224
  & flax, 56, 224
  & garlic, 224
  & ginger, 224
  & ginseng, 224
  & green foods, 223-224
  & green tea, 224
  & guggolipids, 224

INDEX

& hibiscus tea, 224
& iodine, 159, 224
& juicing, 224
& kombucha, 224, 278
& krill oil, 224
& krill, 57
& lecithin, 224
& magnesium, 224
& niacin, 85, 223-224
& oat brain, 224
& olive oil, 224
& omega-3, 224
& policosanol, 224
& pomegranate, 224
& pterostilbene, 237
& red grapes, 224, 230
& reishi mushroom, 224
& resveratrol, 224
& rye bread, 224
& *Seanol®*, 224
& shiitake, 224, 285
& spirulina, 224, 225
& steel cut oats, 224
& *V8®* low sodium veg juice, 224
cholesterol levels & mercury, 319
cholesterol lowering, 187-188
chondroitin sulfate & blood clots, 87
choroid plexus neoplasm, 258
chronic illness & chlorine, 310
   & fluoride, 310
chronic myeloid leukemia & vitamin C, 75
chronic renal failure, 203
cilantro (Chinese parsley), 299:
   & pre-cancerous lesions, 299
   & chelation pesto recipe, 298
   for detox, 154
   for getting rid of mercury, 154, 291, 298
cinnamon & cholesterol, 224
Cipro vs Iodine, 217
circulation problems:
   & flax for, 56
   & garlic for, 130
   & ginger for, 130
   & ginkgo biloba for, 130
   & grape extract for, 234
   & magnesium for, 127
   & niacin for, 130
cirrhosis & selenium, 152
Cisplatin, 149
claiming God's promises, 339, 344-345
clean water & iodine, 216-217

CLL leukemia & green tea, 276-277
clostridium bacteria in dental work, 288
CML leukemia & vitamin A, 285
CNS tumors in children, 250
coconut milk & ulcers, 49
coconut oil, 59
coconut water & colon problems, 49
   & ulcers, 49
cod liver oil, 95
colds, 23 (also, see under common cold):
   & vitamin C for, 63
colitis & magnesium, 127
   & wheat grass, 226
colon cancer:
   & ABM, 280
   & apples, 42
   & calcium, 145
   & chaparral tea, 271
   & chlorophyll, 206-207
   & flax seed, 53
   & lignans, 50
   & magnesium, 121-122, 129
   & molasses, 205-206
   & resveratrol, 234-235
   & soda bicarb, 212
   & sunlight, 104
   & vitamin C, 75
   & vitamin D, 102, 145
colon cancer cure:
   with antineoplastons, 268
   with *Essiac®*, 275
colon health:
   & apple cider vinegar, 49
   & chlorella, 223
   & spirulina, 225
colon problems:
   & aloe vera juice, 49
   & beta-sitosterol, 50
   & bilberry, 49
   & calendula, 49
   & coconut water, 49
   & fish oil, 49
   & ginger, 50
   & green tea, 49
   & krill, 50
   & *Magnascent©* Iodine, 50
   & olive leaf extract, 49
   & oregano, 49
   & propolis, 49
   & raw broccoli, 50
   & spinach juice, 49

INDEX

& white tea, 49
color therapy & healing, 337
colorectal cancer:
   & grape seed extract for, 234
   & magnesium for, 122
   & selenium for, 142-143
comedy & healing, 337
common cold:
   & maitake, 282-283
   & vitamin C, 62
   & *Methotrexate*, 235
concord grapes for breast tumors, 235
conjunctivitis & mag chloride, 127
   & iodine, 127
constipation & flax seed, 56
contamination of polio vaccines, 314
COPD (chronic obstructive pulmonary disease):
   & magnesium, 118-119, 121
copper:
   & zinc ratios, 139
   copper levels, 285
   copper vs zinc, 285
CoQ10, 185-196:
   & breast cancer, 143, 188, 189-190
   & CHF, 191-192
   & diabetes, 185
   & gum disease, 185
   & HTN (hypertension), 185
   & leukemia, 188, 191, 192-193, 194
   & liver cancer, 189-190
   & lung cancer, 189-190
   & melanoma, 193
   & MS, 193-194
   & multiple myeloma, 193
   & pancreatic cancer, 188-189, 194
   & peritoneal cancer, 195, 228-229
   & prostate cancer, 194
   & statins, 187-188
CoQ10 dosing, 190, 191
CoQ10, sources of, 192, 194
Cordyceps sinensis mushroom, 281
   & HIV, 281
   & asthma cure, 281
coriander sativum leaf tincture, 297
Coriolus versicolor (karawatake), 281
   & HIV, 282
corneal transplants, 217
CorOmega® 3, 31
cow's milk & diabetes, 46
C-peptide, 172

cramps & magnesium, 127
cranberries:
   & bladder health, 229
   for leukemia, 229
   for ulcers, 229
craniopharyngioma, 258
C-reactive protein, 122, 125
cretinism, 145, 168, 174
critics threatened by *Vioxx*-maker, 307-308
Crohn's Disease, 23, 284:
   & antibiotic link, 324
   & NSAID usage, 324
   & oil of oregano, 126
   & oral contraceptives, 324
   & vaccines, 301
CRP (C-reactive protein), 122, 125
cruciferous veggies, 223
CSS (chronic subclinical scurvy), 66
CSS Syndrome, 83
cyanide & vitamin C, 62
cysteine, 177
   for heavy metal detox, 298
cystic breasts, 23
   & selenium, 152
cystic fibrosis:
   & selenium, 148-149
   & vaccines, 303
cystine stones, 88
cytomegalovirus (CMV) & vitamin C, 79

D

dairy products:
   & breast cancer link, 109
   & ovarian cancer link, 109
   & prostate cancer link, 109
   & uterine cancer link, 109
damage from *Gardasil*®, 306-307
Dead Sea, 115
deadly mushrooms & vitamin C, 62
deaths from *Gardasil*®, 306-307
declaring God's promises, 339
dementia, 23:
   & magnesium, 120
dengue fever, cure for, 80, 99
   & iodine, 167
   & vitamin C, 79, 80, 99
dental fillings, dangers of, 153-154
dental health & green tea, 276
dental implants, 86
dental revision dentists, 86, 352

INDEX

dental workers & mercury toxins, 290
dentists who remove mercury, 297-298
deodorizers, 295
depression, 23, 85:
   & magnesium, 118-119, 120
   & vitamin D, 106
   vs praise, 346-347
dermatitis & bentonite clay, 296
   & magnesium, 121
detox, 329-338:
   & apple cider vinegar, 209
   & cilantro, 154
   with lemonade, 211
   with seaweed, 333
   safe detox, 327-338
Detoxamin® for lead, 298
DGL & ulcers, 49
DHEA, 118
diabetes:
   & alloxan, 155-156
   & antibiotic link, 324-325
   & CoQ10, 185
   & dairy, 46
   & iodine link, 172
   & magnesium, 118, 122-123
   & pterostilbene, 237-238
   & selenium, 149, 165
   & spirulina, 225
   & vaccines, 301
   & vitamin C, 81-82, 86, 94
   & vitamin D, 102, 105, 106, 107
diabetic neuropathy, 129
diabetic retinopathy & grape extracts, 234
digestion & molasses, 205-206
digestive health & wheat grass, 226
diphtheria & mag chloride, 127
diphtheria & vitamin C, 79
disease:
   & lysine, 92
   & magnesium chloride, 126-127
   & vitamin C, 92
   resistance & iodine, 325
disinfectant, wheat grass juice, 226
dissolving blood clots, 86
distilled water, 216
diuretic (natural), parsley, 278-279
diuretics & magnesium, 118
divine healing & breast cancer, 339-340
divine intervention in healing, 339-350
DOI (*Daily Optimal Intake*), 97
door to the shepherd, 343

Down's Syndrome & selenium, 148-149
Dr. who cured polio, 312
drinking water & lead, 216
drug recalls, 308-309
dry skin, 23
dulse sea vegetable, 244, 333
dysarthria & mercury, 310
dysentery & vitamin C, 79

E

ear infections & dairy link, 46
Ebola, 88, 150-151
   & vitamin C, 79, 97
Ecklonia Cava & cholesterol, 187, 224
eczema:
   & magnesium, 121, 127
   & turmeric, 281
   & vitamin C, 86
   & vitamin D, 106
ellagic acid:
   & grapes, 229
   & immunity, 229
   sources of, 299
Embolization Particle Therapy, 230
encephalitis & vitamin C, 79
ending a detox program, 212
ending a fast, 212, 336-337
endocarditis & chlorophyll, 221
endometriosis & milk thistle, 181
energy:
   & kombucha, 278
   & resveratrol, 236
enoki mushroom & cancer, 282
epilepsy & magnesium, 128
Epsom Salt, 117
   & Alzheimers, 209-210
   & autism, 209-210
   & Parkinson's, 209-210
   & rheumatoid arthritis, 209-210
Epstein-Barr virus, 80
Equal®, 34-35, 210
ergocalciferol, D2, 108
esophageal (& neck) cancer:
   & antineoplastons, 257-258
   & beta carotene, 139
   & Chinese herbs, 286
   & selenium, 286
   & sunlight, 104
   & zinc, 138-139, 286
Essiac® tea, 209, 330:

INDEX

& cancer (overall), 272-276
& colon cancer, 275
& liver cancer, 272
& rectal cancer, 272
& stomach cancer, 272
Essiac, precautions for, 276
estrogen & milk thistle, 181
evening primrose oil, 43, 56
   & leukemia, 52
EVOO, 58
eXcella™ sweetener, 352
excess estrogen & selenium, 152
exercise & cholesterol, 224
eye health & resveratrol, 235-236
eye infections & iodine, 167
   (also, see conjunctivitis)
eye tics & magnesium, 121
eye wash with iodine, 217

F

fat digestion & milk thistle, 181
fatty liver & RM-10, 284
FDA, 146:
   & mercury, 287
   & mercury hearing, 310
   & bromide approval, 319-320
   & Burzynski struggle, 255-258
   admits mercury fillings harmful, 291
   approves toxic ractompamine, 320-321
   denials, 318
   disregard for human life, 320-321
   fights antineoplastons, 255-258
   fights vitamin manufacturers, 260
   hypocrisy of, 307-308, 313
FDA/mercury hearing, 310
female disorders, 23
fenugreek & cholesterol, 224
fever & magnesium chloride, 127
fever blisters & vitamin C, 6
fibrocystic breast disease:
   & cure with iodine, 168-169
   & selenium, 148-149
fibromyalgia, 23, 232:
   & mag malate, 135-135
   & magnesium, 119, 120, 121
   & malic acid, 120
fibrous histiocytoma, 258
fighting battles with worship, 347
fighting bromide, 173-174
fillings, safe removal of, 319

final steps, 345-346
Finasteride, 335
fish, best types of, 96
fish oil:
   & arrhythmias, 119
   & cancer, 56
   & HIV, 56
   & ulcers, 49
fish vs flax, 56
flash-pasteurized juices, 243
flax (also, see under flax oil):
   & blood pressure, 56
   & cancer, 50
   & cholesterol, 56, 224
   & circulation, 56
   & gallstones, 52
   & leukemia, 52
   & lupus nephritis, 54
   & lupus, 52, 54
   & shingles, 52
   varieties of, 51
flax oil, 43-60
   & MS, 55
   & skin health, 106
   & colon cancer, 53
flax seed, 43-60:
   & constipation, 56
   & stomach problems, 49
   varieties of, 51
flax vs fish, 56
Floradix®, 33, 115
Flor-Essence®, 273-274
flu, 23:
   & magnesium chloride, 127
flu season, explanation for, 283
flu shot increases Alzheimer risk, 309
flu vaccines & mercury, 155
flu virus & selenium, 150-151
fluid intake & stones, 231
flukes, 295
fluoride:
   & anemia, 213
   & chronic illness, 310
   & iodine needs, 137, 168
   & liver damage, 213
   & osteosarcoma, 213
   & thyroid problems, cause of, 213
   & vitamin C, 62
fluoride poisoning, 214-216
fluoride water & infant death, 213
Fluorouracil, 174

INDEX

folic acid, 107
  & brain tumors, 99
  & leukemia, 99
  & neural tube defects, 99, 260
  & neuroblastoma, 99
  & spinal cord defects, 99, 260
  for cancer prevention, 259-260
food chemicals, 157
food safety, 219:
  & iodine, 218
foods with pesticides, 218
Fosamax & atrial fib, 119
free radicals, 186, 232-233
freeze-dried broccoli sprouts, 246
French paradox, 234
fresh air, 331
fresh grapes & their juices, 330-331
Fruit/Vegetable Drink (39)
fucoidan & cancer, 333-334
fungal infections & antibiotics, 323, 325
fungus & cancer, 197-198, 204, 212

G

G6PD deficiency, 80
GADF from grapes & CAD, 230
gallbladder & magnesium, 127
gallstones, 230-231:
  & flax, 52
  & lignans, 50
gambling with vaccines, 312
gangrene & magnesium, 130
Gardasil®, 315:
  & *Gullain-Barré*, 306, 307, 313
  deadly statistics for, 306-307
Garden of Life®, 283-284
  & *Primal Defense®*, 324
garlic:
  & cholesterol, 224
  & circulation, 130
  heavy metal remover, 298
gastric cancer & vitamin D, 102
Gentamycin vs iodine, 217
germs & iodine, 244
GSH (glutathione) & premature aging, 179
ginger:
  & cholesterol levels, 224
  & circulation, help for, 130
  & colon problems, 50
  & morning sickness, 50
  & nausea, 50

  & ulcers, 50
ginkgo biloba & circulation, 130
ginseng, 187:
  & cholesterol, 224
GLA oil, 55, 56
glaucoma:
  & glutathione, 177
  & THC, 183
  & vitamin C, 177
glioblastoma:
  & vitamin C, 67
  cure with antineoplastons, 254
glioblastoma multiforme cure, 260
glutamic acid, 177
glutamine, 28, 31
  & cancer, 183
glutathione (GSH), 23, 150, 177-184
  (also, see GSH):
  & asthma, 177
  & cervical cancer, 180-181
  & heavy metals, 177
  & mercury removal, 298
gluten, 156:
  & gluten allergies, 221
  & gluten-free products, 327
glycine, 177
glyconutrients, 284
GMO (genetically-modified foods), atrocity, 146
God's "green thumb" 221-246
God's great heartbreak, 346
God's remarkable provision, 341-342
goiter & breast cancer, 168-169
goiter & iodine, 159
Golden Green Tea, 276
gout, 88-89:
  & oxalates, 230-231
  & soda bicarb, 203-204
  & sour cherries, 231
  & spirulina, 225
  & vitamin C, 231
grape extract for circulation, 234
grape extract for diabetic retinopathy, 234
grape juice, 185-186
grape seed:
  & vitamin C precaution, 234
  & colorectal cancer, 234
  & leukemia, 235
grapes, organic, 236-237:
  & abdominal cancer, 229-230
  & alkalinity, 232-234
  & blood-thinning, 233

INDEX

& caffeic acid, 229
& ellagic acid, 229
& OPCs, 238
& *Pycnogenol®*, 237
& quercetin, 237
grapes vs wine, 237
grapes, best choices, 238
Great Salt Lake & mercury, 295
green drinks & anemia, 227
   & leukemia, 227
green foods & cholesterol, 223-224
   & vitamin K, 221-222
green grasses, 223
green juices, 323
green juices, consumption of, 243
Green Kamut®, 242
Green Miracle juice, 243
green powdered juices, 242-243
green powders, concentrated, 243
green tea, 276-277:
   & arterial plaque, 276
   & bladder cancer, 277
   & cancer (overall), 230
   & cholesterol, 224
   & CLL leukemia, 276-277
   & colon problems, 49
   & dental health, 276
   & halitosis, 276
   & leukemia, 276-277
   & reishi for sarcoma, 277
   & stomach cancer, 277
   & ulcers, 49
green-lipped mussel, 57
greens, juicing of, 240
Grifon®, 35
GSH (also, look under glutathione):
   & bi-polar disorders, 180
   & cataracts, 180
   & liver health, 179
   & Parkinson's, 180
   & schizophremia, 180
   & skin disorders, 181
   how to use, 182
   sources of GSH, 180
guggol & Chinese red yeast rice, 224
guggol & cholesterol, 224
guggulipids & cholesterol, 224
Gullain-Barré & *Gardasil®*, 306, 307, 313
gum disease:
   & alloxan, 155-156
   & CoQ10, 185
   & pancreatic cancer, 299

H

H1N1 vaccine, 46, 80-81, 315-316:
   contaminated with bird flu virus, 316
Haelan, 46
hair color:
   & kombucha, 278
   & molasses, 205-206
   & wheat grass juice, 130
hair growth & kombucha, 278
hairy cell leukemia & vitamin C, 76
halitosis & green tea, 276
hand washing, 219
handling chemo drugs & risks, 299-301
hantavirus & vitamin C, 79
harmony healing, 18
hay fever & magnesium, 127
HCL & hoelen, 282
HDM™, Heavy Metal Detox, 297
headaches & magnesium, 123
headaches & mercury, 310
healing:
   & aroma therapy
   & color therapy, 337
   & comedy, 337
   & divine intervention, 339-350
   & music, 337
healthy fish, 57
heart damage:
   & mercury, 294-295
   & vaccines, 155
heart disease:
   & *Biogel*, 124-125
   & chlorine, 215
   & lysine, 86
   & magnesium, 119, 124
   & proline, 86
   & pterostilbene, 237
   & vitamin C, 81-82, 84-86
   & vitamin D, 105
heart disease protocol, 86, 92
heart failure & mercury, 155
heart health & mag taurate, 134-135
heart problems & mercury, 310-311, 319
heart transplant, 155
heartburn & flax, 49
heavy metal chelator, *Zeolite*, 298
Heavy Metal Detox (HMD™), 297
heavy metal detox, 333:

INDEX

& bladderwrack, 298
& burdock, 298
& chlorella, 222
& cilantro, 154
& cysteine, 298
& garlic, 298
& glutathione, 177
& iodine, 299
& spirulina, 225
hemoglobin & chlorophyll, 227
hemorrhagic fever & vitamin C, 79
Hepatitis B, 146-147:
   the vaccine:
     & autism rates, 303-304
     & baby's death, 304-306
   vaccine video, 317-318
hepatitis:
   & liver cancer, 149
   & vitamin C, 82
hepatitis C & ALA, 149
   & selenium, 149
   & silymarin, 149
herbalene, 279
herbs in bulk orders, 352
herpes & vitamin C, 79
herpes zoster & mag chloride, 127
Herxheimer's reaction, 290-291
hexane, dangers of, 295
hibiscus tea & cholesterol, 224
hiding bromide in flour (*azodicarbonamide*) 320
hiding mercury in consumer products, 309
high blood pressure, 23
   (also, see under HTN & under blood pressure)
high cholesterol, 23
   (also, see cholesterol)
   & magnesium, 120
   & reishi mushroom, 284
   & vitamin C, 84-86
high grade gliomas, 258
Himalayan Salt, 117, 206
himematsutake, (ABM), 280
histamine levels, 85
HIV, 23, 80, 278
   & cordycepin, 281
   & coriolus, 282
   & fish oil, 56
   & kombucha, 278
   & selenium, 150
   & turmeric, 281

& vaccine link, 314
& vitamin C, 83-84
hiziki sea vegetable, 244
HMD™, Heavy Metal Detox, 298, 299
Hodgkin's disease (also see under lymphoma):
   & asparagus, 208
   & Budwig diet, 53
   & vitamin C, 70-71, 75
   cure for, 261-268
Hodgkin's lymphoma testimonial, 352
hoelen mushroom:
   & blood sugar, 282
   & HCL, 282
   & kidney problems, 282
   (Poria cocos) & lupus, 282
homemade liposomal C, 36-38
homeostatic soil organisms, 324
hommacord of cell-decimated chlorella, 297
homocysteine & vitamin C, 86
honey precautions in babies, 244
honey for nausea & vomiting, 334
Host Defense®, 285
household products with mercury, 309
how fluoride kills, 214-216
Hoxsey's famous tea, 277-278
HRT (synthetic), 131-132
HSO Primal Defense, 213
HSO Probiotic Formula, 324
HTN (hypertension; also see under high blood pressure):
   & CoQ10, 185
   & iodine, 167
   & magnesium, 120
   & red grapes, 230
   & sesame oil, 224
   & spirulina, 225
human studies on amalgam fillings, 292
hydrogenated fats, 44-45, 51
hyperkeratosis & mag chloride, 127

I

idiopathic cardiomyopathy, 155
immune system killers, 287-326
immunity:
   & AHCC, 281
   & ellagic acid, 229
   & magnesium, 137
   & mercury fillings, 296
   & shiitake, 285
   & wheat grass juice, 227-228

INDEX

Immunocal, 179
impotence & magnesium, 127
IMVA, 115, 352
Indian deaths from *Gardasil®*, 306
Indian sage, 279
infant botulism, 244
infant death & fluoride water, 213
infected wounds & bentonite clay, 296
inflammation:
    & magnesium, 125-126
    & oil of oregano, 126
    & pepper, 126
    & turmeric, 126
inflammatory breast cancer, 168-169
Innate Response™ selenium, 151
insect bites & Na bicarb, 203
insomnia & magnesium, 118-119
    & mercury, 310
insulin (also, see under diabetes):
    & iodine, 172
    & vitamin C, 81-82, 94
insulin resistance, 122-123
interferon & chlorella, 222
intestinal cancer & selenium, 146
Intracellular Free Magnesium Test, 133
Iodine Protocol, 169, 172-173
iodine, 159-176:
    & ADHD, 174
    & breast cancer, 145, 163-166
    & bromide, 137, 168
    & cancer rates, 161, 167, 170
    & Candida, 161
    & chlorine, 209
    & cholesterol, 159, 224
    & clean water, 160-161, 216-217
    & dengue fever, 167
    & disease resistance, 325
    & eye infections, 167, 217
    & fibrocystic breast disease, 168-169
    & fluoride, 137, 168
    & food safety, 218
    & HTN (hypertension), 167
    & insulin levels, 172
    & lumpy breasts, 174-175
    & mental retardation, 174
    & mercury, 137
    & metabolic syndrome, 159
    & parasites, 161
    & percolate, 137
    & poison ivy, 167
    & prostate cancer, 163, 168-169
    & sinus infections, 167
    & sore throat, 126, 174
    & throat infections, 167
    & thyroid health, 152
    & tumor-shrinking, 170-171
    & urinary infections, 167
    & venereal disease, 167
Magnascent© Iodine, 337
consumption of, 244
deficiency of & cancer, 162
for germs, 244
for heavy metal detox, 299
for the thyroid, 162
in seaweed, 244
kills malaria, 169
kills yeast, 161-162
precautions for using, 160
removes mercury, 166
replaced with toxic bromide, 319-320
sources of, 160
Iodine vs *Cipro*, 217
    vs *Gentamycin*, 217
    vs. bromine, 159-160, 215
    vs. chlorine, 215
iodine diabetes link, 172
Iodoral iodine, 162
IPT therapy (*Insulin Potentiation*), 352
irradiating food, safety of, 217
irritable bowel, 23
isopropyl alcohol & parasites, 295-296
isothyiocyanates (ITC), 246
Issels Treatment Centers, 189
itchy scalp & wheat grass, 226
itchy skin & bentonite clay, 296

J
Jesus is your HEALER, 347
Johanna Brandt, 229-237
Johanna Budwig Formula, 216
juicing, 238-245
juice-fasting & alkalinity, 245
juicers (best), pros & cons, 238-241
juicing & cholesterol, 224
juicing output, 240-241
juicing, what to juice, 241-242
Just Barley™, 242

K
kale, 223:
    & cancer, 230

INDEX

karawatake (*Coriolus versicolor*), 281
Kashin-Beck Disease, 145
kefir, 323
kelp sea vegetable, 244, 333:
  & breast cancer, 333-334
  prevents strontium-90 absorption, 333
Keshan's Disease, 145, 150:
  & selenium, 150
  & vitamin E, 150
kidney cancer & vitamin C, 64-65
kidney damage:
  & carbonated sodas, 231
  & mercury, 292, 295
kidney disease & asparagus, 208
kidney health:
  & asparagus, 208
  & bicarb, 246
  & milk thistle, 181
  & hoelen, 282
  & iodine, 175
kidney stones, 88, 230-232:
  & magnesium, 121
kishiba (yellow reishi), 284
kisshotake (lucky fungus), reishi, 284
knowing Jesus, 340-341
kombu sea vegetable, 244, 333
  & acne, 278
kombucha:
  & arthritis 278
  & blood pressure, 278
  & cholesterol, 224, 278
  & energy, 278
  & hair color, 278
  & hair growth, 278
  & immunity, 278
  & wrinkling, 278
  kombucha tea, 278
krill oil: 55, 59, 187
  & arthritic pain, 57
  & cholesterol, 57, 224
  & colon problems, 50
  & PMS, 57
  & ulcers, 50
kuroshiba (black reishi), 284
Kyasanur Forest Disease, 79

L

Lapatinib (*Tykerb*), 73
L-arginine, 86
lassa fever & vitamin C, 79

lassi (Indian yogurt), 323
lead in drinking water, 216
lead remover, *Detoxamin®*, 298
lecithin & cholesterol, 224
  & vitamin C, 82
lemon grass, 276
lemonade & lemons:
  acidity of, 210
  alkalinity, using for, 210, 245-246
  detox with, 211
  detox with – 7 days, 332
  detox with – 10 days, 333
lemons & limes for alkalinity, 332
lentinan (shiitake) & cancer, 285
leprosy & vitamin C, 79
leukemia, 258:
  & anorexia, 119
  & borage oil, 52
  & chaparral tea, 271
  & CoQ10, 188, 191, 192-193, 194
  & cranberries, 229
  & evening primrose oil, 52
  & flax, 52
  & folic acid, 99
  & grape seed extract, 235
  & green drinks, 227
  & green tea, 276-277
  & magnesium, 119, 128, 129
  & resveratrol, 234-235
  & spirulina, 225
  & thymulin, 285
  & vitamin C, 70
  & zinc, 285
leukemia (ALL) & thymulin, 139
  & zinc, 139
leukemia (APL) & vitamin A, 139
leukemia (CML) & vitamin A, 139
leukemia prevention, 259-260
leukoplasia & magnesium chloride, 127
Life Mel Honey, 25
LifeStraw®, 216-217
LifeWorks Wellness Center, 352
lignans:
  & bad estrogen, 51
  & breast cancer, 50
  & colon cancer, 50
  & gallstones, 50
  & prostate cancer, 50
  & uterine cancer, 50
lime juice acidity, 210
limes for rapid alkalinity, 210

INDEX

linol acids, 49
Lipitor injuries, 308
liposomal C, 29, 65, 93, 130, 142, 178
liposomal glutathione (GSH), 177-178
liver & ascorbyl palmitate, 62
liver cancer:
  & ABM, 280
  & chlorophyll, 206-207
  & CoQ10, 189-190
  & *Essiac* tea, 272
  & hepatitis, 149
  & resveratrol, 237
  & selenium, 146-147
  & shiitake, 285
liver damage & fluoride, 213
liver health & GSH, 179
liver transplants & ALA, 149
  & selenium, 149
  & silymarin, 149
Lodamin & cancer, 230
Lou Gehrig's & mercury, 309
  & selenium, 152
Lugol's Iodine, 31-32, 160-161, 165, 166
  & breast cancer, 161
Lugol's, homemade, 161, 353
lumpy breasts & iodine, 174-175
lung cancer:
  & ABM, 280
  & asparagus, 208
  & CoQ10, 189-190
  & glutathione (GSH), 180
  & PSK, 281-282
  & resveratrol, 234-235
  & selenium, 142-143, 147
  & vitamin C, 71-72, 74
lupus, 23, 182, 258
  & alfalfa precaution, 221
  & flax, 52, 54
  & hoelen mushroom, 282
  & vitamin D, 106-107
lupus nephritis & flax, 54
lymphoma:
  & cure with antineoplastons, 257
  & magnesium & zinc for, 128-129
  & vitamin C, 64-65, 72-73, 147-148
lymphosarcoma & vitamin C, 75
Lypo-Spheric™ C, 29, 178
Lyprinol®, 55, 57-58:
  & asthma, 58
  & CFS, 58
  & rheumatoid arthritis, 58

  vs *Celebrex,* 58
Lyrica injuries, 308
lysine & disease, 92
  & heart disease, 86

M

mad cow disease & selenium, 150-151
mag chloride, 127 (also look under
  magnesium:
mag chloride & boils, 127
  & bronchitis, 127
  & CFS, 127
  & chronic mastitis, 127
  & conjunctivitis, 127
  & diphtheria, 127
  & fever, 127
  & flu, 127
  & herpes zoster, 127
  & hyperkeratosis, 127
  & leukoplasia, 127
  & mumps, 127
  & optic neuritis, 127
  & osteomyelitis, 127
  & pneumonia, 127
  & polio, 127
  & rheumatic disease, 127
  & rubella, 127
  & scarlet fever, 127
  & snake bites, 127
  & tetanus, 127
  & tonsillitis, 127
  & urticaria, 127
  & whooping cough, 127
  & wound healing, 127
mag chloride to kill diseases, 126-127
mag malate & CFS, 135-136
  & fibromyalgia, 135-136
mag taurate & heart health, 134-135
Magnascent© Iodine, 28, 31-32, 161, 166, 171, 337
  & colon problems, 50
  & periodontal disease, 299
  URL for, 353
magnesium, 113-140:
  & acne, 121, 127
  & aging, 133-134
  & Alzheimer's, 127
  & arrhythmias, 110
  & asthma, 118-119, 127
  & atrial fib. 119

INDEX

& autism, 118-119, 121, 123-124
& best supplements, 115-116
& blood pressure, 134
& breast cancer, 129
& calcium, 134-135
& cancer, 167
& CFS, 119, 120
& cholesterol, 224
& circulation, 127
& colitis, 127
& colon cancer, 121-122, 129
& colorectal cancer, 122
& COPD, 119
& cramps, 127
& deficiency symptoms, 114
& dermatitis, 121
& diabetes, 122-123
& dosing, 115, 116, 118
& eczema, 121, 127
& epilepsy, 128
& fibromyalgia, 119, 120
& gallbladder, 127
& gangrene, 130
& hay fever, 127
& headaches, 123
& heart disease, 119, 124
& immunity, 137
& impotence, 127
& inflammation, 125-126
& insomnia, 118-119
& leukemia, 119, 128, 129
& migraines, 119
& nephropathy, 122
& ocean water, 138
& oil digestion, 54
& osteoporosis, 87, 113
& PAD, 129-130
& Parkinson's, 127
& precautions for, 136
& psoriasis, 121, 127
& PVD, 129-130
& retinopathy, 122
& sources for, 114, 128
& statins, 188
& stomach cancer, 119
& stones, 129, 231
& strokes, 123
& suicide levels, 128
& supplements, 114-115
& testing for, 132-133
& warts, 127
& wasting of, 118, 120
& zinc, 128
magnesium aspartate, 116
magnesium, B6 & zinc, 128
magnesium chloride, 115, 117
magnesium glycinate, 86
magnesium hydroxide, 115, 116
Magnesium Loading Test, 132-133
magnesium spray, 115-116, 129, 137-138, 161, 177
magnesium stearate, 329
magnesium taurate, 117
magnesium, zinc & lymphoma, 128-129
maitake mushroom:
  & blood-thinners, 283
  & cancer, 230, 282-283
  & common cold, 282-283
  & MS, 283
  precautions for, 283
Maitake D-fraction & cancer, 28, 35, 283
malaria:
  & iodine, 169
  & vitamin C, 79
malic acid & CFS, 120
malic acid & fibromyalgia, 120
mantle zone lymphoma, 258
mantle-cell non-Hodgkin's lymphoma, 267
Manuka Honey & ulcers, 49
maple syrup, 202:
  & soda bicarb cure, 201
  & soda-bicarb recipe, 334
mastitis (chronic) & mag chloride, 127
matsuka mushroom, 284
MB (merbromin), (mercury), 309
MD Anderson resveratrol research, 233
measles:
  & autism from vaccine, 304
  & bentonite clay, 296
  & vitamin C, 79
  vaccine found with avian bird flu, 311-312
mecury & Parkinson's, 309
mecury removal with glutathione, 298
media bias & vitamins, 89-90
media bias against alternative medicine, 312-313
Medulloblastoma & antineoplastons 250
melanoma, 144:
  & chaparral tea, 271
  & CoQ10, 193
  (stage IV) cure, 267-268
memory & ptcrostilbene, 237

INDEX

meningitis, 313
mental capacity & resveratrol, 236
mental retardation & iodine, 174
mercury:
  & Alzheimer's, 309
  & antibiotic use, 304
  & blurred vision, 310
  & calcium bentonite clay, 296
  & Candida, 290
  & chlorella growth factor, 297
  & cholesterol levels, 319
  & dangers of, 155
  & dysarthria, 310
  & FDA hearing, 310
  & headaches, 310
  & heart damage, 294-295
  & heart death, 155
  & heart problems, 310-311
  & human saliva tests, 292
  & insomnia, 310
  & iodine, 137, 166
  & kidney damage, 295
  & *Lou Gehrig's*, 309
  & mercuric acetate, 309
  & mercuric oxide yellow, 309
  & mercurochrome, 309
  & neurotoxic effects, 290
  & parasites, 295-296
  & personality changes, 310
  & polyneuropathy, 310
  & *Reynaud's* syndrome, 319
  & saliva testing, 292
  & selenium, 137
  & T-cell suppression, 292
  & testosterone, 304
  & the heart, 319
  & triglycerides, 319
  & unsteady gait, 310
  & vapors & antibiotics, 322-323
  & vitamin C, 62
  & warning signs, 294
  & weakness, 310
mercury chelators, 297:
  chlorella, 291
  cilantro, 291
  selenium, 291
mercury contamination in dental offices, 290
mercury contamination in homes, 290
mercury detox with cilantro, 154
mercury fillings:
  & children, 296
  & immunity, 296
  & kidney damage, 292
  & MS (multiple sclerosis), 293
  endorsed by ADA, 297
mercury health crisis, 288
  in flu vaccines, 155
  in *Great Salt Lake*, 295
  in household products, 309
  in the bones, 318-319
mercury kills white blood cells, 292
mercury poisoning:
  & fillings, 287-294
  & selenium, 153-154
  symptoms of, 318-319
mercury removed by selenium, 319
mercury removers (also see chelators), 154, 297
  with cilantro recipe, 298
  with selenium, 298
mercury-free dentists, 353
mercury-removing dentists, 297-298
mesima mushroom & cancer, 280
mesothelioma, 258, 295:
  & antineoplastons, 268
  & vaccine link, 314
  & vitamin C, 76
metabolic syndrome:
  & iodine, 159
  & magnesium, 125
  & seaweed, 159
methanol (wood alcohol), 210
methiolate, 309
Methotrexate & concord grapes, 235
migraines, 23:
  & magnesium spray, 129
  & magnesium, 119
milk thistle:
  & endometriosis, 181
  & estrogen, 181
  & fat digestion, 181
  & instructions for use, 181-182
  & kidney cell regeneration, 181
  & skin health, 106, 181
Mineral Rich®, 164-165, 209, 211, 328, 332
mixed olioma, 258
molasses:
  & bowel growth, 205-206
  & breast growths, 205-206
  & colon cancer, 205-206
  & digestion, 205-207
  & hair color, 205-206

INDEX

& pyorrhea, 205-206
& sinus problems, 205-206
& tongue growth, 206
& uterine growths, 205-206
molasses, how to take, 206
molasses/soda bicarb recipe, 335-337
monkey virus contaminates vaccine, 314
mononucleosis & vitamin C, 63
MONSANTO, 146
Morgellon's Disease cure, 353
morning sickness & ginger, 50
mouth cancer:
  & Chinese herbs, 286
  & riboflavin (B2), 286
  & selenium, 286
  & spirulina, 225
  & vitamin A, 286
  & zinc, 286
mouth washes & chlorophyll, 227
Moxxor, 58
MRM®, 32-33
MRSA:
  & antibiotic resistance, 325
  & bentonite clay, 296
  & vitamin C, 77
MS (Multiple Sclerosis), 23:
  & CoQ10, 193-194
  & flax oil, 55
  & magnesium, 118-119, 120
  & maitake, 283
  & mercury fillings, 293
  & selenium, 152
  & vegetarian diets, 194
  & vitamin D deficiency, 102, 107, 283
MS in Scotland, 107
multiple myeloma:
  & AHCC, 281
  & antineoplastons, curing with, 257
  & CoQ10, 193
  & spirulina, 225
mumps:
  & mag chloride, 127
  & vitamin C, 79
murasakishiba (purple reishi), 284
muscle spasms & magnesium, 120
muscular dystrophy & selenium, 148-149
mushrooms (see specific mushrooms):
  for cancer, 280-285
  precautions for, 284
music for healing, 337
mustard greens, 223

mycosis fungoides-sezary syndrome, 258:
  & vitamin C, 76
myelogenous leukemia & vitamin C, 66, 78
myxedematous endemic cretinism, 145
  (also, see under cretinism)
myxopapillary ependymoma, 254
NAC, 180
NAFTA, 219
Nanocolloidal Detox Factors, 291
Nascent iodine, 324
NATREN® probiotic, 353
natto, 323
natural cancer-killers, 247-286
natural estrogens, 50
natural HRT, 131-132
natural progesterone & osteoporosis, 113
nausea & ginger, 50
nephropathy & magnesium, 122
neural tube defects (spina bifida), 99
neuroblastoma, 257:
  & antineoplastoms, 259
  & folic acid, 99
  prevention of, 99, 259-260
neuro-endocrine tumors, 258
neuropathy, 23
  & ALA, 149
neutropenia, 25
New Chapter® products, 281, 285

N

niacin (natural):
  & cholesterol, 85, 223-224
  & circulation, 130
  & the skin, 130-131
  precautions for, 224
niacinamide & cancer, 70
Niaspan, 131
nigela sativa oil (black seed), 59
night vision & resveratrol, 235-236
NMR – *Nuclear Magnetic*
   Resonance Test, 133
non-GMO lecithin, 84
Non-Hogkin's lymphoma testimonial, 353
nordihydroguaiaretic acid (NDGA), 271
nori sea vegetable, 244, 333
Novartis AG & atrial fib, 119
NSAIDs link to Crohn's Disease, 324
nutmeg & cancer, 230
Nutra-Sweet™, 210
NutriCology®, 115-116, 118

INDEX

nutrition in the womb, 99

O

oat bran & cholesterol, 224
obesity & resveratrol, 233
obesity & selenium, 152
obeying God, 346
ocean water & blood, 138
ocean water & magnesium, 138
oil of oregano (wild):
 & autoimmunity, 126
 & Crohn's Disease, 126
 & inflammation, 126
 & osteoporosis, 126
Ola Loa®, 209, 211, 328, 332
oligomeric proanthocyanidins, (OPCs), 238
olioma (mixed), 258
olive leaf:
 & ulcers, 49
 & colon problems, 49
olive oil, 43, 55, 58
 & cholesterol, 224
omega-3 oil sources, 55
 & cholesterol, 224
Omegasentials™, 53
Omsk Fever & vitamin C, 79
onions, heavy metal removers, 298
OPCs & grapes, 238
optaflexx (ractopamine), 321-322
optic neuritis & mag chloride, 127
optic pathway gliomas, 259
oral contraceptives & Crohn's Disease, 324
Orange Wunder Formula, 19, 23, 24, 26, 27-35, 53-54, 64, 117, 130, 216, 246
oregano (also, see under oil of oregano):
 & colon problems, 49,
 & ulcers, 49
organic food, 52, 217-218
 & grapes, 236-237
 vs conventional food, 322
organic selenium, 154
organic *V8®* juice, 224
orphan drugs, 249
Orthomolecular Medicine, 95
OSHA & chemo safety, 300-301
osteoarthropathy, 145
osteomyelitis & mag chloride, 127
osteopenia, 232
osteoporosis:
 & magnesium, 87, 113, 121

 & natural progesterone, 113
 & oil of oregano, 126
 & selenium, 152
 & sunshine, 109
 & vitamin C, 82
 & vitamin D, 109
osteosarcoma & fluoride, 213
ovarian cancer, 257:
 & ABM, 280
 & dairy, 109
 & polyporus, 283-284
 & selenium, 144
 & sunlight, 104
 & vitamin C, 67, 71-72, 75
 (advanced) & *RM-10*, 283-284
oxalates, 88
 sources of, 230-231
 & calcium, 231
 & raw foods, 230-231
oxygen levels & alkalinity, 246

P

P4-D1 & sun protection, 222
Paclitaxel, 149
PAD & magnesium, 129-130
palpitations & selenium, 152
pancreatic cancer:
 & antineoplastons, 269
 & CoQ10, 188-189, 194
 & gum disease, 299
 & resveratrol, 234-235
 & selenium, 152, 148-149
 & vaccine link, 314
 & vitamin C, 67, 76, 77
 & vitamin D, 103
pancreatic disease & selenium, 148-149
pancreatic health & chlorophyll, 221
paralysis from *Gardasil®*, 306-307
parasites:
 & iodine, 161
 & isopropyl alcohol, 295-296
 & mercury, 295-296
 & pets, 295
 & vitamin C, 79
Parkinson's Disease:
 & Epsom Salt, 209-210
 & GSH, 180
 & magnesium, 121, 127
 & mercury, 309
parsley:

INDEX

& cancer, 230, 278-279
& stone formation, 278
(for diuretic), 278-279
precautions for using, 278-279
pawpaw & cancer, 230
paylean (ractopamine), 321
PBs (sodium phenylbutrates), 247, 268
PCN vs chlorophyll, 221
PCP & vitamin C, 62
peace of mind, 346
PEARLS™, 36
pectin (citrus) & cholesterol, 224
pepper & inflammation, 126
percolate & iodine, 137
perfumes, 295
perilla oil, 58, 59
periodontal disease & *Magnascent*©, 299
peripheral neuropathy & statins, 187
peritoneal cancer:
 & bovine cartilage, 229
 & CoQ10, 195, 228-229
 & wheat grass juice, 228-229
pernicious anemia, 189
personality changes & mercury, 310
pertussis & vitamin C, 79
pesticides in food, 218
pets & parasites, 295
pH:
 & bladder cancer, 245-246
 & urine testing, 336
 balance, 197-220
pharmacist risk for handling chemo, 300-301
pharyngitis, 167
phenol-soluble modulin (PSM), 325
phenylalanines, 210
phenylmercuric acetate, 309
phenylmercuric nitrate, 309
pheochromocytoma & vitamin C, 76
phycocyanin in spirulina, 225
phyto-estrogens, 52
pigs & the swine flu, 315-316
pigs blood in vaccines, 303
pigs poisoned, 321-322
pilocytic astrocytoma & antineoplastons, 249
pine bark, 233-234
pineoblastoma cure, 255
Plasmodium falciparum parasite, 79
PMS & krill, 57
PMT, premenstrual tension, 133-134
pneumonia:
 & mag chloride, 127

& vitamin C, 79, 83-84
poison in turkey & pork, 321-322
poison ivy & bentonite clay, 296
poison ivy & iodine, 167
pokeweed root, 278
policosanol & cholesterol, 187, 224
polio, 80:
 & mag chloride, 127
 & magnesium, 121
 & vitamin C cure, 79, 312
polio vaccines contaminated, 314
Poly-MVA cancer survivors, 353
polyneuropathy:
 & mercury, 310
 & statins, 187
polyporus umbellatus mushroom:
 & bladder cancer, 283-284
 & ovarian cancer, 283-284
polysaccharides, 284
pomegranate & cholesterol, 224
posion oak & bentonite clay, 296
power in worship, 347
Power Seed Mix, 42
praise vs depression, 346-347
praising God, 345
pranthocyanidins, 233
prayer & worship, 340
pre-cancerous lesions & cilantro, 299
premature aging, 113
 & GSH, 179
premature baldness, 213
pre-menstrual tension, 133-134
premies & magnesium, 121
preparing your soul, 341-342
PRESCRIPT-ASSIST® probiotic, 323
PRIMA-1 & cancer, 230
probiotics:
 HSO, 213, 324
 NATREN®, 353
 PEARLS™, 36
 PRESCRIPT-ASSIST®, 323
probiotic resources, 324
products with mercury, 302
proline & heart disease, 86
propolis & colon problems, 49
prostate & pumpkinseed oil, 59
prostate cancer, 257:
 & antineoplastons, 269-270
 & calcium, 135
 & CoQ10, 194
 & dairy, 109

INDEX

   & iodine, 163, 168-169
   & lignans, 50
   & magnesium, 127
   & molasses formula, 335-337
   & *Orange Wunder Formula* (Ch. 2)
   & resveratrol, 234-235
   & selenium, 142
   & soda bicarb protocol, 335-337
   & vitamin C, 74
prostate problems & magnesium, 127
protein & vegans, 223
PSK (from coriolus mushroom):
   & cancer, 282-283
   & gastric cancer, 281-282
   & injections with, 213
psoriasis, 23
   & magnesium, 121, 127
   & turmeric, 106, 281
   & vitamin D, 106
psychosis, 23
pterostilbene:
   & blood sugar, 237
   & breast cancer 237-238
   & cancer, 237-238
   & cholesterol, 237
   & diabetes, 237-238
   & heart disease, 237
   for memory, 237
   in blueberries, 237
pulmonary diseases, 168
pumpkinseed oil, 59
   & prostate, 59
   & urinary health, 59
purines & stones, 231
purpose of detox, 327-328
PVD & magnesium, 129-130
Pycnogenol®, 233-234
   & allergies, 237
   & arthritis, 237
   & CAD, 237
   & cancer, 237
   & stress, 237
   in grapes, 237
pyorrhea & molasses, 205-206

Q

quark, 46
quercetin & grapes, 237

R

rabies & vitamin C, 79
ractopamine:
   approved by FDA, 320-321
   (optaflexx), 321-322
   (paylean), 321
radiation & bentonite clay, 296
radiation & vitamin C, 62
raising glutathione levels, 178-179
rapid alkalinity:
   & apple cider vinegar, 207-208, 332
   & lemons, 210
   & limes, 210
   & soda bicarb, 211
raw cabbage juice & ulcers, 49
raw foods:
   & alkalinity, 216
   & bacteria, 217-218
   & oxalates, 230-231
   diet & B12, 231-232
   how to clean, 218
   in cancer diet, 227
   safety of, 217-218
Raynaud's Syndrome & magnesium, 120
RDA for iodine, 162, 169
Real Salt, 117
recombinant monkey viruses, 303
recombinant virology, 314
rectal cancer:
   & *Essiac* tea, 272
   & selenium, 146
   & sunlight, 104
Red Blood Cell Magnesium Test, 132-133
red blood cells & spirulina, 225
red clover, 279
red grapes:
   & cholesterol, 224, 230
   & HTN, 230
   for fighting cancer, 230
red wine & cataracts, 236
refined sugar precautions, 232
regenerating brain cells, 277
reishi mushrooms (*kisshotake,* the lucky
     fungus):
   & vitamin C, 284
   for high cholesterol, 224, 284
   for cancer, 284
reishi, blood-thinner, 284
reishi, natural antihistamine, 284
RELOX procedure, 121
removing amalgam fillings, 319
renal stones, 203

INDEX

renal tubular acidosis, 203
Rene Caisse, 272-276
Resperin Canada Essiac® tea, 274
restless leg syndrome & magnesium, 120
resveratrol, 187:
    & breast cancer, 234-235, 237
    & CAD, 236
    & cancer, 230, 233-238
    & cholesterol, 224
    & colon cancer, 234-235
    & energy, 236
    & eye health, 235-236
    & grapes, 233-238
    & killing bacteria, 236
    & leukemia, 234-235
    & liver cancer, 237
    & lung cancer, 234-235
    & mental capacity, 236
    & night vision, 235-236
    & obesity, 233
    & pancreatic cancer, 234-235
    & prostate cancer, 234-235
    & research with, 233
    & sources of, 237
reticulum cell sarcoma & vitamin C, 75
retina problems & borage oil, 55
retinal, 285
retinoic acid, 285
retinopathy:
    & magnesium, 122
    & selenium, 148-149
retrovirus found in *Rotateq* vaccine, 311-312
Revelation of God, 341-341
Revici, Dr. Emanuel, 151
Reynaud's Syndrome & mercury, 319
rhabdoid brain tumor cure, 251
rheumatic disease & mag chloride, 127
rheumatic disease & soda bicarb, 203-204
rheumatic fever & vitamin C, 79
rheumatoid arthritis:
    & Epsom Salt, 209-210
    & Lyprinol®, 58
    & selenium, 148-149
riboflavin (B2) & mouth cancer, 286
rickets, 103
Rift Valley Fever & vitamin C, 79
RM-10 Formula:
    & advanced ovarian cancer cure, 283-284
    & fatty liver, 284
Rocky Mtn Spotted Fever & Vit C., 79
room air fresheners, 295

root canal, dangers of, 85, 288
root canals & children, 296
Rotarix vaccine contamination, 311-312
royal jelly, 213
RSV & vitamin C, 79
rubella & mag chloride, 127
rye bread & cholesterol, 224

S

safe detox, 327-338
salba oil, 58
saliva & mercury levels, 292
Salk vaccine, 312
salt in the Bible, 211-212
Salt Loading Protocol, 173
sample prayer, Appendix I, 349-350
sarcoma, green tea & reishi, 277
sauerkraut, 323
saving fresh-squeezed juices, 330
scarlet fever & mag chloride, 127
    & vitamin C, 79
scented candles, 295
schizophrenia, 23
    & GSH, 180
    & selenium, 148-149
Scotland & MS cases, 107
scurvy, 63, 83, 77-78, 97
Sea Salt (sun-dried), 117, 206
sea vegetables, 244
Seanol® & cholesterol, 224
seaweed:
    & blood pressure, 334
    & breast cancer rates, 163-164
    & cancer, 333
    & metabolic syndrome, 159
    & strokes, 334
    for detox, 333
    for the heart, 124-125
    how to use, 244
seborrheic dermatitis & selenium, 148-149
seeking God in prayer first, 330
    for healing, 339-350
    for spiritual guidance, 329
seizures & magnesium, 121
selenium, 141-158:
    & acne, 148-149, 152
    & asthma, 147
    & birth defects, 148-149
    & BRCA-1 gene, 144
    & breast cancer, 143, 144, 145

INDEX

& breast tumors, 137
& cancer, 150, 151
& cancer risk, 318
& cataracts, 148-149
& cervical cancer, 145-146
& cirrhosis, 152
& colorectal cancer, 142-143
& cystic breasts (also, see fibrocystic breasts), 148-149, 152
& cystic fibrosis, 148-149
& diabetes, 149, 165
& Down's Syndrome, 148-149
& esophageal cancer, 286
& excess estrogen, 152
& fibrocystic breasts, 148-149, 152
& flu virus, 150-151
& heavy metal detox, 148-149
& hepatitis C, 149
& HIV, 150
& inorganic forms of, 147, 151
& intestinal cancer, 146
& Keshan's Disease, 150
& liver cancer, 146-147
& liver transplants, 149
& *Lou Gehrigs*, 152
& lung cancer, 142-143, 147
& mad cow disease, 150-151
& mercury poisoning, 153-154
& mercury, 137
& mouth cancer, 286
& MS (multiple sclerosis), 152
& muscular dystrophy, 148-149
& obesity, 152
& organic forms of, 142, 143, 151
& ovarian cancer, 144, 145-146
& palpitations, 152
& pancreatic disease, 148-149
& pancreatitis, 152
& prostate cancer, 142
& rectal cancer, 146
& research, 68-69
& retinopathy, 148-149
& rheumatoid arthritis, 148-149
& safe amounts of, 157
& schizophrenia, 148-149
& seborrheic dermatitis, 148-149
& sickle cell, 152
& SIDS, 148-149
& sources of, 142, 143, 151, 189, 297
& T3, 152
& thyroid function, 148-149, 152

selenium, dosing of, 142, 149
  for fighting mercury, 155, 291, 319
  for killing viruses, 150-151
  levels & cancer risk, 318
  poisoning & vitamin C, 62
  removing mercury, 298
selenium, vit A & bone cancer, 144
selenium, vit C & lymphoma, 147-148
selenium, vit E & ALA, 147
senility, 23:
  & magnesium, 120
Serum Ionized Magnesium Test, 133
sesame oil & HTN, 224
sesame sprouts & calcium, 226
seven-day detox program, 331-332
shark cartilage & cancer, 230
sheep sorrel, 272
shiitake mushrooms, 187
  & cholesterol, 224, 285
  & immunity, 285
  & liver cancer, 285
shingles:
  & flax, 52
  & vitamin C, 63
shiroshiba (white reishi), 284
sick pets & wheat grass, 226
sickle cell disease, 80:
  & selenium, 152
SIDS (sudden infant death syndrome), 81, 313:
  & magnesium, 121
  & selenium, 148-149
  & vitamin C, 63, 78
  statistics for, 317
Siegel, Maryjo, 261-268
  & lymphoma cure, 261-268
silymarin (from milk thistle):
  & hepatitis C, 149
  & liver transplants, 149
  & sun exposure, 181
Simoncini, Dr. T., URL, 352
Singapore fines bromide-users, 320
sinus infections & iodine, 167
sinus problems & molasses, 205-206
Sir Jason Winter's tea, 279
skin cancer:
  & asparagus, 208
  & barley juice, 222
  & surgery, 222
skin disorders:
  & flax oil, 106
  & GSH, 181

INDEX

& milk thistle, 106
& wheat grass, 226
skin treatment discovery, 130-131
Sleep Minerals, 110
slippery elm & ulcers, 49
slippery elm bark, 272
snake bites & mag chloride, 127
SOD, 181
sodium bicarbonate:
   & alkalinity, 166-167, 211
   & arthritis, 203-204
   & cancer, 334
   & colon cancer, 200, 212
   & gout, 203-204
   & insect bites, 203
   & maple syrup cure, 201
   & maple syrup recipe, 334
   & molasses recipe, 335-337
   & prostate cancer protocol, 335-337
   & rheumatic disease, 203-204
   & ulcers, 50
sodium ascorbate:
   homemade, 71, 95, 97-98, 148
sodium pyroglutamate from ABM, 280
solid cancers & ABM, 280
sore gums & wheat grass, 226
sore throat:
   & iodine, 126, 174
   & wheat grass, 226
soul, what is it? 340-341
sour cherries for gout, 231
spinach, 223
spinach juice & ulcers, 49
spinal cord defects & folic acid, 260
spirulina:
   & anemia, 225
   & B12, 225
   & blindness, 225
   & blood disorders, 225
   & cancer, 225
   & cholesterol, 224, 225
   & colon health, 225
   & diabetes, 225
   & gout, 225
   & HTN, 225
   & heavy metals, removal of: 225
   & leukemia, 225
   & mouth cancer, 225
   & multiple myeloma, 225
   & red blood cells, 225
   & tobacco chewers, 225

   & viruses, 225
split-gill mushroom & cancer, 280
sprouts, 55, 226-229
   rinsing of, 226
statins:
   CoQ10, 187-188
   & magnesium, 188
   & peripheral neuropathy, 187
   & polyneuropathy, 187
steel cut oats & cholesterol, 224
Stevia®, 34-35, 332
stomach cancer:
   & Essiac tea, 272
   & green tea, 277
   & magnesium, 119
   & sunlight, 104
stomach problems & flax seed, 49
stone formation, 232
   & B vitamins, 231
   & carbonated sodas, 231
   & fluid intake, 231
   & magnesium, 129, 231
   & parsley tea, 278
strawberries fight cancer, 230
strep & dairy, 46
stress & magnesium, 119
stress & *Pycnogenol*®, 237
strokes & magnesium, 120, 123
strokes & seaweed, 334
strontium for bone health, 87, 333
strontium-90:
   & bone marrow, 333
   & removal of, 333
   & kelp, 333
struvite stones, 88, 231
Sublingual Magnesium Assay (Exatest), 133
subversive groups, 316-317
suicidal tendencies, 85
suicide in the dental profession, 290
suicide levels & magnesium, 128
sulfa drugs & vitamin C, 62
sulfa vs chlorophyll, 221
sun exposure, 96
sunflower seeds & calcium, 226
sunlight (also, see under sunshine):
   & bladder cancer, 104
   & breast cancer, 104
   & colon cancer, 104
   & ovarian cancer, 104
   & vitamin D, 96
sunlight exposure, 105, 331

INDEX

sunscreen, safe forms, 111
sunshine, 331:
  & osteoporosis, 109
  & vitamin D, 102
sunshine levels, 102
Super Nuthera for autism, 210
supplement choices, 328-329
surgery & skin cancer, 222
sushi, 333
SV-40 monkey virus, 314
Swanson Health Products, 222
swimming pools & chlorine, 215
swine flu & the pigs, 315-316
synthetic HRT, 131-132
synthetic vitamin D, 108-109

T

T cells:
  & chlorella, 222
  & mercury, 292
  & vitamin D, 105
T3 & selenium, 152
TB & vitamin C, 79
tea & cancer, 270-279
terminal cancers & antineoplastons, 248
  (also, see under Burzynski)
testosterone & mercury, 304
tetanus & mag chloride, 127
THC & cancer, 183
The Grape Cure, 229-237
thimerosal:
  & autism, 302, 304
  & neuro injury, 302
  in vaccines, 302, 304
THREELAC™ & Candida, 199
throat infections & iodine:
(also, see under sore throats)
    167
thrombocytopenia, 25
thymulin & ALL (leukemia), 139, 285
thyroid disorders & hormones:
  & breast cancer, 163, 165
  & fluoride, 213
  & iodine, 152
  & selenium, 148-149,152
timed-release niacin, precautions for, 224
timed-release vitamin C, 98
tinder polypore mushroom & cancer, 280
titanium dioxide additive, 329
tobacco chewers & spirulina, 225

tobacco smoke, 295
tomatoes & cancer, 230
tongue growth & molasses, 206
tonsillitis & mag chloride, 127
toulene, dangers of, 295
Tourette's Syndrome & magnesium, 120
toxicity of chemo, 299-300, 301
trichinosis & vitamin C, 79
trigeminal neuralgia, 294
triglycerides & mercury, 319
Triodide iodine, 162
trypanosomal infections & vitamin C, 79
tuckahoe bread & hoelen, 282
Tulsi tea, 276
tumors & anti-angiogenesis foods, 230
tumors & chlorella, 223
tumor-shrinking with iodine, 170-171
turkey poisoned meat, 321-322
Turkish rhubarb, 272
turmeric:
  & autism, 281
  & cancer, 230
  & eczema, 281
  & HIV, 281
  & inflammation, 126
  & psoriasis, 106, 281
TwinLab® & *B12 Dots®*, 232
Tykerb (Lapatinib), 73
Tylenol® recalls, 308-309
typhoid & vitamin C, 79

U

ubiquinone, 188
Ukrain for curing cancer, 230
ulcers, 23
  & bee propolis, 49
  & beta-sitosterol, 50
  & bilberry, 49
  & calendula, 49
  & carrot juice, 49
  & chia seeds, 49
  & chlorophyll, 221
  & coconut milk, 49
  & coconut water, 49
  & cranberries, 229
  & DGL, 49
  & fish oil, 49
  & ginger, 50
  & green tea, 49
  & krill oil, 50

INDEX

& *Manuka Honey*, 49
& olive leaf, 49
& oregano, 49
& raw broccoli, 50
& raw cabbage juice, 49
& slippery elm, 49
& soda bicarb, 50
& spinach juice, 49
& water, 49
& white tea, 49
umbelliferae & cancer, 230
UnbllqLOH (chromosome), 259
undenatured whey protein isolate, 178-9
undifferentiated connective tissue disease (UCTD), 269
unfermented soy, 175
Universal Pathogen Killer, Iodine, 168-169
unsteady gait & mercury, 310
uric acid, 203
urinary health & pumpkinseed oil, 59
urinary infections:
   & iodine, 167
   & vitamin C, 70
urine pH testing, 336
urticaria & mag chloride, 127
USANA products, 353
uterine cancer & dairy, 109
   & lignans, 50
   & sunlight, 104
uterine growths & molasses, 205-206

V

V8® low sodium veg juice & cholesterol, 224
V8® organic juice, 224
vaccines:
   & aluminum levels, 303-304, 315
   & autism link, 301, 313
   & autistic children, 301
   & bi-polar disorder link, 303
   & brain tumors, 301
   & contamination of, 303, 311-312
   & Crohn's Disease link, 301
   & cystic fibrosis link, 303
   & diabetes link, 301
   & HIV link, 314
   & heart damage link, 155
   & mesothelioma link, 314
   & pancreatic cancer link, 314
   & pigs blood, 303
   & safety of, 317-318
   & thimerosal in, 302, 304
   & vitamin C, help with, 63
   contamination by monkey virus, 314
   effectiveness of, 317
   gambling with, 312
   horrors of, 311-316
   makers of, amorality of, 302
vaccines with aluminum, 303-304, 315
valuable links, Appendix II, 351-354
vanadium & vitamin C, 62
VD & iodine, 167
vegans & protein, 223
vegetables (raw) & alkalinity, 232
vegetarian diets & MS, 194
venom & vitamin C, 62
Viagra injuries, 308
Vioxx®, 256, 318, 320
Vioxx® maker threatens critics, 307-308
viruses, 23
   & selenium, 150-151
   & spirulina, 225
visual pathway gliomas, 258-259
vitamin A:
   & APL leukemia, 139, 285
   & breast cancer, 95
   & CML leukemia, 139, 285
   & mouth cancer, 286
   sources of, 144
vitamin C, 187, 61-100:
   & arsenic, 62
   & asthma, 87
   & benzene, 62
   & bladder cancer, 75
   & bladder tumors, 64-65
   & blood clots, 86
   & bone density, 113
   & botulism, 79
   & brain tumor, 75
   & breast cancer, 72, 74, 95, 137
   & brucellosis, 79
   & cancer, 94
   & carcinoma, 75, 76
   & cardiomyopathy, 86
   & Chediak-Higashi Disease, 83-84
   & chicken pox, 63
   & chronic Myeloid leukemia C, 75
   & colds, 63
   & colon cancer, 75
   & common cold, 62
   & cyanides, 62
   & cytomegalovirus, 79

INDEX

& deadly mushrooms, 62
& dengue fever, 79-80, 99
& diabetes, 81-82, 94
& diphtheria, 79
& disease, 92
& dosing, 66, 87, 93-95, 108
& dysentery, 79
& ebola, 79, 97
& edema, 86
& encephalitis, 79
& fever blisters, 63
& fluoride, 62
& glioblastoma, 67
& gout, 231
& grape seed precaution, 234
& hairy cell leukemia, 76
& hantavirus, 79
& heart disease, 84-86
& hemorrhagic fever, 79
& hepatitis, 82
& herpes, 79
& high cholesterol, 84-86
& HIV, 83-84
& Hodgkin's, 70-71, 75
& homocysteine, 86
& how much to take, 66, 87, 93-95, 108
& insulin, 94
& kidney cancer, 64-65
& kidney stones, 88
& lassa fever, 79
& lecithin combo, 82
& leprosy, 79
& leukemia, 70
& lung cancer, 71-72, 74
& lymphoma, 64-65, 73-74
& lymphosarcoma, 75
& malaria, 79
& measles, 79
& mercury, 62
& mesothelioma, 75
& mono, 63
& MRSA, 79
& mumps, 79
& mycosis fungoides, 76
& myelogenous leukemia, 66, 78
& *Omsk Fever*, 79
& *Orange Wunder Formula*, 20, 22, 23, 27-31, 35-38
& osteoporosis, 82
& ovarian cancer, 67, 71-72, 75
& pancreatic cancer, 67, 76, 77

& parasites, 79
& PCP, 62
& pertussis, 79
& pesticides, 62
& pheochromocytoma, 76
& pneumonia, 79, 83-84
& polio, cure for, 79
& prostate cancer, 74
& rabies, 79
& radiation, 62
& reishi mushrooms, 284
& research involving, 67-69, 71
& RSV, 79
& reticulum cell sarcoma, 75
& rheumatic fever, 79
& *Rift Valley Fever*, 79
& *Rocky Mtn Spotted Fever*, 79
& scarlet fever, 79
& selenium poisoning, 62
& shingles, 63
& SIDS, 63, 78
& stones, 231
& strychnine, 62
& sulfa drugs, 62
& TB, 79
& test strips, 83, 96
& timed-release form, 98
& trichinosis, 79
& trypanosomal infections, 79
& typhoid, 79
& UTIs, 79
& vaccines, 63
& vanadium, 62
& venom, 62
& *West Nile Fever*, 79, 97
& *Yellow Fever*, 79
&toxin relief, 62
vitamin C dosing, 66, 87, 93-95, 108
vitamin C, polio cure, 312
vitamin D, 101-112:
   & amounts needed, 105
   & asthma, 106
   & autoimmune disorders, 106
   & bathing, 96
   & breast cancer, 95, 102, 110
   & cancer, 101-103
   & colon cancer, 102, 145
   & depression, 106
   & diabetes link, 102, 105, 107
   & eczema, 106
   & gastric cancer, 102

INDEX

& heart disease, 105
& how it works, 105
& levels of (safety), 101, 107, 108
& lupus, 106-107
& MS (multiple sclerosis), 102, 107, 283
& osteoporosis, 109
& pancreatic cancer, 103
& psoriasis, 106
& sources of, 101, 108
& sunlight, 96, 102
& synthetic forms of, 108-109, 144
& T-cells, 105

vitamin E:
& best forms of, 153, 165, 180-181
& best sources for, 153
& bladder cancer, 153
& breast cancer, 95
& cervical cancer, 180-181
& fighting mercury levels, 155
& Keshan's Disease, 150
& selenium, 144
in sprouts, 226

vitamin K in green foods, 221-222
Vytorin, 187

W

wakame sea vegetable, 244, 333:
& lung cancer, 334
Waldenstrom's macroglobulinemia, 258
Wall Street Reform Bill, 322
walnut oil, 59
warts & magnesium, 127
water:
& detox, 329-330
& ulcers (cure for), 49
vs juice-fasting, 245
weakness & mercury link, 310
West Nile Virus, 80
& vitamin C, 79, 97
wheat grass juice, 195:
& breast cancer, cure for, 228
& colitis, 226
& digestive health, 226
& itchy scalp, 226
& peritoneal cancer, 228-229
& sick pets, 226
& sore gums, 226
& sore throat, 226
wheat grass juice for immunity, 227-228
wheat grass Juice/disinfectant, 226

wheat grass juicing, 241-242
Whey Protein Shake (40-41)
whey protein source, 354
Whitaker Wellness Center, 189, 354
white bread & bromide (bromine) poison, 319-320
white tea & colon problems, 49
white tea & ulcers, 49
whole foods, 182
whooping cough, 317
& mag chloride, 127
Wilm's tumor, 258
wine & bacteria, 217-218
wine vs grapes, 237
Wolfe-Chaikoff Effect, 164
world deficient in iodine, 170
world population growth, 316-317
worship:
& prayer, 340
learning how, 347
your future, 346
wound healing:
& chlorophyll, 221
& magnesium, 120
& mag chloride, 127
wrinkling & kombucha, 278

X - Y

yeast & iodine, 161-162
yeast infections:
& antibiotics, 325
& cancer, 325
& iodine for, 161-162
Yellow Fever & vitamin C, 79
yogurt, 323
your uniqueness, 340-341

Z

Zeolite, heavy metal chelator, 298
resources for, 298, 354
Zetia, 187
zinc 113-140
& abdominal cancer, 138-139
& ALL leukemia, 139, 285
& copper ratios, 139, 285
& esophageal cancer, 138-139, 286
& magnesium, 128
& mouth cancers, 286

Author Bio

Deanna Loftis is a licensed RN in several states. She spent many years working with med-surg and orthopedic patients in a clinical setting before returning to school for a B.B.A. (major in Managed Care), graduating Summa Cum Laude from Northwood University. She also worked many years in a managed care staff and supervisory position, which included following solid organ transplant patients and bone marrow (or stem cell) transplant patients in case management for a major insurance company. Because of losing three family members to cancer, and the horrendous side effects that they (and many of her patients) suffered from chemo and radiation, she began an intensive study into alternative cancer therapies, which resulted in her first award-winning book in 2005: *Painless Cancer Cures & Preventions Your Doctor May Not Be Aware Of* and her second award-winning book in 2009, *Gentle Cures for Tough Cancers*.

Deanna continues to research and study all forms of alternative cancer therapies and now updates her readers with her newest book: *Designer Cancer Killers & Orange Wunder God-Designed, God-Inspired To Kill Your Cancer, Not You!* This newest book describes the formulas that Deanna developed after yet another close family member was diagnosed with a Stage IV cancer and was told that he was inoperable. It will tell you exactly what she did to help him get well and stay well even during the time that he decided to go through chemo treatments and beyond. There is also information on many other natural, effective treatments for health disorders besides cancer. Whether you decide to use alternative therapies, conventional medicine, or a combination of both, Deanna's newest book and formulas will give you important tips to help you learn to trust in God through prayer and worship, prolong your life, and restore your health or the health of a loved one.